Respiratory Medicine

Series Editor:
Sharon I.S. Rounds

More information about this series at http://www.springer.com/series/7665

Laura M. Sterni • John L. Carroll
Editors

Caring for the Ventilator Dependent Child

A Clinical Guide

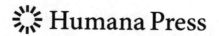 Humana Press

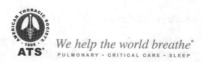
We help the world breathe®
PULMONARY · CRITICAL CARE · SLEEP

Editors
Laura M. Sterni, MD
Eudowood Division of Pediatric
  Respiratory Sciences
The Johns Hopkins University
  School of Medicine
Baltimore, MD, USA

John L. Carroll, MD
Division of Pediatric Pulmonary
  and Sleep Medicine
University of Arkansas for Medical
  Sciences
Little Rock, AR, USA

ISSN 2197-7372   ISSN 2197-7380   (electronic)
Respiratory Medicine
ISBN 978-1-4939-8128-1   ISBN 978-1-4939-3749-3   (eBook)
DOI 10.1007/978-1-4939-3749-3

Printed on acid-free paper

This Humana Press imprint is published by Springer Nature
The registered company is Springer Science+Business Media LLC New York

*This book is dedicated to the patients
who require chronic home ventilator support
and the families and professionals who care
for them. We are inspired by your resilience,
creativity, and dedication.*

*And to our families:
To my husband Hank and sons Colin
and Mark, with gratitude and love. (LS)
To my wife Tiziana and children, Maggie,
Molly, and Maddy, with love
and appreciation. (JC)*

Preface

Children with chronic respiratory failure are living longer, healthier lives than ever before due to advances in medical care, respiratory-related technologies, and respiratory equipment for home use. Over the last several decades, emphasis on the importance of family and community in the care of children with special healthcare needs has resulted in a major shift from institutional/residential care settings to long-term care in the home. Very few children with chronic medical conditions and special healthcare needs are more complex and challenging than children with chronic respiratory failure, who often are dependent for life support on mechanical ventilation. The precise number is unknown, but it has been estimated that thousands of children receive home mechanical ventilation in the United States and the prevalence of home mechanical ventilation for children is likely to be similar in Europe and elsewhere [1].

Children with disorders leading to respiratory insufficiency can be supported in the home with invasive or noninvasive ventilator support. These children often have multiple medical problems, they are supported by complex equipment, and their high risk of complications demands the constant attention of caregivers. Families are faced with a herculean task, made more challenging by the lack of care coordination, lack of expert practice guidelines, and wide variations in practice. At the time of this writing (2016), there are no evidence-based guidelines for the care of children on home mechanical ventilation, and overall the quality of evidence provided by the scant research literature in this area is poor. In addition to a lack of research-derived guidelines for this population, there is also no comprehensive information resource covering all relevant aspects of pediatric home ventilator management.

The goal of this book is to provide, based on literature review and the extensive experience of the expert authors, a single volume with chapters covering all major aspects of caring for children on home mechanical ventilation. In a very real sense, this book is intended to fill a gap until research is sufficient to provide high-quality, evidence-based practice guidelines. Unfortunately, given the profound lack of high-grade research studies in this area, it clearly will be many years and perhaps more than a decade before evidence-based guidelines are even possible. In the meantime, we hope this volume will be a worthwhile resource for the diverse groups of practitioners who care for these children, including nurses, respiratory therapists, discharge planners, social workers, physicians, and others. It is intended to be useful, not only for pediatric pulmonologists but also for pediatric intensivists, cardiologists, physical medicine/rehabilitation specialists, and the primary care physicians involved in the complexities of managing care for this unique group of special needs children.

Baltimore, MD, USA   Laura M. Sterni
Little Rock, AR, USA   John L. Carroll

1. King AC. Long-term home mechanical ventilation in the United States. Respir Care. 2012;57:921–930; discussion 930–922.

Acknowledgments

We thank the outstanding authors who contributed to this book. The authors invited to participate were chosen due to their positions as academic leaders in this field and their extensive experience in the management of children on home mechanical ventilation. We are grateful for their scholarship, commitment, and expertise.

Contents

Contributors

Raanan Arens, MD Division of Pediatric Respiratory and Sleep Medicine, The Children's Hospital at Montefiore, Albert Einstein College of Medicine, Bronx, NY, USA

Sherry L. Barnhart, RRT-NPS, FAARC Respiratory Care Discharge Planner, Respiratory Care Services, Arkansas Children's Hospital, Little Rock, AR, USA

Ariel Berlinski, MD College of Medicine, Arkansas Children's Hospital, University of Arkansas for Medical Sciences, Little Rock, AR, USA

Deborah S. Boroughs, RN, MSN Bayada Home Health Care, Pediatric Specialty Practice, Logan Township, NJ, USA

April Carpenter, APRN Arkansas Children's Hospital, University of Arkansas for Medical Sciences, Little Rock, AR, USA

John L. Carroll, MD Division of Pediatric Pulmonary and Sleep Medicine, University of Arkansas for Medical Sciences, Little Rock, AR, USA

J. Michael Collaco, MD, MPH Eudowood Division of Pediatric Respiratory Sciences, Johns Hopkins University School of Medicine, Baltimore, MD, USA

Joan Dougherty, BSN, CPN, CSN Pennsylvania Ventilator Assisted Children's Home Program (VACHP), Philadelphia, PA, USA

Jeffrey D. Edwards, MD, MA, MAS Division of Pediatric Critical Care Medicine, Columbia University College of Physicians and Surgeons, New York, NY, USA

Fiona Healy, MBBCh Department of Respiratory Medicine, Children's University Hospital, Dublin, Ireland

Thomas G. Keens, MD Division of Pediatric Pulmonology and Sleep Medicine, Children's Hospital Los Angeles, Keck School of Medicine of the University of Southern California, Los Angeles, CA, USA

Sheila Kun, RN, MS Division of Pediatric Pulmonology and Sleep Medicine, Children's Hospital Los Angeles, Keck School of Medicine of the University of Southern California, Los Angeles, CA, USA

Dennis Z. Kuo, MD, MHS Center for Applied Research and Evaluation, Arkansas Children's Hospital, Little Rock, AR, USA

Ian MacLusky Children's Hospital of Eastern Ontario, University of Ottawa, Ottawa, ON, Canada

Carole L. Marcus, MBBCh Sleep Center, Children's Hospital of Philadelphia, University of Pennsylvania, Philadelphia, PA, USA

Brian McGinley, MD Pediatric Pulmonary and Sleep Medicine, University of Utah, Salt Lake City, UT, USA

Sharon A. McGrath-Morrow, MD, MBA Eudowood Division of Pediatric Respiratory Sciences, Johns Hopkins University School of Medicine, Baltimore, MD, USA

Kiran Nandalike, MD Division of Pediatric Respiratory and Sleep Medicine, The Children's Hospital at Montefiore, Albert Einstein College of Medicine, Bronx, NY, USA

Gillian M. Nixon The Ritchie Centre, Department of Paediatrics and The Hudson Institute of Medical Research, Monash University, Melbourne, VIC, Australia

Melbourne Children's Sleep Centre, Monash Children's Hospital, Melbourne, VIC, Australia

Howard B. Panitch, MD Division of Pulmonary Medicine, Technology Dependence Center, The Children's Hospital of Philadelphia, University of Pennsylvania Perelman School of Medicine, Philadelphia, PA, USA

Iris A. Perez, MD Division of Pediatric Pulmonology and Sleep Medicine, Children's Hospital Los Angeles, Keck School of Medicine of the University of Southern California, Los Angeles, CA, USA

Walter M. Robinson, MD, MPH Vanderbilt University School of Medicine, Nashville, TN, USA

Anita K. Simonds, MD FRCP NIHR Respiratory Biomedical Research Unit, Royal Brompton & Harefield NHS Foundation Trust, London, UK

Laura M. Sterni, MD Eudowood Division of Pediatric Respiratory Sciences, The Johns Hopkins University School of Medicine, Baltimore, MD, USA

Sally L. Davidson Ward, MD Division of Pediatric Pulmonology and Sleep Medicine, Children's Hospital Los Angeles, Keck School of Medicine of the University of Southern California, Los Angeles, CA, USA

Denise Willis, BS, RRT-NPS Respiratory Care Services, Pulmonary Medicine Section, Arkansas Children's Hospital, Little Rock, AR, USA

Nanci Yuan, MD Stanford Children's Health Sleep Center, Palo Alto, CA, USA

Chapter 1
Chronic Ventilator Support in Children: Why, Who, and When

Ian MacLusky

Introduction

Until around 25 years ago, there were limited options for long-term ventilation of children, requiring either cumbersome equipment ("iron lung") or invasive ventilation (via a tracheostomy). Consequently the majority of children on long-term ventilation were cared for either in general hospitals or specific long-term ventilation facilities. With improving technology, particularly in the delivery of noninvasive ventilation [2], there has been a marked increase in the number of children being placed on long-term ventilation [2–5], to the point that it is currently regarded as a standard of care for children with conditions that were previously thought to be inevitably fatal, the majority of whom are now cared for in their home. Despite its widespread use, however, there remains very little comparative literature on the optimal indications and patient selection process, optimal timing, or most effective process for initiation of chronic ventilation in children. Moreover most of the available evidence is either from adult populations or mixed populations of adults and children with, unfortunately, a paucity of pediatric specific data. This is reflected by the marked variability in frequency, types of patients, and differing modes of ventilation reported between different centers [1, 6, 7], with ongoing evolution in the conditions deemed appropriate for long-term ventilation [3, 6, 8, 9].

Most long-term ventilation programs have developed their own criteria and protocols for the initiation of long-term ventilation, based largely on logic and empiric experience. Although these protocols are generally similar, being based on similar experience and therapeutic goals, there is still a lack of agreement as to precisely

I. MacLusky (✉)
Children's Hospital of Eastern Ontario, University of Ottawa,
401 Smyth Rd, Ottawa, ON, Canada, K1H 8L1
e-mail: imaclusky@cheo.on.ca

© Springer Science+Business Media New York 2016
L.M. Sterni, J.L. Carroll (eds.), *Caring for the Ventilator Dependent Child*,
Respiratory Medicine, DOI 10.1007/978-1-4939-3749-3_1

who would benefit from long-term home ventilation, or exactly when in the child's disease process it should be initiated [1]. Ideally we would have clear evidence to guide us in our approach to initiation of home ventilation. What literature there is, however, generally describes which individuals were placed on long-term ventilation, how ventilation was initiated, and some outcome data, the majority of this data, as noted, covering populations of all ages. Given that children placed on long-term ventilation, by definition, are commonly facing life-limiting illnesses and that caring for these children has a major impact on family functioning and family finances, the relative absence of objective data providing support for these protocols is a significant deficit of our knowledge.

In order to address which children require chronic ventilator support, it is easiest to first consider the "why," the rationale for placing a child on long-term ventilator support.

Why?

When considering the indications for initiating chronic ventilation, the mode of ventilation required or available has a significant impact on the decision-making process. Simplistically there are two options for delivering chronic ventilation:

1. Noninvasive positive pressure ventilation (NIPPV) by an oral or nasal interface such as a mask, or negative pressure ventilation such as with a cuirass (though this commonly also requires a tracheotomy).
2. Invasive positive pressure ventilation by a tracheotomy.
   Phrenic nerve pacing is a third option for selected patients. It is usually regarded as invasive in that it requires surgical implantation, with many children continuing to require tracheostomy post insertion.

As will be discussed in Chap. 2 and Chap. 3, these different methodologies have their particular advantages and disadvantages. Compared to invasive ventilation, noninvasive ventilation is, however, more readily discontinued in that it simply requires placement of an interface, such as nasal or full face mask. It is therefore amenable to use as a "therapeutic trial," since it can be easily discontinued if found to be ineffective, poorly tolerated, or actually detrimental to the child's respiratory status or quality of life. In a neurologically intact child, with milder degrees of hypoventilation such that ventilatory support is not required for survival, even relatively young children can therefore themselves decide when or whether to use the device. Invasive ventilation, in contrast, not only requires surgical intervention but also, due to the increased complexity of the equipment and the level of care required, necessitates a significantly greater family commitment, both in terms of increased risks associated with initiation and greater caregiver time and education to allow for safe care of the child at home. At the more severe end of the clinical spectrum, however, where patients are dependent on ventilatory support for survival, both patients and family need to understand the rationale for assisted ventilation, whether invasive or noninvasive, and the important role it plays in the care plan of the child.

A variety of reasons exist for initiation of long-term ventilation in children:

1. Prolongation of life. A child with end-stage respiratory failure, as evidenced by persisting daytime hypercapnia, has limited life expectancy. This is therefore the simplest scenario in terms of justification and decision making, since, in the absence of a definitive treatment, long-term ventilation is the only option for continued survival (though assisted ventilation can be a component of palliative care, below). Ideally the patient (where appropriate) and their family will have had sufficient time and education to make an informed decision, in agreement with the child's medical team, as to whether initiation of chronic ventilation is an appropriate therapy for their child (Chap. 4). For example, parents of a neonate with profound hypoventilation as the presenting indicator of congenital central hypoventilation syndrome have little option other than invasive ventilation for their child's survival. In contrast, parents of a child with progressive neuromotor disease, such as spinal muscle atrophy, will hopefully have had sufficient time and counseling to decide in advance the appropriate therapeutic plan in order to delay or ameliorate the onset of overt hypoventilation.

2. Increased life expectancy. It is an oxymoron that a child in end-stage respiratory failure needs assisted ventilation to maintain life. There is good evidence, however, that initiating long-term ventilation earlier in the disease course can significantly improve life expectancy in selected populations. Perhaps the best evidence is in patients with progressive neuromotor disease. For example, with initiation of noninvasive ventilation, there has been almost a doubling in life expectancy of patients with Duchenne muscular dystrophy [10]. Although this is not randomized controlled data, the improvement in life expectancy is so striking, and reported by multiple centers [11–13], to believe that it is a consequence of the initiation of ventilation.

3. Improvement in quality of life. One common concern, and a reason for not initiating ventilation in patients with terminal illness, was the concern that this was merely "prolonging their suffering." It has, however, been realized that, although many patients perceive themselves as asymptomatic [14], not only does the resulting hypercapnia and hypoxemia produce significant symptoms in their own right, but the associated sleep fragmentation also causes significant symptoms, such as morning headaches, daytime somnolence, and generalized fatigue. Correcting these sequelae by initiating nocturnal ventilatory support, even if this were not to increase longevity, can result in significant improvements in quality of life and is sufficient to warrant its use in selected patients. Moreover it has been realized that individuals with progressive disease adapt to their medical condition, which becomes their "normal," for example, individuals with neuromotor disease.

   (a) Perceive their quality of life as being significantly better than either their parents or their medical team [15, 16].

    (b) May actually see their ventilator in a positive light since, by improving their ventilation, they feel better and consequently perceive a resulting improved quality of life [17].

4. Treatment of hypoventilation.

    (a) Nocturnal. Most children with progressive respiratory impairment will develop episodes of nocturnal hypoventilation years before they progress to daytime hypoventilation. Rapid eye movement sleep (REM) is classically associated with loss of skeletal muscle tone and hence loss of accessory muscles of respiration (though diaphragmatic function is preserved), whereas slow wave sleep (SWS or stage 3) is associated with loss of respiratory stimulation from the frontal cortex and hence relative loss of respiratory drive [18]. Consequently hypoventilation in diseases associated with loss of neuromotor function or respiratory muscle fatigue (end-stage pulmonary disease or disturbance of thoracic cage function) is typically worse during REM sleep, whereas patients with disorders of respiratory drive show worse sleep-disordered breathing in SWS. Although there may be a reduction in respect to respiratory function, the arousal response is commonly relatively well preserved and the sleep-related hypoventilation frequently triggers an arousal. This can happen repeatedly through the night, resulting in significant sleep fragmentation. Since, however, its onset is frequently insidious, many patients remain relatively asymptomatic [19, 20]. It is only with correction of the sleep-related hypoventilation that the patients may become aware of the severity of the symptoms arising secondary to their nocturnal hypoventilation and separate them from the symptoms associated with their underlying disease [21].

    (b) Diurnal. As discussed above, once children with progressive disease become hypercapnic even while awake, they generally have a very limited life expectancy, with assisted ventilation (in the absence of any curative lesion) being their only hope for prolonged survival.

5. Improvement in clinical status.

    (a) Lung clearance/cough. Efficient clearance of endobronchial matter requires an effective cough. Both progressive pulmonary and neuromotor diseases in particular are associated with reduced respiratory motor function resulting in reduced inspiratory (for generation of elastic recoil) and expiratory effort and hence reduced ability to generate a forceful expiration [22]. This adversely affects cough generation, with increasing risk of mucous plugging and opportunistic infections [22, 23]. A variety of techniques are therefore routinely employed to increase lung volumes [23]. Even in normal individuals, sleep suppresses cough [24], with the loss of skeletal muscle tone seen in REM sleep likely compounding the already elevated risk of mucous plugging and opportunistic infections. There is evidence to suggest that assisted nocturnal ventilation may reduce this risk [25, 26], presumably by increasing respiratory volume, as well as respiratory muscle rest [22], and hence improved cough effectiveness during sleep.

(b) Progressive loss of lung volume. In patients with progressive neuromotor disease, there is typically an associated, progressive restrictive defect, with progressive loss of lung volumes (see below). This is frequently due to associated reductions in tidal volume [27]. This appears to be ameliorated by the regular use of devices that induce maximal insufflation capacity (lung volume recruitment, or LVR) [27]. Whether a similar benefit can be obtained by using assisted ventilation to maintain lung volumes during sleep remains speculative in neuromotor disease, though this has been found in obesity hypoventilation syndrome [28].

6. Cost efficiency. Whatever healthcare system funding may be in place, caring for a child on chronic ventilation in an acute healthcare setting, such as a hospital, remains an extremely expensive treatment option. Although dependent upon a number of factors, most importantly being the level of externally funded supports provided in the community [1, 29], in general caring for a ventilator-dependent child at home versus in a long-term healthcare institution results in a significant cost saving to the healthcare system [30]. Discharging a patient home on chronic ventilation, however, although saving the healthcare system, transfers the costs of their care onto the family [1, 31]. There is marked variability worldwide in respect to the community resources provided to assist families in caring for these children. In even the most well-resourced healthcare system, however, a large proportion of the cost of these children's care within the home, not merely financial but also in terms of time and emotional investment, is borne by the family, especially the mothers [32]. At the same time, most parents, if given the option, would care for their child at home, with the necessity of ventilation usually adding little, if any, to the caregiver stress already created by the child's primary illness [33].

7. "Prophylaxis." Particularly in respect to noninvasive ventilation, which can be readily discontinued (above), it is attractive to believe that chronic ventilation might, if used early, be of value in ameliorating or at least delaying the progression of at least the respiratory component of a patient's disease. There is, however, unfortunately little data to support this hypothesis. In a 1994 study by Raphael et al. [34], a group of adolescents with Duchenne muscular dystrophy and forced vital capacities between 20 and 50 % of predicted but without daytime hypercapnia were randomly assigned to receive either "conventional treatment" or conventional treatment plus intermittent nocturnal noninvasive positive pressure ventilation (NIPPV) by nasal mask. The aim of the study was to prevent the progressive pulmonary restriction typically seen in these patients and therefore prolong survival. The authors, however, terminated this study early since NIPPV appeared to confirm no advantage on deterioration in pulmonary function, but paradoxically was associated with a fourfold higher death rate in the treatment population (eight patients versus two patients). In comparison, however, in a subsequent controlled study, 26 patients were randomized to receive either NIPPV or standard care without respiratory support [35]. Patients with NIPPV had improvements in nocturnal gas exchange and appeared to reduce the risk of acute deteriorations with daytime hypercapnia.

8. Parental and family wishes. Obviously in the ideal situation, there will be complete agreement between the parents, the child's medical team, and (where appropriate) the child themselves as to the necessity and appropriateness of initiation of long-term ventilation. Unfortunately this is frequently not the case, with relatively few families given adequate anticipatory information [36]. Despite our best efforts, and even with appropriate guidance, there inevitably will still be the (hopefully rare) situation where, even though the child's physicians may feel this is not in the child's best interests, the parents insist on initiating or continuing ventilation (usually, in this case, invasive). Generally, however the medical team may feel, the general rule in most Western healthcare systems is that the final decision rests with the family and (if able) the child (Chap. 4).

9. Temporizing device. Placing a child on chronic ventilation generally presupposes that the child is suffering from a chronic respiratory disease for which ongoing respiratory support is necessary. There are situations, however, where ventilator support (primarily noninvasive) might be used as a "temporizing" device.

   (a) Respiratory support. Ventilatory support in the home can be used until definitive treatment (such as lung transplantation for patients with end-stage pulmonary disease), or spontaneous recovery (such as phrenic neuropraxia or axonotmesis following cardiac surgery) can occur.

   (b) Palliative care. In patients in end-stage respiratory failure, for whatever cause, short-term ventilation is an option to be used as a temporizing device to allow the child to be discharged home, allowing (if that is the parents' wishes) to be cared for and die at home rather than in hospital. An example would be extubation to noninvasive ventilation (even if required 24 h/day) to allow for discharge home where the family's wishes are for the child to spend their remaining time at home (Chap. 5).

Who?

Once the rationale for chronic ventilation is accepted, consideration of which patients are most likely to benefit from chronic ventilation then follows. It should be noted, however, that there is actually no consensus on how much of a role the above factors should play in deciding precisely which child should be offered long-term ventilation. Consequently there is marked variability in both modes of ventilation employed and types of patients offered long-term ventilation, as well as in the criteria to use to determine exactly when chronic ventilation should be initiated. In simple terms children requiring long-term ventilation generally fall into five broad disease categories.

The most common cause of chronic hypoventilation is respiratory muscle failure, due either to a primary disorder of respiratory muscle or neuromotor function or failure of normal respiratory muscles in the presence of excess load due to primary pulmonary or thoracic cage disorders.

1. Progressive neuromotor disease (Chap. 14). These disorders are characterized by progressive loss of skeletal muscle function. With involvement of thoracic cage and respiratory motor function, these patients inevitably develop a variety of respiratory sequelae.

   (a) Progressive pulmonary restrictive defect. This commonly arises in association with disturbances in thoracic cage and spinal anatomy (scoliosis), as well as the decreased range of motion of the chest wall, resulting in progressive deterioration in respiratory system compliance and loss of lung volumes [27].

   (b) Increasing risk of opportunistic infections. Due to decrements in respiratory muscle strength, as well as reduced ability to achieve maximal inspiration, these patients have deterioration in cough effectiveness, and hence reduced ability to clear retained secretions, associated with increasing risks of opportunistic infections [23].

   (c) Increasing hypoventilation. Patients with respiratory muscle weakness, particularly if involving diaphragmatic function, may be able to "compensate" (at least initially) by use of accessory muscles of respiration. They may, however, show hypoventilation specifically in REM sleep, due to the relative loss of skeletal motor activity associated with REM-related alpha premotor neuron inhibition. Infants are particularly at risk, due to both the fact that, due to their increased thoracic cage compliance [37], they are more dependent upon diaphragmatic function for normal respiration, but also due to the significantly greater quantity of REM sleep required by infants [38].

These disorders can be divided into two groups, based on their primary pathophysiology.

- Diseases primarily affecting respiratory motor neuron function, either specifically to respiratory motor neurons, such as due to phrenic nerve damage from surgery or trauma, or as part of a more generalized disorder of spinal motor neurons, such as spinal muscle atrophy (SMA). SMA is characterized by progressive skeletal muscle weakness consequent to atrophy of spinal alpha motor neurons [39]. It is divided into four categories, based on age of presentation and rapidity of progression, with type 1 having the worst prognosis (death occurring usually, without respiratory support, in the first 2 years of life). In the more severe types, hypoventilation is to be expected, with initiation of respiratory support (primarily noninvasive) resulting in significant improvements in life expectancy [40]. Specifically for type 1 patients, since invasive ventilation does not appear to add to life expectancy (compared to noninvasive) while contributing to the loss of ability to communicate [41], invasive ventilation is generally considered inappropriate as a therapeutic option for this patient population [42, 43].
- Diseases primarily affecting respiratory muscle function, such as the muscular dystrophies, with Duchenne muscular dystrophy (DMD) comprising the largest population [44].

2. Severe respiratory disease. Compared to adults (e.g., COPD), there are relatively few clinical scenarios where a child can be expected to have chronic, stable hypercapnia secondary to a primary pulmonary disease.

   (a) Cystic fibrosis. Noninvasive ventilation has not been shown to increase the life expectancy of patients with cystic fibrosis, while invasive ventilation (due to the adverse consequences of tracheostomy on the ability to cough and clear secretions) is rarely employed. There is some evidence, admittedly in small numbers, that noninvasive ventilation may help in terms of airway clearance, as well as nocturnal gas exchange and quality of life [45], in patients with severe pulmonary disease [2, 46]. It has also been employed for patients with end-stage cystic fibrosis awaiting lung transplant and has been successful in maintaining reasonably good health until a donor organ becomes available [47]. Given its limited success in patients with cystic fibrosis, invasive ventilation is rarely employed [48].

   (b) Bronchopulmonary dysplasia (BPD). Consequent to the appreciation of the role oxygen and ventilation play in the generation of BPD in general, efforts are now made to limit as much as possible the initiation or maintenance of ventilator support in children born prematurely [49]. Despite these efforts, there remains a small population, however, with chronic, severe lung disease that requires ongoing ventilation for survival. For example, 7 % of children in the Massachusetts population of home-ventilated children had chronic lung disease due to prematurity [4] (Chap. 15).

3. Static or progressive disease affecting thoracic cage.

   (a) Scoliosis. Scoliosis is probably the most common skeletal deformity resulting in respiratory impairment. The lateral curvature of the spine in scoliosis results in compression of the ribs, and thereby the lung, on the concave side, with spreading of the ribs on the convex side, resulting in overstretched muscles, with reduced respiratory muscle efficiency and thoracic cage compliance [50]. The impact of scoliosis on respiratory function is directly affected by both the severity of the scoliosis and whether it is idiopathic, with otherwise normal respiratory muscle function, or developing in the context of a progressive neuromotor disorder, such as DMD [51, 52]. Both the reduced thoracic cage compliance and (if starting early enough in lung development) the associated reduction in lung growth increase the work of breathing, in severe cases sufficient to overload the respiratory muscles, resulting in hypoventilation (initially during REM sleep, but, if severe enough, eventually resulting in daytime hypoventilation). Treatment is primarily surgical, mainly to prevent progression since it rarely is associated with subsequent improvement in lung function [50]. In more severe cases, particularly patients with associated neuromotor disease, ongoing ventilatory support may be required [50].

   (b) Primary chest wall disorders. This comprises a diverse, and generally rare, group of disorders [50], which can include:

- Restrictive defects, such as asphyxiating thoracic dystrophy (Jeune's syndrome) [53]
- Disorders of loss of intrinsic rigidity of the chest wall, such as in traumatic flail chest [50], or following thoracoplasty, historically used for treatment of advanced tuberculosis [50], now rarely employed, and more likely for resection of chest wall malignancies [54]

4. Excess loading of the respiratory system (obstructive sleep apnea, obesity hypoventilation).

   (a) Obstructive sleep apnea (OSA). OSA typically causes nocturnal desaturations associated with significant sleep fragmentation, though usually, except in the more severe cases, without significant or persisting hypoventilation [55]. In more severe cases, or if associated with other disorders (such as Duchenne muscular dystrophy or morbid obesity), the resulting disturbance in respiratory drive may be sufficient to require initiation of ventilatory support (Chap. 13).

   (b) Obesity hypoventilation. With the increasing incidence of obesity (even in children) reported in most societies, there is an increasing incidence of obesity hypoventilation syndrome [56]. Obesity hypoventilation arises as a consequence of a combination of impaired mechanics due to excess respiratory muscle loading and impaired compensatory mechanisms associated with sleep-disordered breathing (many patients also having at least elements of obstructive sleep apnea) [56]. Consequently with increasing obesity, these patients initially develop sleep-related hypoventilation. If respiratory drive is preserved while awake, these patients will be able to maintain daytime normocapnia, explaining why many morbidly obese patients maintain adequate daytime ventilation. A subgroup will, however, develop blunted respiratory drive and consequently daytime hypoventilation. This may be due to individual susceptibility [57], but can occur as a primary hypothalamic disorder, with both hyperphagia and intrinsic blunting of respiratory drive (below) [58].

5. Disorders affecting respiratory drive (central hypoventilation syndromes). Respiratory control can be divided into voluntary (cerebral cortex) and involuntary (brainstem). Normal respiration is dependent upon a complex integration of a rhythmic pattern of respiratory motor activity, generated by the central pattern generator (CPG) within the pons and medulla, with ongoing adaptation to afferent information from the peripheral arterial chemoreceptors (carotid and aortic bodies), central chemoreceptors (brainstem), intrapulmonary receptors, and respiratory muscle mechanoreceptors [59]. The CPG is comprised of a complex network of neuron groups that control and drive respiratory muscle activity, including the upper airway muscles, during discrete phases of the respiratory cycle: pre-inspiration, inspiration, active expiration, and passive expiration [60]. The major CPG neuron groups are the pontine respiratory group, the medullary neuron groups including the pre-Botzinger complex and Botzinger

complex, and the ventral respiratory neuron groups. CPG activity is modulated in part via inputs from neurons in the dorsal medulla (dorsal respiratory group), including the nucleus tractus solitarius (NTS), which relays pulmonary mechanoreceptor, peripheral chemoreceptor, and other visceral afferent sensory inputs [61]. Located in the ventral medulla, neurons in the retrotrapezoid nucleus (RTN) are modulated by CO_2 and receive input from other CO_2-sensitive areas as well as input from the peripheral chemoreceptors. The RTN interacts with pre-Botzinger and Botzinger neurons to modulate CPG activity, and it appears to serve as an important site for integration of CO_2 and O_2 chemosensory drive. Under normal circumstances, this results in a three-phase respiratory pattern: inspiration (abduction of upper airway and diaphragmatic contraction), post-inspiration (adduction of the larynx, thereby increasing airway resistance and hence slowing of expiratory airflow), and stage 2 (late) expiration (with, in normal circumstances, low levels of internal intercostal and abdominal muscle activity) [61]. Feedback from afferent neurons which respond to changes in respiratory system mechanics, such as with cardiorespiratory disease, induces adaptive changes in respiratory patterns [62]. Any disorder that results in impairment of this interaction of internal rhythm generation with adaptation to external stimuli will therefore result in disturbed ventilatory control and hence central hypoventilation.

(a) Primary dysfunction of the respiratory nuclei, such as congenital central hypoventilation syndrome (CCHS) (Chap. 17)

- CCHS arises due to mutations (primarily polyalanine repeat expansions) in the *PHOX2B* gene [63]. Although congenital, CCHS can present at any age, the degree clinical involvement being linked to the number of polyalanine repeats [63]. CCHS is associated with a variety of disorders of autonomic function, as well as increased risk of neural crest tumors [63]. The primary respiratory disorder is alveolar hypoventilation due blunted central respiratory drive [64], necessitating lifelong respiratory support, the degree of involvement determining whether invasive versus noninvasive. Individuals presenting in infancy (the more severely affected) generally require invasive ventilation, though, as with those presenting later in life, with improvements in spontaneous ventilation with age, they may later be weaned to noninvasive ventilation solely during sleep [63].
- Other. A variety of other congenital disorders involving both autonomic and hypothalamic function have been associated with varying degrees of central hypoventilation [58]. Some are static and some rapidly progressive, with ventilatory support necessary depending upon the degree of nocturnal hypoventilation. A number of these syndromes are associated with abnormalities in appetite regulation, with the hyperphagia and resulting obesity increasing the risk of hypoventilation (above).

b. Secondary to trauma to the respiratory nuclei (Chiari malformation, brainstem tumor, spinal cord trauma) or to respiratory motor function (spinal cord trauma, with damage to phrenic nerve nuclei) (Chap. 16)

When?

Although the need for long-term ventilation can arise as a consequence of a sudden, catastrophic illness, most children requiring long-term ventilation suffer from a progressive disease where the development of respiratory failure is an expected and inevitable sequel of their disease. This does, therefore, allow for anticipatory guidance, giving the family, patient, and their medical team time to discuss and plan for the future and thereby have a clear understanding and preparation for what chronic ventilation entails before it becomes a necessary treatment. Eventual hypoventilation is predictable in many patients with progressive neuromuscular or pulmonary disease. The optimal time, and particularly what criteria to be used to determine exactly when ventilator support should be initiated, remains somewhat controversial and almost certainly has to be individualized for each patient [65].

1. Blood gases.
   (a) Arterial/capillary blood gas. Although this is the "gold standard" for measuring ventilatory status, it is invasive, difficult to do while the patient is asleep, and only gives values for one moment in time (though bicarbonate level provides an estimate of chronicity of hypoventilation). It is therefore primarily of use to document awake hypercapnia.
   (b) Pulse oximetry. Pulse oximetry has the attraction that it provides a continuous, noninvasive record that can be obtained during sleep. It is also a surrogate for hypercapnia, since, at a constant inspired oxygen concentration, any rise in arterial carbon dioxide level, as described by the alveolar gas equation, results in a reduction in alveolar oxygen pressure (pAO_2) and hence a proportionate fall in arterial oxygen pressure (paO_2) [66]. Consequently any elevation in arterial carbon dioxide above 50 mmHg pressure (so long as the child is breathing room air) will perforce cause a fall in saturation. There are, however, a number of situations where it can provide erroneous information [67], as well as not providing information on sleep state (i.e., whether SWS or REM sleep was ever achieved).
   (c) Noninvasive carbon dioxide (CO_2) monitoring (transcutaneous or end tidal). Both of these methodologies allow for continuous monitoring of carbon dioxide levels. They both, however, have their limitations in terms of ease of obtaining and reliability of data obtained [68].
   (d) Combination. Allowing for their limitations, combining both CO_2 and O_2 can be used as a home-based tool in evaluating sleep-related hypoventilation

[69, 70], though, again, limited by the absence of any information on sleep state.

2. Clinical. Most patients requiring chronic ventilation suffer from a progressive disease, the hypoventilation arising insidiously as a result of slow deterioration of their clinical status. Consequently these patients may adapt to this deterioration and become tolerant of the resulting impact on their respiratory function and, as a result, be remarkably (at least perceived) asymptomatic [14, 71]. Clinical assessment is therefore notoriously unreliable in this patient population. Despite this, a number of authorities have, however, suggested using clinical assessment to determine both need for, and also adequacy of ventilatory support, primarily in patients with neuromotor disease.

   (a) Symptoms of nocturnal hypoventilation. As noted, because of the REM-associated skeletal hypotonia, sleep-related hypoventilation is most likely to occur, at first, during REM sleep. Associated symptoms include frequent awakenings, night sweats, nightmares, nocturnal enuresis, morning headaches, daytime hypersomnolence, and decreased daytime performance [72].
   (b) Respiratory pattern. The diaphragm is the primary muscle of inspiration in normal individuals at rest, with the external intercostals being adjunct inspiratory muscles and the internal intercostals being expiratory muscles and usually only active during exercise or forced expiration [22]. With respiratory muscle fatigue, there may become evidence of recruitment of accessory muscles of respiration (intercostals and shoulder girdle) even at rest. Moreover, with increasing muscle weakness, paradoxical respiration may become apparent. Normally chest and abdominal compartments move in synchrony during respiration. With intercostal muscle weakness, particularly if the upper airway is also involved, increasing upper airway resistance, then on inspiration the abdomen moves out, but the chest wall moves in. In contrast, with predominantly diaphragmatic weakness, where the accessory muscles become the primary muscles of respiration, the chest wall moves out on inspiration, yet the abdomen is sucked in. Consequently evaluation of the patient's respiratory pattern can provide a significant amount of information regarding their respiratory reserve and muscle groups involved [22].

3. Polysomnography. Nocturnal polysomnography (where available) is the "gold standard" for diagnosing sleep-related breathing disorders and in particular nocturnal hypoventilation not associated with daytime hypoventilation [23, 42]. It is really the only methodology to ensure that all sleep stages were in fact seen, since patients who never get below light (stage 2) sleep may have very different ventilation patterns compared to patients with long period of REM or slow wave sleep [18] (above). It is also the only methodology of quantifying the impact therapeutic maneuvers (e.g., nocturnal ventilation) have on sleep architecture. Since pulse oximetry and continuous CO_2 monitoring are also integral components, polysomnography therefore provides a continuous evaluation of respiratory status, not only in response to changing sleep state but also to therapeutic maneuvers. Polysomnography is, however, labor intensive (and hence relatively

expensive) and, in many centers, of limited availability. Moreover, given the complexity of sensors employed, and the adverse impact the sleep laboratory environment may have on sleep, as well as the fact that only 1, perhaps 2, nights can be studied, some authorities have questioned whether polysomnography is either reliable or necessary and recommended using symptoms, supported by oximetry and carbon dioxide monitoring instead to assess adequacy of nocturnal ventilation [73].

4. Pulmonary function. Pulmonary function testing is a readily available, noninvasive, standardized method of measuring both progression of respiratory status and respiratory muscle function. It can be performed by most cognitively intact children aged 6 years and over. It therefore holds attraction as a potential method (especially in patients with slowly progressive neuromotor or pulmonary disease) for predicting the necessity for initiation of ventilation.

   (a) Pulmonary disease. Most of the data linking pulmonary function to respiratory status comes from patients with cystic fibrosis (CF), the severity of which, as a primarily airways disease, is best assessed using the forced expiratory volume in 1 s (FEV_1). As a general rule, the probability of survival of greater than 2 years of patients whose FEV_1 is less than 30 % predicted is under 50 % [74]. This is a relatively old data, but gives a value at which hypercapnic respiratory failure (either due to progression of the disease or, as is commonly seen, acute deterioration associated with an additional viral infection) becomes increasingly likely. Although influenced by many factors (age, nutritional status, rapidity of progression, opportunistic infection) in patients with progressive pulmonary disease, formal evaluation of nocturnal ventilatory status (oximetry or polysomnography) should be considered once their FEV_1 falls below 40 % predicted [75].

   (b) Neuromotor disease. Most of the data linking pulmonary function to respiratory status comes from patients with DMD, as a disease where patients are cognitively intact, and survival expected well past the age where the patients can perform reliable pulmonary function testing. Since these disorders cause primarily a restrictive pulmonary defect, the inspiratory vital capacity (IVC) provides the most reliable predictor of nocturnal hypoventilation, with increasing risk once IVC falls below 40 % predicted [14, 65, 76], though an FEV_1 of less than 40 % has also been suggested as a useful predictor of sleep-related hypoventilation [77]. Alternatively, at least in adults, peak cough flow has been shown to be a useful indicator, with flows of less than 160 L per minute being predictors for the need for assisted ventilation [65, 78]. Appropriate values for children have not, however, been established. Part of the problem with the above tests is that they require maintenance of an oral seal to perform the test, which can be difficult in individuals with neuromotor disease. Since this is not required for sniff nasal inspiratory pressure (SNIP), this may offer a useful alternative [79], though again values predictive of the need for ventilation, particularly in children, have yet to be determined.

Conclusion

Long-term ventilation, primarily with the aim for discharge to home, has become a routine therapeutic option for children with nocturnal or persisting hypoventilation. Even though it has now essentially become a standard of care for many clinical situations, there still remains debate about the precise indications (which patients are most likely to benefit), the criteria for its initiation, and what is the optimal methodology to use in individual patients. Despite these limitations, clinical experience, born out by patient and parental reports, is that for many children, it has resulted in dramatic improvements in not only longevity but also quality of life, allowing safe discharge to home for many children who previously faced spending the remainder of their life in hospital. With its apparent effectiveness, it is difficult to ethically justify randomized controlled trials. Despite this, with its resulting increasing use, and resulting longitudinal evaluation of larger populations, we will hopefully be better placed to answer exactly which patients would most benefit and the optimal timing for its initiation.

References

1. Lloyd-Owen SJ, Donaldson GC, Ambrosino N, Escarabill J, Farre R, Fauroux B, et al. Patterns of home mechanical ventilation use in Europe: results from the Eurovent survey. Eur Respir J. 2005;25:1025–31.
2. Hess DR. The growing role of noninvasive ventilation in patients requiring prolonged mechanical ventilation. Respir Care. 2012;57(6):900–18.
3. Wallis C, Paton JY, Beaton S, Jardine E. Children on long-term ventilatory support: 10 years of progress. Arch Dis Child. 2011;96(11):998–1002.
4. Graham RJ, Fleegler EW, Robinson WM. Chronic ventilator need in the community: a 2005 pediatric census of Massachusetts. Pediatrics. 2007;119(6):e1280–7.
5. Paulides FM, Plotz FB, den Oudenrijn LP V-v, van Gestel JP, Kampelmacher MJ. Thirty years of home mechanical ventilation in children: escalating need for pediatric intensive care beds. Intensive Care Med. 2012;38(5):847–52.
6. King AC. Long-term home mechanical ventilation in the United States. Respir Care. 2012;57(6):921–30.
7. Simonds AK. Home ventilation. Eur Respir J. 2003;22 Suppl 47:38–46.
8. Chatwin M, Bush A, Simonds AK. Outcome of goal-directed non-invasive ventilation and mechanical insufflation/exsufflation in spinal muscular atrophy type I. Arch Dis Child. 2011;96(5):426–32.
9. Simonds AK. Ethical aspects of home long term ventilation in children with neuromuscular disease. Paediatr Respir Rev. 2005;6(3):209–14.
10. Passamano L, Taglia A, Palladino A, Viggiano E, D'Ambrosio P, Scutifero M, et al. Improvement of survival in Duchenne Muscular Dystrophy: retrospective analysis of 835 patients. Acta Myol. 2012;31(2):121–5.
11. Curran FJ, Colbert AP. Ventilator management in Duchenne muscular dystrophy and postpoliomyelitis syndrome: twelve years' experience. Arch Phys Med Rehabil. 1989;70:180–5.
12. Eagle M, Bourke J, Bullock R, Gibson M, Mehta J, Giddings D, et al. Managing Duchenne muscular dystrophy—the additive effect of spinal surgery and home nocturnal ventilation in improving survival. Neuromuscul Disord. 2007;17(6):470–5.

13. Yasuma F, Sakai M, Matsuoka Y. Effects of noninvasive ventilation on survival in patients with Duchenne's muscular dystrophy. Chest. 1996;109(2):590.
14. Katz SL, Gaboury I, Keilty K, Banwell B, Vajsar J, Anderson P, et al. Nocturnal hypoventilation: predictors and outcomes in childhood progressive neuromuscular disease. Arch Dis Child. 2010;95(12):998–1003.
15. Bach JR, Campagnolo DI, Hoeman S. Life satisfaction of individuals with Duchenne muscular dystrophy using long-term mechanical ventilatory support. Am J Phys Med Rehabil. 1991;70(3):129–35.
16. Bach JR, Vega J, Majors J, Friedman A. Spinal muscular atrophy type 1: Quality of life. Am J Phys Med Rehabil. 2003;82(2):137–42.
17. Noyes J. Health and quality of life of ventilator-dependent children. J Adv Nurs. 2006;56(4):392–403.
18. Xie A. Effect of sleep on breathing—why recurrent apneas are only seen during sleep. J Thorac Imaging. 2012;4(2):194–7.
19. Chokroverty S. Sleep dysfunction in neuromuscular disorders. Scweizer Archiv fur Neurologie und Psychiatrie. 2003;154(7):400–6.
20. Arens R, Muzumdar H. Sleep, sleep disordered breathing, and nocturnal hypoventilation in children with neuromuscular diseases. Paediatr Respir Rev. 2010;11(1):24–30.
21. Windisch W. Impact of home mechanical ventilation on health-related quality of life. Eur Respir J. 2008;32(5):1328–36.
22. Allen J. Pulmonary complications of neuromuscular disease: a respiratory mechanics perspective. Paediatr Respir Rev. 2010;11(1):18–23.
23. Finder JD, Birnkrant D, Carl J, Farber HJ, Gozal D, Iannaccone ST, et al. Respiratory care of the patient with Duchenne muscular dystrophy: ATS consensus statement. Am J Respir Crit Care Med. 2004;170(4):456–65.
24. Lee KK, Birring SS. Cough and sleep. Lung. 2010;188 Suppl 1:S91–4.
25. Gomez-Merino E, Bach JR. Duchenne muscular dystrophy: prolongation of life by noninvasive ventilation and mechanically assisted coughing. Am J Phys Med Rehabil. 2002;81(6):411–5.
26. Katz S, Selvadurai H, Keilty K, Mitchell M, MacLusky I. Outcome of non-invasive positive pressure ventilation in paediatric neuromuscular disease. Arch Dis Child. 2004;89(2):121–4.
27. McKim DA, Katz SL, Barrowman N, Ni A, LeBlanc C. Lung volume recruitment slows pulmonary function decline in Duchenne muscular dystrophy. Arch Phys Med Rehabil. 2012;93(7):1117–22.
28. Heinemann F, Budweiser S, Dobroschke J, Pfeifer M. Non-invasive positive pressure ventilation improves lung volumes in the obesity hypoventilation syndrome. Respir Med. 2007;101(6):1229–35.
29. Loorand-Stiver L. Transitioning long-term ventilator-dependent patients out of the intensive care unit—an environmental scan. Ottawa: Canadian Agency for Drugs and Technologies in Health; 2012.
30. Bach JR, Intintola P, Alba AS, Holland IE. The ventilator-assisted individual. Cost analysis of institutionalization vs rehabilitation and in-home management. Chest. 1992;101(1):26–30.
31. Lewarski JS, Gay PC. Current issues in home mechanical ventilation. Chest. 2007;132(2):671–6.
32. Toly VB, Musil CM, Carl JC. Families with children who are technology dependent: normalization and family functioning. West J Nurs Res. 2012;34(1):52–71.
33. Mah JK, Thannhauser JE, Kolski H, Dewey D. Parental stress and quality of life in children with neuromuscular disease. Pediatr Neurol. 2008;39(2):102–7.
34. Raphael JC, Chevret S, Chastang C, Bouvet F. Randomised trial of preventive nasal ventilation in Duchenne muscular dystrophy. French Multicentre Cooperative Group on Home Mechanical Ventilation Assistance in Duchenne de Boulogne Muscular Dystrophy. Lancet. 1994;343(8913):1600–4.
35. Ward S, Chatwin M, Heather S, Simonds AK. Randomised controlled trial of non-invasive ventilation (NIV) for nocturnal hypoventilation in neuromuscular and chest wall disease patients with daytime normocapnia. Thorax. 2005;60(12):1019–24.

36. Sritippayawan S, Kun SS, Keens TG, Davidson Ward SL. Initiation of home mechanical ventilation in children with neuromuscular diseases. J Pediatr. 2003;142(5):481–5.
37. Sly PD, Flack FS, Hantos Z. Respiratory mechanics in infants and children. In: Hamid Q, Shannon J, Martin J, editors. Physiologic basis of respiratory disease. Hamilton: BC Decker; 2005. p. 49–54.
38. Crabtree VM, Williams NA. Normal sleep in children and adolescents. Child Adolec Psychiatric Clin N Am. 2009;18:799–811.
39. Lunn MR, Wang CH. Spinal muscular atrophy. Lancet. 2008;371(9630):2120–33.
40. Gregoretti C, Ottonello G, Chiarini Testa MB, Mastella C, Rava L, Bignamini E, et al. Survival of patients with spinal muscular atrophy type 1. Pediatrics. 2013;131(5):e1509–14.
41. Bach JR, Saltstein K, Sinquee D, Weaver B, Komaroff E. Long-term survival in Werdnig-Hoffmann disease. Am J Phys Med Rehabil. 2007;86(5):339–45.
42. Wang CH, Finkel RS, Bertini ES, Schroth M, Simonds A, Wong B, et al. Consensus statement for standard of care in spinal muscular atrophy. J Child Neurol. 2007;22(8):1027–49.
43. Roper H, Quinlivan R. Implementation of "the consensus statement for the standard of care in spinal muscular atrophy" when applied to infants with severe type 1 SMA in the UK. Arch Dis Child. 2010;95(10):845–9.
44. Flanigan KM. The muscular dystrophies. Semin Neurol. 2012;32(3):255–63.
45. Noone PG. Non-invasive ventilation for the treatment of hypercapnic respiratory failure in cystic fibrosis. Thorax. 2008;63(1):5–7.
46. Moran F, Bradley JM, Piper AJ. Non-invasive ventilation for cystic fibrosis. Cochrane Database Syst Rev. 2013;4, CD002769.
47. Efrati O, Modan-Moses D, Barak A, Boujanover Y, Augarten A, Szeinberg AM, et al. Long-term non-invasive positive pressure ventilation among cystic fibrosis patients awaiting lung transplantation. Isr Med Assoc J. 2004;6(9):527–30.
48. Sheikh HS, Tiangco ND, Harrell C, Vender RL. Severe hypercapnia in critically ill adult cystic fibrosis patients. J Clin Med Res. 2011;3(5):209–12.
49. Kugelman A, Durand M. A comprehensive approach to the prevention of bronchopulmonary dysplasia. Pediatr Pulmonol. 2011;46(12):1153–65.
50. Donath J, Miller A. Restrictive chest wall disorders. Semin Respir Crit Care Med. 2009;30(3):275–92.
51. Tsiligiannis T, Grivas T. Pulmonary function in children with idiopathic scoliosis. Scoliosis. 2012;7(1):7.
52. Leger P, Bedicam JM, Cornette A, Reybet-Degat O, Langevin B, Polu JM, et al. Nasal intermittent positive pressure ventilation. Long-term follow-up in patients with severe chronic respiratory insufficiency. Chest. 1994;105(1):100–5.
53. Baujat G, Huber C, El HJ, Caumes R, Do Ngoc TC, David A, et al. Asphyxiating thoracic dysplasia: clinical and molecular review of 39 families. J Med Genet. 2013;50(2):91–8.
54. Eng J, Sabanathan S, Mearns AJ. Chest wall reconstruction after resection of primary malignant chest wall tumours. Eur J Cardiothorac Surg. 1990;4(2):101–4.
55. Marcus CL, Brooks LJ, Draper KA, Gozal D, Halbower AC, Jones J, et al. Diagnosis and management of childhood obstructive sleep apnea syndrome. Pediatrics. 2012;130(3):576–84.
56. Chau EH, Lam D, Wong J, Mokhlesi B, Chung F. Obesity hypoventilation syndrome: a review of epidemiology, pathophysiology, and perioperative considerations. Anesthesiology. 2012;117(1):188–205.
57. Berger KI, Goldring RM, Rapoport DM. Obesity hypoventilation syndrome. Semin Respir Crit Care Med. 2009;30(3):253–61.
58. Carroll MS, Patwari PP, Weese-Mayer DE. Carbon dioxide chemoreception and hypoventilation syndromes with autonomic dysregulation. J Appl Physiol. 2010;108(4):979–88.
59. Caruana-Montaldo B, Gleeson K, Zwillich CW. The control of breathing in clinical practice. Chest. 2000;117(1):205–25.
60. Bianchi AL, Gestreau C. The brainstem respiratory network: an overview of a half century of research. Respir Physiol Neurobiol. 2009;168(1–2):4–12.

61. Smith JC, Abdala AP, Borgmann A, Rybak IA, Paton JF. Brainstem respiratory networks: building blocks and microcircuits. Trends Neurosci. 2013;36(3):152–62.
62. Molkov YI, Bacak BJ, Dick TE, Rybak IA. Control of breathing by interacting pontine and pulmonary feedback loops. Front Neural Circuits. 2013;7:16.
63. Weese-Mayer DE, Berry-Kravis EM, Ceccherini I, Keens TG, Loghmanee DA, Trang H. An official ATS clinical policy statement: congenital central hypoventilation syndrome: genetic basis, diagnosis, and management. Am J Respir Crit Care Med. 2010;181(6):626–44.
64. Perez IA, Keens TG. Peripheral chemoreceptors in congenital central hypoventilation syndrome. Respir Physiol Neurobiol. 2013;185(1):186–93.
65. Birnkrant DJ, Bushby KM, Amin RS, Bach JR, Benditt JO, Eagle M, et al. The respiratory management of patients with duchenne muscular dystrophy: a DMD care considerations working group specialty article. Pediatr Pulmonol. 2010;45(8):739–48.
66. Cruickshank S, Hirschauer N. The alveolar gas equation. Contin Educ Anaesth Crit Care Pain. 2004;4(1):24–7.
67. Chan ED, Chan MM, Chan MM. Pulse oximetry: Understanding its basic principles facilitates appreciation of its limitations. Respir Med. 2013;107(6):789–99.
68. Wollburg E, Roth WT, Kim S. End-tidal versus transcutaneous measurement of PCO_2 during voluntary hypo- and hyperventilation. Int J Psychophysiol. 2009;71(2):103–8.
69. Bauman KA, Kurili A, Schmidt SL, Rodriguez GM, Chiodo AE, Sitrin RG. Home-based overnight transcutaneous capnography/pulse oximetry for diagnosing nocturnal hypoventilation associated with neuromuscular disorders. Arch Phys Med Rehabil. 2013;94(1):46–52.
70. Nardi J, Prigent H, Adala A, Bohic M, Lebargy F, Quera-Salva MA, et al. Nocturnal oximetry and transcutaneous carbon dioxide in home-ventilated neuromuscular patients. Respir Care. 2012;57(9):1425–30.
71. Mellies U, Ragette R, Schwake C, Boehm H, Voit T, Teschler H. Daytime predictors of sleep disordered breathing in children and adolescents with neuromuscular disorders. Neuromuscul Disord. 2003;13(2):123–8.
72. Benditt JO, Boitano LJ. Pulmonary issues in patients with chronic neuromuscular disease. Am J Respir Crit Care Med. 2013;187(10):1046–55.
73. Bach JR, Zhitnikov S. The management of neuromuscular ventilatory failure. Semin Pediatr Neurol. 1998;5(2):92–105.
74. Kerem E, Reisman J, Corey M, Canny GJ, Levison H. Prediction of mortality in patients with cystic fibrosis [see comments]. N Engl J Med. 1992;326:1187–91.
75. Fauroux B, Pepin JL, Boelle PY, Cracowski C, Murris-Espin M, Nove-Josserand R, et al. Sleep quality and nocturnal hypoxaemia and hypercapnia in children and young adults with cystic fibrosis. Arch Dis Child. 2012;97(11):960–6.
76. Ragette R, Mellies U, Schwake C, Voit T, Teschler H. Patterns and predictors of sleep disordered breathing in primary myopathies. Thorax. 2002;57(8):724–8.
77. Hukins CA, Hillman DR. Daytime predictors of sleep hypoventilation in Duchenne muscular dystrophy. Am J Respir Crit Care Med. 2000;161(1):166–70.
78. Tzeng AC, Bach JR. Prevention of pulmonary morbidity for patients with neuromuscular disease. Chest. 2000;118(5):1390–6.
79. Fitting JW. Sniff nasal inspiratory pressure: simple or too simple? Eur Respir J. 2006;27(5):881–3.

Chapter 2
Non-Invasive Mechanical Ventilation in Children: An Overview

Brian McGinley

Hypoventilation

Ventilatory control is a precisely tuned physiologic process that maintains systemic oxygen and carbon dioxide levels within very narrow ranges required for appropriate cellular function. This delicate balance has resulted in a complex system that senses changes in oxygen (O_2), carbon dioxide (CO_2), and pH in arterial blood and in the brain and responds to these changes through compensatory responses in the upper airway and respiratory pump muscles to maintain ventilation (see Fig. 2.1). Oxygen levels are primarily sensed by the peripheral chemoreceptors, the carotid bodies, and the aortic bodies. CO_2 is sensed mainly by central chemoreceptors that are widely distributed in the brainstem and, along with the peripheral chemoreceptors, input to the medullary respiratory centers in the brainstem. Perturbations in O_2, CO_2, and pH will prompt precise changes in the depth of respiration (tidal volume), respiratory rate, and/or the breathing pattern via diaphragmatic, accessory chest wall and abdominal muscular contraction. Upper airway musculature also receives input from central and peripheral chemoreceptors resulting in contraction to maintain patency.

When alveolar ventilation is insufficient and oxygen levels become too low and/or carbon dioxide levels too high, cellular function is impaired. The alveolar ventilation equation is useful in understanding the physiologic processes leading to hypoventilation and indicates that systemic carbon dioxide levels (pCO_2) are proportional to the ratio between systemic carbon dioxide production (VCO_2) and alveolar ventilation (VA) as follows:

B. McGinley, M.D. (✉)
Pediatric Pulmonary and Sleep Medicine, University of Utah,
81 N Mario Capecchi Dr., Salt Lake City, UT 84113, USA
e-mail: brian.mcginley@hsc.utah.edu

© Springer Science+Business Media New York 2016
L.M. Sterni, J.L. Carroll (eds.), *Caring for the Ventilator Dependent Child*,
Respiratory Medicine, DOI 10.1007/978-1-4939-3749-3_2

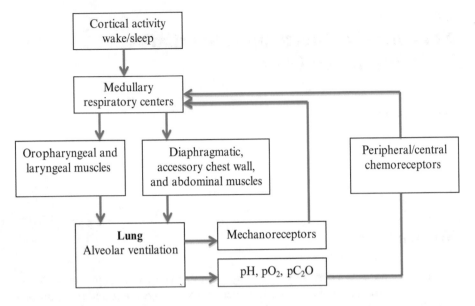

Fig. 2.1 Ventilatory control

$$pCO2 =\propto \frac{VCO2}{VA}$$

Children who hypoventilate can usually be divided into one of two general categories, as follows: children with lung disease, abnormal upper airway, and/or respiratory pump impairment but normal respiratory drive versus children with normal lung, upper airway, and respiratory pump function but abnormal respiratory drive. The first category (abnormal lungs/airways/respiratory pump, normal drive) includes those with upper airway obstruction (e.g., obstructive sleep apnea), insufficient respiratory pump strength to maintain adequate minute ventilation (e.g., Duchenne muscular dystrophy), and severe lung disease (e.g., end-stage cystic fibrosis). In contrast, the second category (normal lungs/upper airway/respiratory pump, abnormal drive) includes those with inadequate sensation or responses to perturbations of CO_2, O_2, or pH, which commonly manifest as central sleep apnea. This group includes children with peripheral or central nervous system impairment and children given medications that decrease respiratory drive (see Table 2.1). It is important to note that some patients may fall into both categories of hypoventilation mechanisms, having impaired pulmonary/respiratory pump function and abnormal respiratory drive. For example, blunting of respiratory drive may occur in patients with long-standing muscle weakness and chronic CO_2 retention.

Table 2.1 Factors and diseases that may result in hypercapnia

Disturbance of respiratory mechanics	Causes and diseases
Normal respiratory system but abnormal respiratory drive	
Reductions in respiratory drive	Sedation/anesthesia and sleep
	Prematurity
	Congenital central hypoventilation syndrome
	Obesity hypoventilation syndrome
	Cerebral blood flow disturbance
	Chiari malformation
	Metabolic alkalosis
	Prader-Willi syndrome
	Hypothyroidism
	Sedation/anesthesia and sleep
Lung, airway, or respiratory pump impairment with normal respiratory control	
Disorders of oropharyngeal and laryngeal muscles	Obstructive sleep apnea
	Vocal cord dysfunction
Respiratory muscles	Muscular dystrophy
	Spinal muscular atrophy
	Spinal trauma
	Diaphragmatic paresis
	Myasthenia gravis
	Poliomyelitis
	Amyotrophic lateral sclerosis
Chest wall	Kyphoscoliosis
	Postthoracotomy, spondyloplastic
Lungs	Rheumatic diseases
	Cystic fibrosis
	Bronchopulmonary dysplasia
	Chronic lung disease
	Asthma
	Kartagener syndrome
Increased CO_2 production (relevant in advanced respiratory disease)	Fever
	Excess carbohydrate intake

Children with Normal Lung and Respiratory Pump Function with Abnormal Respiratory Drive

When central chemoreceptors and the brainstem respiratory controller are not intact, perturbations in O_2 and CO_2 will arise due to decreased respiratory drive and most commonly manifest during sleep. Examples are children administered sedating medications, infants with apnea of prematurity, and patients with congenital central hypoventilation syndrome (CCHS), metabolic alkalosis,

Prader-Willi syndrome, and CNS disorders such as a Chiari malformation. Mechanisms underlying the association of hypoventilation with sleep state in this group are numerous and vary by disorder. For example, patients with CCHS have genetically determined abnormalities in central CO_2 sensing, with profound effects on central chemoreceptor function and breathing rhythm generation during sleep [1]. Children with Prader-Willi syndrome may hypoventilate during sleep due to obstructive sleep apnea, abnormal ventilatory sensitivity to CO_2, and/or obesity-related hypoventilation [2].

Obesity hypoventilation is defined as a weight and/or BMI greater than the 95th percentile associated with daytime symptoms of sleepiness, daytime hypercapnia with CO_2 greater than 45 mmHg, or serum bicarbonate greater than or equal to 27 meq/L and/or oxygen saturation less than 92 % on room air during wakefulness in the absence of other causes of hypoventilation [3]. Obesity hypoventilation is associated with decreased quality of life, cardiovascular comorbidity, pulmonary hypertension, and increased mortality.

Children with Lung Disease and/or Respiratory Pump Impairment with Normal Respiratory Drive

For children in this category, hypoventilation also most commonly manifests during sleep. The transition from wake to sleep is associated with a number of physiologic changes that result in a fall in minute ventilation. Specifically, sleep as compared to wake is associated with decreased ventilation predominantly through a reduction in tidal volume [4]. Additionally, during sleep when neuromuscular tone wanes, the upper airway is prone to collapse leading to obstructive sleep apnea [5–8]. Taken together, sleep compared to wake is a more vulnerable state for hypoventilation.

Decreased neuromuscular strength, underlying lung disease, and cardiac disease independently contribute to hypoventilation and are included in the group of children who typically have normal respiratory drive but respiratory system impairment. Children with neuromuscular disease have an increased incidence of upper airway obstruction and are also susceptible to pathophysiologic processes in the lungs that compromise minute ventilation. While diaphragm strength is retained in most neuromuscular disorders, the progressive loss of skeletal muscle tone in the intercostal and expiratory respiratory muscles results in a slow onset of hypoventilation in many patients that often manifests first during sleep [9]. The development of scoliosis, which is common in children with neuromuscular disease, further worsens hypoventilation as a result of decreases in both lung volumes and chest wall compliance [10]. Children with neuromuscular weakness who lose the ability to cough effectively are vulnerable to increased mucous impaction and resultant atelectasis. Finally, lower lung volumes have been shown to increase pharyngeal collapsibility during sleep, posited to be largely a result of decreased caudal traction on the pharynx [11]. These factors individually or in combination can lead to an inability to meet ventilatory requirements over time.

Evaluation of Ventilation and CO_2 Homeostasis

Evaluation of ventilation during sleep should begin with a detailed history and physical examination. Symptoms of hypoventilation during sleep include frequent awakenings, headaches on awakening, difficulty concentrating, decreased energy, fatigue, and sleepiness during the day. It is recommended that a discussion of these symptoms occurs at clinic visits for children with suspected obstructive sleep apnea and for all children with neuromuscular disease or other conditions associated with hypoventilation. It should be noted that symptoms obtained during history and physical exam can underestimate polysomnography findings [12]. Thus, there should be a low threshold to perform polysomnography in children at high risk for hypoventilation.

When suspicion for hypoventilation during sleep arises, polysomnography is recommended to assess for the presence and severity of sleep disordered breathing and if present to differentiate between potential etiologies such as upper airway obstruction, decreased respiratory drive, or lung disease leading to gas exchange abnormalities. Hypoventilation during sleep in children is defined as CO_2 greater than 50 mmHg for greater than 25 % of total sleep time [13]. Figure 2.2 shows a 12-year-old male with achondroplasia and severe obstructive sleep apnea (apnea-hypopnea index of 112 events/h of sleep) following adenotonsillectomy. As can be seen the patient exhibited ongoing thoracic and abdominal effort associated with an absence of inspiratory airflow associated with oxyhemoglobin desaturations to 83 %

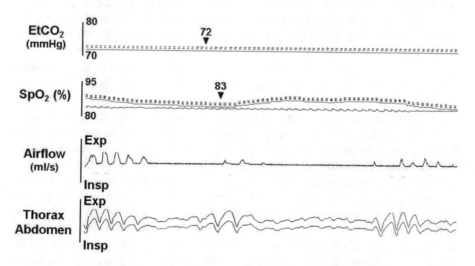

Fig. 2.2 Obstructive sleep apnea on polysomnography

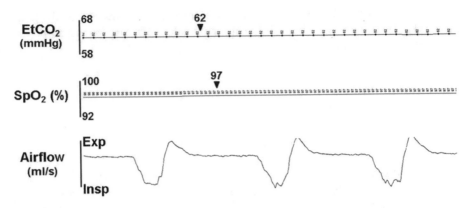

Fig. 2.3 Central hypoventilation on polysomnography

indicating obstructive apneas. The high rate of obstructive apneas in this patient was associated with transcutaneous CO_2 levels that were greater than 50 mmHg for approximately 70 % of the total sleep time and were as high as 72 mmHg.

In contrast, Fig. 2.3 shows a polysomnographic tracing of the breathing pattern during sleep of a 12-year-old female with a Chiari malformation who complained of headaches on awakening. Her apnea-hypopnea index was 0 events/h. Her end-tidal CO_2 levels, however, were greater than 50 mmHg for 50 % of her sleep time and were as high as 62 mmHg. The patient had a respiratory rate of eight breaths per minute and the inspiratory flow contour was round consistent with a non-obstructed breathing pattern. These findings are consistent with hypoventilation secondary to a decreased respiratory drive.

If polysomnography is not available, additional methods to evaluate ventilation during sleep include pulse oximetry, end-tidal or transcutaneous CO_2 devices, or blood gas performed during wake or sleep. It should be noted that while recommendations for the assessment of CO_2 during polysomnography by the American Academy of Sleep Medicine do not distinguish between end-tidal and transcutaneous devices, there are potential shortcomings with both devices [13]. Both end-tidal and transcutaneous CO_2 measurements are well tolerated by children during sleep, readily available, and commonly employed to assess CO_2 during polysomnography. Sidestream end-tidal CO_2 accurately reflects arterial CO_2 under normal breathing conditions when adequate expiratory airflows are entrained, which can be seen when the CO_2 waveform plateaus reflecting exhalation of gas from the alveoli. The sidestream end-tidal method can underestimate CO_2 levels, however, when the plateau in CO_2 concentration is not attained [14]. Underestimation of CO_2 with the end-tidal device will occur during rapid shallow breathing, when nasal airflow is reduced or absent such as when the cannula is removed or if the patient is mouth breathing. The transcutaneous CO_2 method has also been used to assess arterial CO_2 levels during sleep. There are well-described gradients between arterial and transcutaneous levels during sleep; however, transcutaneous measurements of CO_2 may underestimate systemic levels if contact with skin is impaired or overestimate if the heated probe is in contact with the same area of skin for a prolonged period leading to elevated localized temperature and thereby local increases in CO_2 production [15, 16].

In children with lung disease or neuromuscular disorders, lung function tests should also be considered as a part of their routine assessment. Lung volumes can be particularly helpful identifying patients at risk for hypoventilation. Decreases in residual volume are commonly seen prior to a reduction in total lung capacity. Lung function in patients with Duchenne muscular dystrophy has been correlated with findings of gas exchange perturbations during polysomnography [9]. In general, ventilation during sleep should be evaluated when FVC falls below 60 % predicted [17]. If the patient has additional comorbidities such as heart disease or lung disease, ventilatory failure might occur with milder degrees of neuromuscular weakness.

Noninvasive Treatment of Hypoventilation

Noninvasive positive pressure ventilation is the delivery of air from a compressor to the patient without use of an endotracheal tube, with patient interfaces that include nasal or full face mask, nasal prongs, nasal cannula, or mouthpiece. The most common noninvasive ventilation modalities are continuous positive airway pressure (CPAP) and bi-level positive airway pressure. For both modalities air is delivered from a compressor via tightly fitting nasal or full face mask attached by headgear or straps that fit around the head and increases pressure in the upper airway. Noninvasive ventilation treatment during wake can be effectively achieved with the use of a ventilator that delivers large tidal volumes to the patient by a mouthpiece often referred to as sip and puff ventilation. A relatively new noninvasive ventilation positive pressure modality is high-flow nasal therapy (HFNT), which delivers air at high flow rates via nasal cannula and can be used during wake and sleep [18, 19]. Effective treatment of hypoventilation requires an understanding of the underlying pathophysiology responsible for an elevation of systemic CO_2 and the mechanisms of different noninvasive positive pressure ventilation modalities on gas exchange.

The goal of ventilatory support is to increase minute ventilation and thereby reduce systemic CO_2 levels. As discussed above systemic CO_2 is proportional to the ratio of CO_2 production (VCO_2) to alveolar ventilation, which is equivalent to tidal volume (Vt) minus physiologic dead space (Ds). Thus, reducing systemic CO_2 levels can be achieved by increasing tidal volumes and/or decreasing physiologic dead space as follows:

$$pCO2 =\propto \frac{VCO2}{Vt - Ds}$$

For children with obstructive sleep apnea who hypoventilate due to upper airway obstruction, CPAP can effectively alleviate upper airway obstruction, and when respiratory drive is intact, inspiratory tidal volumes increase and gas exchange improves [20]. For children with insufficient respiratory pump strength or lung disease as well as for children with decreased respiratory drive, bi-level positive airway pressure can augment tidal volumes to normalize gas exchange during sleep. High-flow nasal therapy produces a small amount of positive pressure in the upper airway, thereby decreasing upper airway obstruction [21]. The high flow of air also washes out gas in the upper airway decreasing dead space. It should be noted that while correction of hypoxia can be achieved with supplemental oxygen, caution must be used in children who hypoventilate such as children with neuromuscular disease because of the potential for worsening hypercapnia when hypoxic ventilatory drive is decreased. Thus, when supplemental oxygen is administered to children who hypoventilate, CO_2 levels should always be monitored.

Continuous Positive Airway Pressure

The most common indication for noninvasive positive pressure ventilation in children is obstructive sleep apnea. Obstructive sleep apnea is the result of pharyngeal collapse during sleep due to the combination of increased mechanical loads (anatomic upper airway properties) and insufficient compensatory neuromuscular responses to obstruction [8, 22–26]. During sleep when neuromuscular tone falls, the upper airway is prone to collapse [5, 27, 28]. Manipulations of nasal CPAP to assess nasal pressure maximal flow relationships are considered the gold standard to assess upper airway collapsibility, termed the critical closing pressure or Pcrit. Utilizing the Starling resistor to model airflow through a collapsible tube, airflow through the pharynx is dependent on the relationships between the surrounding pressure of the pharynx and pressure downstream in the lower airways and upstream at the nose. When Pcrit is more positive than upstream pressure, complete collapse occurs and there is no airflow (apnea). When pressure downstream falls below Pcrit, partial airway occlusion occurs and airflow is dependent on the gradient between pressure upstream and the collapsible segment in the pharynx. To alleviate upper airway obstruction, either the Pcrit must be lowered (more negative) or nasal pressure increased. Adenotonsillectomy is the first line of treatment recommended by the American Academy of Pediatrics for children for obstructive sleep apnea children, which reduces mechanical loads in the pharynx and decreases Pcrit [29]. Additional factors that can reduce Pcrit include a change in body position, for example, from supine to side, and weight loss [30]. Following adenotonsillectomy approximately 35 % of children have residual sleep apnea [31]. For children with residual sleep apnea, children who refuse surgery, or children who are not deemed appropriate surgical candidates, noninvasive positive pressure ventilation is recommended. The primary effect of CPAP is to increase nasal pressure and create a positive pressure gradient upstream between the nose and the point of airway collapse in the pharynx. In addition to improving pharyngeal patency, CPAP also has been shown to improve gas exchange by increasing lung volumes and decreasing atelectasis [32].

Because patient comfort is correlated with adherence with noninvasive positive pressure ventilation [32–34], selecting an appropriately sized mask the patient finds comfortable is important. There are a number of patient interfaces including nasal masks, full face masks, and nasal pillows. If treatment of upper airway obstruction is the goal, caution should be used with a full face mask. At the same level of pressure, a full face mask compared to a nasal mask is often associated with decreased efficacy in restoring upper patency and in some cases will not restore upper airway patency at high pressure levels or require increased pressure levels resulting in discomfort to the patient [26]. The mechanisms that decrease the efficacy of a full face mask for treating obstructive sleep apnea are not clear; however, investigators speculate that when breathing through the nose and mouth, a full face mask does not create an adequate pressure gradient across the oropharynx or hypopharynx to restore patency and that increased pressure applied to the chin may force the mandible and tongue posteriorly and increase pharyngeal collapse. Moreover, a full face mask should be used with great caution in young patients and those with neuromuscular weakness because the patient has to be able to remove the mask in event of emesis to avoid aspiration or during machine or power failure to prevent an asphyxic event. Polysomnography is recommended to assess the appropriate pressure settings because it effectively demonstrates the relationship between nasal pressure on upper airway obstruction, gas exchange, and sleep quality [35].

Bi-level Positive Airway Pressure

For patients who hypoventilate without evidence of upper airway obstruction or have ongoing impairment in gas exchange after upper obstruction is alleviated with CPAP, bi-level positive airway pressure has been shown to effectively restore appropriate oxygen and carbon dioxide levels in children. The therapeutic mechanisms to increase minute ventilation are similar to invasive mechanical ventilation; most bi-level devices provide an ability to alter expiratory pressure, inspiratory pressure, respiratory rate, and inspiratory time. In contrast to invasive mechanical ventilation, when using noninvasive positive pressure ventilation to increase minute ventilation, the upper airway must be taken into consideration. If upper airway obstruction is present, expiratory positive airway pressure (EPAP) should be adjusted first to restore upper airway patency so that adjustments of inspiratory positive airway pressure (IPAP), respiratory rate, and inspiratory times can effectively increase minute ventilation and restore normal gas exchange. In patients without upper airway obstruction, a full face mask can be used effectively to restore ventilation; however, the same concerns for young patients and patients with neuromuscular disease above persist. The bi-level settings required to restore gas exchange should be assessed while monitoring oxygen and carbon dioxide levels using the lowest pressures that effectively alleviate upper airway obstruction and normalize gas exchange, which like CPAP are best assessed with polysomnography

[35]. Once noninvasive positive pressure ventilation is established during sleep, reevaluation with polysomnography should occur regularly, with intervals dependent on age and clinical features. For example, the evaluation of ventilation during sleep in older children can occur yearly if stable, while reevaluation of ventilation during sleep in younger children might be scheduled more frequently as requirements may change with growth.

High-Flow Nasal Therapy

High-flow nasal therapy (HFNT) has been used in the hospital setting particularly on pediatric intensive care units and has recently become commercially available for home use. High-flow nasal therapy delivers air through a nasal cannula that is heated and humidified at flow rates ranging from 5 to 50 L/min. In contrast to CPAP or bilevel airway pressure devices, high-flow nasal therapy does not require formation of a seal at the nose and/or mouth. High-flow nasal therapy has proven efficacious in the treatment of children and adults with mild to moderate OSA [21, 36]. While there is a slight increase in nasal pressure, the lack of a seal limits the amount of nasal pressure to approximately 2 cm H_2O at 20 L/min in adults, suggesting that there are additional mechanisms of action that stabilize the breathing pattern and normalize gas exchange [21]. Figure 2.4 is a 15-year-old female with cystic fibrosis who underwent

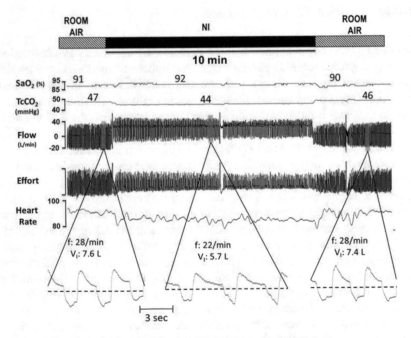

Fig. 2.4 Trial of high-flow nasal therapy in a patient with cystic fibrosis

trial off and on HFNT at 20 L/min alternating over 10 min periods. HFNT at 20 L/min was associated with a reduction in both CO_2 from 47 to 44 mmHg and minute ventilation from 7.6 to 5.7 L/min. The alveolar ventilation equation (see "Children with Normal Lung and Respiratory Pump Function with Abnormal Respiratory Drive") indicates that the reduction in systemic CO_2 associated with a decrease in minute ventilation is due to either decreased dead space ventilation by washing CO_2 out of the upper airway or decreased production of CO_2 suggesting decreased energy expenditure from the work of breathing. The effects of HFNT on CO_2 levels in children without upper airway obstruction suggest a potential role for children with lung disease and neuromuscular disorders, including those with mild disease, or as a bridging therapy until more aggressive noninvasive ventilatory support (e.g., bi-level positive airway pressure) or tracheostomy is required. HFNT might also be particularly helpful for young children including infants with OSA and children who have significant difficulty tolerating CPAP or bi-level noninvasive ventilation due to the patient interface. Studies evaluating effectiveness of HFNT in the home setting have not been performed, and the role of HFNT in both children with OSA and children who hypoventilate without OSA has not been adequately determined.

Noninvasive Positive Pressure Ventilation During Wakefulness

Hypoventilation can develop acutely during wakefulness in patients with neuromuscular disorders or in otherwise healthy children, for example, with pneumonia or status asthmaticus. The use of noninvasive positive pressure ventilation in the intensive care unit setting for children with an acute onset of hypoventilation during wakefulness has been shown effective at reducing intubation and length of stay and should be considered as the first approach to support ventilation particularly for children with neuromuscular disorders. Treatment with noninvasive positive pressure ventilation in the critical care setting, however, is outside of the scope of this book chapter. For children with chronic hypoventilation during wakefulness, noninvasive ventilation has been shown to effectively restore oxygen and carbon dioxide levels and might decrease the need for mechanical ventilation [37]. For short periods of time, noninvasive positive pressure ventilation via mask can be well tolerated during wake without significant complication. Because noninvasive positive pressure ventilation by mask requires a tight seal and if use is required for more than 24 h consecutively, the risk of skin breakdown increases, which needs to be taken into consideration for children requiring ventilator support for prolonged periods [38].

When hypoventilation is present during wakefulness, assessing hypoventilation during sleep and if present treating can improve daytime gas exchange and reverse hypercapnia when awake [39–42]. Several studies in children with neuromuscular disease have demonstrated decreased development of hypercapnia during wakefulness and improvement in diurnal oxygenation and carbon dioxide levels when gas exchange was normalized during sleep [40, 43–45]. Reversal of daytime hypoventilation with nocturnal noninvasive positive pressure ventilation treatment suggests that patients develop a loss of sensitivity to elevated carbon dioxide and hypoxia that can be restored and improve ventilation during wakefulness when gas exchange is normalized during sleep. In children with neuromuscular disorders, rest of respiratory musculature during sleep might also play a role in restoring daytime gas exchange.

For patients requiring chronic noninvasive positive pressure ventilation during wakefulness and sleep, a commercially available mouthpiece can be attached to a ventilator for use when awake, which is often referred to as mouthpiece ventilation or sip and puff ventilation [46, 47]. One approach is to set the ventilator in assist control cycling at high volumes in a timed mode with the alarms turned off. The mouthpiece should be placed next to the patient's mouth allowing them to place it between their lips and inhale at regular intervals to augment inspiratory tidal volumes as needed. Mouthpiece ventilation is well tolerated and does not interfere with eating or speaking. If patients have an aversion to noninvasive positive pressure ventilation, if it is contraindicated, or if hypoventilation cannot be corrected by noninvasive positive pressure ventilation, invasive mechanical ventilation should be considered.

Alternatively, high-flow nasal therapy (HFNT) when heated and humidified has been shown to improve oxygenation and comfort in children with respiratory distress in an intensive care setting [48]. In adults, HFNT during wakefulness increased tidal volumes and lowered respiratory rate [18]. These studies suggest a possible role for HFNT in children with chronic hypoventilation during wakefulness. Taken together the data suggest the use of heated and humidified air delivered through a nasal cannula has the potential for treatment of chronic hypoventilation in children during wakefulness; however, further studies assessing its specific role are needed.

Introducing Noninvasive Positive Pressure Ventilation

Initiation of noninvasive positive pressure ventilation should be considered in children with diurnal or nocturnal hypoventilation and obstructive sleep apnea as noted above. Discussion of the need for and the goals of noninvasive positive pressure ventilatory support should occur with patients and their families and the medical team on a routine basis and should begin as early as possible. For most patients with progressive and slow onset of hypoventilation, ventilatory support can be effectively initiated in the outpatient setting. Initiation of noninvasive positive pressure ventilatory support can be difficult for families and when possible should be done slowly and carefully because experience with noninvasive positive pressure ventilation in the first 1–2 weeks of use is strongly associated with long-term adherence [33, 49]. Introduction of the device during wakefulness for young children and children resistant to initiation can be helpful. One approach is to introduce the mask alone without airflow during wakefulness and when tolerated add a low level of pressure. Once airflow is tolerated during wakefulness, it can be incorporated into the bedtime routine slowly increasing the duration of use. For patients unable to tolerate the initiation of noninvasive positive pressure ventilation, psychologists trained in cognitive behavioral therapy can be helpful [50]. Tracheostomy may be considered in children who are unable to tolerate noninvasive positive pressure ventilation or when noninvasive positive pressure ventilation is inadequate to meet the patient's ventilatory needs.

Benefits of Noninvasive Positive Pressure Ventilation

In children with neuromuscular disorders, such as Duchenne muscular dystrophy, who have hypercapnia, the use of noninvasive positive pressure ventilation has been associated with improved survival [51–53]. In children with spinal muscular atrophy treatment, noninvasive positive pressure ventilation and invasive mechanical ventilation via tracheostomy were similar in regard to mortality [37]. It should be noted that most studies assessing effects of noninvasive positive pressure ventilation in children with neuromuscular disease on mortality are limited by their retrospective design and small numbers of patients studied.

In addition to effects on mortality, noninvasive positive pressure ventilation has also been associated with reduced comorbidities in children with neuromuscular disease. Specifically, noninvasive positive pressure ventilation has been associated with decreased incidence of hospital admission [45]. Use during sleep has been shown to improve quality of sleep, decrease daytime sleepiness, increase sense of well-being and independence, improve concentration, and reduce the incidence of morning headaches [40, 52–54].

Decreased neuromuscular tone is associated with impairment of chest wall shape and growth, which might also be mitigated with noninvasive positive pressure ventilation. As a result of intercostal and expiratory muscle weakness, respiratory movement can become asynchronous ultimately resulting in a bell-shaped chest wall. There is some evidence that chest wall shape can be maintained when noninvasive ventilation is introduced early in life and pressure levels are titrated to prevent asynchronous respiratory motion [55]. While underlying mechanisms responsible for maintaining chest wall shape are unclear, possibilities include alleviation of lower airway obstruction and the reduction of atelectasis. The effects of noninvasive positive pressure ventilation on chest wall shape and growth is an active area of study that has the potential to slow the rate of decline of pulmonary function and thereby significantly improve respiratory health of children with neuromuscular disorders.

Complications of Noninvasive Ventilation

The most common complication of noninvasive positive pressure ventilation is skin breakdown and ulceration. As discussed previously, the risk is increased with use over prolonged periods of time. The risk of skin breakdown also increases with excessive tightening of headgear straps and increased pressure applied to the face [38, 56]. When initiating CPAP, the medical team can be very helpful in demonstrating appropriate amount of pressure required to create an effective seal. The mask should be cleaned daily to remove oils that adhere to the mask from the face and contribute to skin breakdown. When skin irritation begins, it can be effectively alleviated with use of hydrocolloid tape to prevent skin irritation while maintaining a good seal and minimizing air leak. These complications can be decreased with assessments of mask fit and adjustments of mask fit and type when needed. Other common complications include nasal dryness and irritation which can result in nasal bleeding. This can be effectively treated with application of heat and humidity [57–59]. If irritation continues despite adequate heat and humidity, nasal steroids can effectively reduce nasal irritation. Use of positive pressure during sleep can result in gaseous distention of the abdomen, the risk of which is increased with higher levels of pressure. If a G-tube is present, venting the abdomen through the G-tube during sleep can help to decrease the risks associated with gastric distention. As discussed previously, there is risk of aspiration associated with emesis into a full face mask. Introduction of tightly sealed mask with pressure applied to rapidly developing facial bony structures has been associated with significant maxillary hypoplasia. Fauroux et al. assessed 40 children who had been using noninvasive positive pressure ventilation for a minimum of 4 weeks and found facial flattening in 68 % of children, with severity correlated with hours per day of mask use [60]. The risk of maxillary hypoplasia might be reduced with alternative patient interfaces or by altering masks to apply pressure at different points on the face and could include use of nasal pillows when possible; however, there are no studies assessing these interventions.

Future Considerations

Noninvasive positive pressure can effectively support the ventilatory needs for many children who hypoventilate. Understanding the etiology responsible for hypoventilation and choosing the appropriate modality and settings are critical to restore ventilation. Many questions regarding noninvasive ventilation, however, remain. Adherence with noninvasive ventilation remains suboptimal in some patient populations including children with obstructive sleep apnea. While advances in patient interfaces have improved comfort, adherence has not improved markedly. Of particular concern are young children and infants, for whom options for noninvasive patient interfaces are limited. Moreover, the roles of newer noninvasive ventilation modalities including the high-flow nasal cannula system for children who hypoventilate have not been adequately determined.

References

1. Guyenet PG. Regulation of breathing and autonomic outflows by chemoreceptors. Compr Physiol. 2014;4:1511–62.

2. Nixon GM, Brouillette RT. Sleep and breathing in Prader-Willi syndrome. Pediatr Pulmonol. 2002;34:209–17.
3. Tulaimat A, Littleton S. Defining obesity hypoventilation syndrome. Thorax. 2014;69:491.
4. Colrain IM, Trinder J, Fraser G, Wilson GV. Ventilation during sleep onset. J Appl Physiol. 1987;63:2067–74.
5. Fogel RB, Trinder J, White DP, Malhotra A, Raneri J, Schory K, Kleverlaan D, Pierce RJ. The effect of sleep onset on upper airway muscle activity in patients with sleep apnoea versus controls. J Physiol. 2005;564:549–62.
6. Katz ES, White DP. Genioglossus activity during sleep in normal control subjects and children with obstructive sleep apnea. Am J Respir Crit Care Med. 2004;170:553–60.
7. Lo YL, Jordan AS, Malhotra A, Wellman A, Heinzer RA, Eikerman M, Schory K, Dover L, White DP. The influence of wakefulness on pharyngeal airway muscle activity. Thorax. 2007;62(9):799–805.
8. McGinley BM, Schwartz AR, Schneider H, Kirkness JP, Smith PL, Patil SP. Upper airway neuromuscular compensation during sleep is defective in obstructive sleep apnea. J Appl Physiol. 2008;105:197–205.
9. Suresh S, Wales P, Dakin C, Harris MA, Cooper DG. Sleep-related breathing disorder in Duchenne muscular dystrophy: disease spectrum in the paediatric population. J Paediatr Child Health. 2005;41:500–3.
10. Katz SL, Gaboury I, Keilty K, Banwell B, Vajsar J, Anderson P, Ni A, Maclusky I. Nocturnal hypoventilation: predictors and outcomes in childhood progressive neuromuscular disease. Arch Dis Child. 2010;95:998–1003.
11. Squier SB, Patil SP, Schneider H, Kirkness JP, Smith PL, Schwartz AR. Effect of end-expiratory lung volume on upper airway collapsibility in sleeping men and women. J Appl Physiol. 2010;109:977–85.
12. Carroll JL, McColley SA, Marcus CL, Curtis S, Loughlin GM. Inability of clinical history to distinguish primary snoring from obstructive sleep apnea syndrome in children. Chest. 1995;108:610–8.
13. Berry RB, Budhiraja R, Gottlieb DJ, Gozal D, Iber C, Kapur VK, Marcus CL, Mehra R, Parthasarathy S, Quan SF, et al. Rules for scoring respiratory events in sleep: update of the 2007 AASM Manual for the Scoring of Sleep and Associated Events. Deliberations of the Sleep Apnea Definitions Task Force of the American Academy of Sleep Medicine. J Clin Sleep Med. 2012;8:597–619.
14. Russell GB, Graybeal JM. Reliability of the arterial to end-tidal carbon dioxide gradient in mechanically ventilated patients with multisystem trauma. J Trauma. 1994;36:317–22.
15. Berlowitz DJ, Spong J, O'Donoghue FJ, Pierce RJ, Brown DJ, Campbell DA, Catcheside PG, Gordon I, Rochford PD. Transcutaneous measurement of carbon dioxide tension during extended monitoring: evaluation of accuracy and stability, and an algorithm for correcting calibration drift. Respir Care. 2011;56:442–8.
16. Clark JS, Votteri B, Ariagno RL, Cheung P, Eichhorn JH, Fallat RJ, Lee SE, Newth CJ, Rotman H, Sue DY. Noninvasive assessment of blood gases. Am Rev Respir Dis. 1992;145:220–32.
17. Hull J, Aniapravan R, Chan E, Chatwin M, Forton J, Gallagher J, Gibson N, Gordon J, Hughes I, McCulloch R, et al. British Thoracic Society guideline for respiratory management of children with neuromuscular weakness. Thorax. 2012;67 Suppl 1:i1–40.
18. Mundel T, Feng S, Tatkov S, Schneider H. Mechanisms of nasal high flow on ventilation during wakefulness and sleep. J Appl Physiol. 2013;114:1058–65.
19. Nilius G, Franke KJ, Domanski U, Ruhle KH, Kirkness JP, Schneider H. Effects of nasal insufflation on arterial gas exchange and breathing pattern in patients with chronic obstructive pulmonary disease and hypercapnic respiratory failure. Adv Exp Med Biol. 2013;755:27–34.
20. Sullivan CE, Issa FG, Berthon-Jones M, Eves L. Reversal of obstructive sleep apnoea by continuous positive airway pressure applied through the nares. Lancet. 1981;1:862–5.
21. McGinley BM, Patil SP, Kirkness JP, Smith PL, Schwartz AR, Schneider H. A nasal cannula can be used to treat obstructive sleep apnea. Am J Respir Crit Care Med. 2007;176:194–200.
22. Patil SP, Schneider H, Marx JJ. Differences in the control of upper airway (UA) collapsibility in obstructive sleep apnea and normal subjects. Am J Respir Crit Care Med. 2002;165:A39.

23. Patil SP, Schneider H, Marx JJ, Gladmon E, Schwartz AR, Smith PL. Neuromechanical control of upper airway patency during sleep. J Appl Physiol. 2007;102:547–56.

24. Schwartz AR, Eisele DW, Smith PL. Pharyngeal airway obstruction in obstructive sleep apnea: pathophysiology and clinical implications. Otolaryngol Clin North Am. 1998;31:911–8.

25. Schwartz AR, Patil SP, Laffan AM, Polotsky V, Schneider H, Smith PL. Obesity and obstructive sleep apnea: pathogenic mechanisms and therapeutic approaches. Proc Am Thorac Soc. 2008;5:185–92.

26. Smith PL, Wise RA, Gold AR, Schwartz AR, Permutt S. Upper airway pressure-flow relationships in obstructive sleep apnea. J Appl Physiol. 1988;64:789–95.

27. Fogel RB, Trinder J, Malhotra A, Stanchina M, Edwards JK, Schory KE, White DP. Within-breath control of genioglossal muscle activation in humans: effect of sleep-wake state. J Physiol. 2003;550:899–910.

28. Pierce R, White D, Malhotra A, Edwards JK, Kleverlaan D, Palmer L, Trinder J. Upper airway collapsibility, dilator muscle activation and resistance in sleep apnoea. Eur Respir J. 2007;30:345–53.

29. Farber JM. Clinical practice guideline: diagnosis and management of childhood obstructive sleep apnea syndrome. Pediatrics. 2002;110:1255–7.

30. Schwartz AR, Gold AR, Schubert N, Stryzak A, Wise RA, Permutt S, Smith PL. Effect of weight loss on upper airway collapsibility in obstructive sleep apnea. Am Rev Respir Dis. 1991;144:494–8.

31. Friedman M, Wilson M, Lin HC, Chang HW. Updated systematic review of tonsillectomy and adenoidectomy for treatment of pediatric obstructive sleep apnea/hypopnea syndrome. Otolaryngol Head Neck Surg. 2009;140:800–8.

32. Al-Mutairi FH, Fallows SJ, Abukhudair WA, Islam BB, Morris MM. Difference between continuous positive airway pressure via mask therapy and incentive spirometry to treat or prevent post-surgical atelectasis. Saudi Med J. 2012;33:1190–5.

33. Budhiraja R, Parthasarathy S, Drake CL, Roth T, Sharief I, Budhiraja P, Saunders V, Hudgel DW. Early CPAP use identifies subsequent adherence to CPAP therapy. Sleep. 2007;30:320–4.

34. van Zeller M, Severo M, Santos AC, Drummond M. 5-years APAP adherence in OSA patients—do first impressions matter? Respir Med. 2013;107:2046–52.

35. Kushida CA, Chediak A, Berry RB, Brown LK, Gozal D, Iber C, Parthasarathy S, Quan SF, Rowley JA. Clinical guidelines for the manual titration of positive airway pressure in patients with obstructive sleep apnea. J Clin Sleep Med. 2008;4:157–71.

36. McGinley B, Halbower A, Schwartz AR, Smith PL, Patil SP, Schneider H. Effect of a high-flow open nasal cannula system on obstructive sleep apnea in children. Pediatrics. 2009;124:179–88.

37. Bach JR, Saltstein K, Sinquee D, Weaver B, Komaroff E. Long-term survival in Werdnig-Hoffmann disease. Am J Phys Med Rehabil. 2007;86:339–45.

38. Gregoretti C, Confalonieri M, Navalesi P, Squadrone V, Frigerio P, Beltrame F, Carbone G, Conti G, Gamna F, Nava S, et al. Evaluation of patient skin breakdown and comfort with a new face mask for non-invasive ventilation: a multi-center study. Intensive Care Med. 2002;28:278–84.

39. Annane D, Orlikowski D, Chevret S, Chevrolet JC, Raphaël JC. Nocturnal mechanical ventilation for chronic hypoventilation in patients with neuromuscular and chest wall disorders. Cochrane Database Syst Rev. 2007, (4):CD001941.

40. Mellies U, Ragette R, Dohna SC, Boehm H, Voit T, Teschler H. Long-term noninvasive ventilation in children and adolescents with neuromuscular disorders. Eur Respir J. 2003;22:631–6.

41. Nickol AH, Hart N, Hopkinson NS, Moxham J, Simonds A, Polkey MI. Mechanisms of improvement of respiratory failure in patients with restrictive thoracic disease treated with non-invasive ventilation. Thorax. 2005;60:754–60.

42. Piper AJ, Sullivan CE. Effects of long-term nocturnal nasal ventilation on spontaneous breathing during sleep in neuromuscular and chest wall disorders. Eur Respir J. 1996;9:1515–22.

43. Ward S, Chatwin M, Heather S, Simonds AK. Randomised controlled trial of non-invasive ventilation (NIV) for nocturnal hypoventilation in neuromuscular and chest wall disease patients with daytime normocapnia. Thorax. 2005;60:1019–24.
44. Simonds AK, Ward S, Heather S, Bush A, Muntoni F. Outcome of paediatric domiciliary mask ventilation in neuromuscular and skeletal disease. Eur Respir J. 2000;16:476–81.
45. Young HK, Lowe A, Fitzgerald DA, Seton C, Waters KA, Kenny E, Hynan LS, Iannaccone ST, North KN, Ryan MM. Outcome of noninvasive ventilation in children with neuromuscular disease. Neurology. 2007;68:198–201.
46. Garuti G, Nicolini A, Grecchi B, Lusuardi M, Winck JC, Bach JR. Open circuit mouthpiece ventilation: concise clinical review. Rev Port Pneumol. 2014;20:211–8.
47. Toussaint M, Steens M, Wasteels G, Soudon P. Diurnal ventilation via mouthpiece: survival in end-stage Duchenne patients. Eur Respir J. 2006;28:549–55.
48. Spentzas T, Minarik M, Patters AB, Vinson B, Stidham G. Children with respiratory distress treated with high-flow nasal cannula. J Intensive Care Med. 2009;24:323–8.
49. Weaver TE, Kribbs NB, Pack AI, Kline LR, Chugh DK, Maislin G, Smith PL, Schwartz AR, Schubert NM, Gillen KA, et al. Night-to-night variability in CPAP use over the first three months of treatment. Sleep. 1997;20:278–83.
50. Slifer KJ, Kruglak D, Benore E, Bellipanni K, Falk L, Halbower AC, Amari A, Beck M. Behavioral training for increasing preschool children's adherence with positive airway pressure: a preliminary study. Behav Sleep Med. 2007;5:147–75.
51. Gomez-Merino E, Bach JR. Duchenne muscular dystrophy: prolongation of life by noninvasive ventilation and mechanically assisted coughing. Am J Phys Med Rehabil. 2002;81:411–5.
52. Simonds AK, Muntoni F, Heather S, Fielding S. Impact of nasal ventilation on survival in hypercapnic Duchenne muscular dystrophy. Thorax. 1998;53:949–52.
53. Vianello A, Bevilacqua M, Salvador V, Cardaioli C, Vincenti E. Long-term nasal intermittent positive pressure ventilation in advanced Duchenne's muscular dystrophy. Chest. 1994;105:445–8.
54. Baydur A, Layne E, Aral H, Krishnareddy N, Topacio R, Frederick G, Bodden W. Long term non-invasive ventilation in the community for patients with musculoskeletal disorders: 46 year experience and review. Thorax. 2000;55:4–11.
55. Petrone A, Pavone M, Testa MB, Petreschi F, Bertini E, Cutrera R. Noninvasive ventilation in children with spinal muscular atrophy types 1 and 2. Am J Phys Med Rehabil. 2007;86:216–21.
56. Munckton K, Ho KM, Dobb GJ, Das-Gupta M, Webb SA. The pressure effects of facemasks during noninvasive ventilation: a volunteer study. Anaesthesia. 2007;62:1126–31.
57. Ballard RD, Gay PC, Strollo PJ. Interventions to improve compliance in sleep apnea patients previously non-compliant with continuous positive airway pressure. J Clin Sleep Med. 2007;3:706–12.
58. Nilius G, Domanski U, Franke KJ, Ruhle KH. Impact of a controlled heated breathing tube humidifier on sleep quality during CPAP therapy in a cool sleeping environment. Eur Respir J. 2008;31:830–6.
59. Weaver TE. Adherence to positive airway pressure therapy. Curr Opin Pulm Med. 2006;12:409–13.
60. Fauroux B, Lavis JF, Nicot F, Picard A, Boelle PY, Clement A, Vazquez MP. Facial side effects during noninvasive positive pressure ventilation in children. Intensive Care Med. 2005;31:965–9.

Chapter 3
Chronic Invasive Mechanical Ventilation

Howard B. Panitch

Introduction

Chronic mechanical ventilation via tracheostomy is commonly employed in children with craniofacial abnormalities that cause obstruction that cannot be overcome by noninvasive means, infants and some children with chronic respiratory failure who require continuous ventilatory support, infants and children with congenital heart disease, and those with severe developmental delay who cannot adapt to noninvasive ventilation [1–4]. Compared with those children with chronic respiratory failure who use noninvasive ventilation, children requiring invasive ventilatory support tend to be younger at the time that they first require chronic ventilatory support [2, 5], have more complex disease [6], or require more hours per day of support [5]. Invasive ventilation is also used when noninvasive support does not correct respiratory failure or when a child cannot tolerate noninvasive ventilation [7]. Ventilation via tracheostomy is also occasionally employed transiently to facilitate rehabilitation in a child with chronic respiratory failure recovering from a catastrophic illness or injury.

H.B. Panitch, M.D. (✉)
Division of Pulmonary Medicine, Technology Dependence Center, The Children's Hospital of Philadelphia, University of Pennsylvania Perelman School of Medicine,
11054 Colket Translational Research Building, 3501 Civic Center Boulevard, Philadelphia, PA 19104, USA
e-mail: panitch@email.chop.edu

© Springer Science+Business Media New York 2016
L.M. Sterni, J.L. Carroll (eds.), *Caring for the Ventilator Dependent Child*,
Respiratory Medicine, DOI 10.1007/978-1-4939-3749-3_3

Ventilator Settings and Mechanics of Breathing

Ventilators used for children with tracheostomies assist breathing by providing positive pressure to assume some or all of the respiratory work. The way a ventilator controls a delivered breath is derived from the Equation of Motion of the Respiratory System. Briefly, the pressure needed to move air from the atmosphere into the alveolus must be used to overcome elastic forces to inflate the lung and chest wall, and resistive forces to stretch tissues and to move air through the airways. At very high respiratory rates (i.e., as seen during high-frequency oscillatory ventilation), there is also a pressure cost associated with accelerating gas particles. This inertance pressure is negligible over the range of breathing frequencies of conventional ventilators, however, and can be ignored when considering breathing frequencies of less than 100 breaths/min.

The simplified equation of motion is written $P = \Delta VE + R\dot{V}$, where P is the pressure above end-expiratory pressure required to achieve an adequate breath, ΔV is the volume change desired (tidal volume), E is the elastance (the reciprocal of compliance, describing the tendency of the lung tissue to resist stretch), R is resistance, and $\dot{V}$ is the inspiratory flow. The pressure required to achieve the breath can be generated by a ventilator alone (in which case all of the pressure is positive or above airway opening pressure), by the patient's respiratory muscles alone (where all inspiratory pressure is below airway opening pressure), or by a combination of the two.

Depending on how the ventilator is set to interact with the patient, resulting breaths can either be mandatory or spontaneous (Table 3.1). If the ventilator *either* initiates *or* ends (cycles) an inspiration based on operator settings, it is termed a "mandatory" breath. If, however, the patient both initiates (triggers) *and* cycles a breath, it is termed a "spontaneous" breath [8] (Fig. 3.1). Note that in this scheme, a breath can be considered spontaneous even if the ventilator provides some of the pressure for the breath, as long as the breath is started and stopped by patient effort or respiratory system mechanics.

According to the equation of motion, for any given breath only one variable at a time (pressure, volume, or flow) can be made an independent variable and therefore set by an operator (Table 3.1). The other variables are dependent and will be determined by how the independent variable is set and by the patient's respiratory mechanics. This is exactly how ventilators work, by controlling either pressure, volume, or flow for a given breath. Early home ventilators were equipped to control only volume, but newer generation machines can be set up to control either pressure or volume.

When a ventilator is set in pressure control (PC) mode (sometimes called pressure preset ventilation), each breath delivered by the ventilator provides a preset pressure for a set duration (inspiratory time). The size of the resulting breath will depend on respiratory system resistance and compliance; if these change between breaths, i.e., because of bronchospasm, leak in the system, pneumothorax, mucous plug, etc., so too will the volume of the resulting breath. The inspiratory flow is determined by the

Table 3.1 Type of ventilator breath

Mode	Inspiratory trigger	Expiratory cycle	Inspiratory time	Peak inspiratory pressure	Tidal volume	Inspiratory flow
VC-CMV	T or patient	V or T	Set or function of rate and $\dot{V}$	Variable: changes with respiratory mechanics or patient effort	Set; remains constant	Set or function of rate and $\dot{V}$ settings; remains constant
PC-CMV	T or patient	T	Set; remains constant	Set; remains constant	Variable: changes with respiratory mechanics or patient effort	Variable: changes with respiratory mechanics or patient effort; decelerating waveform
PC-CSV	Patient	$\dot{V}$	Function of rate and $\dot{V}$ or respiratory mechanics	Set; remains constant	Variable: changes with respiratory mechanics or patient effort	Variable: changes with respiratory mechanics or patient effort; decelerating waveform
VC-IMV	M: T S: patient	M: V or T S: P or $\dot{V}$	M: see VC-IMV S: see PC-CSV	M: see VC-IMV S: see PC-CSV	M: see VC-IMV S: see PC-CSV	M: see VC-IMV S: see PC-CSV
PC-IMV	M: T S: patient	M: T S: P or $\dot{V}$	M: see PC-IMV S: see PC-CSV	M: see PC-IMV S: see PC-CSV	M: see PC-IMV S: see PC-CSV	M: see PC-IMV S: see PC-CSV

VC volume control, *PC* pressure control, *CMV* continuous mandatory ventilation, *CSV* continuous spontaneous ventilation, *IMV* intermittent mandatory ventilation, *T* time, *V* volume, $\dot{V}$ flow, *M* mandatory, *S* spontaneous

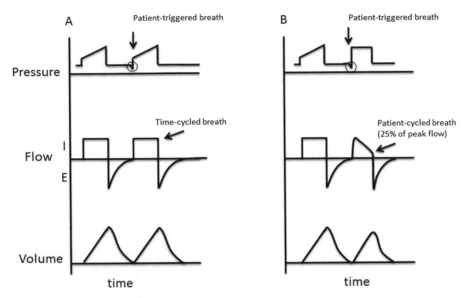

Fig. 3.1 Mandatory and spontaneous ventilation. (**a**) A patient is receiving volume control-continuous mandatory ventilation (VC-CMV). The airway pressure tracing of the first breath shows that it is a machine (time)-triggered breath, based on the rate set by the clinician. The second breath is triggered by the patient, as seen by the drop in airway opening pressure, but it is cycled based on the inspiratory time set by the clinician. Since both breaths are either triggered *or* cycled by the ventilator settings, they are considered mandatory breaths. (**b**) A patient is receiving volume control intermittent mandatory ventilation with pressure support ventilation (VC-IMV+PSV). As in the first example, the first breath is machine triggered and cycled. The second breath is patient triggered and cycles when inspiratory flow falls below 25 % of the peak inspiratory flow. Since the second breath is triggered by patient effort and cycled by patient respiratory system mechanics, it is a spontaneous breath; thus, the mode is IMV. (*I* inspiration, *E* exhalation)

mechanics of the patient's respiratory system and decreases as the airway-alveolar pressure difference decreases with lung filling. Although the flow rate is not set by the operator, the time required to reach the desired inspiratory pressure (called "rise time," "slope," or "profile") can be adjusted and so can alter the initial flow.

A ventilator set in volume control (VC) mode will deliver the desired tidal volume even when compliance or resistance of the respiratory system changes: it merely changes the pressure used to deliver the breath. The inspiratory flow of the breath is constant throughout the breath, but the flow rate can be set by the operator. A higher inspiratory flow will fill the lung faster but at a higher pressure.

Combining the factor being controlled with the type of breathing pattern desired, ventilator breaths can therefore be classified as either pressure or volume controlled and continuous mandatory ventilation (CMV), continuous spontaneous ventilation (CSV), or intermittent mandatory ventilation (IMV) where mandatory breaths are interspersed with spontaneous ones [9].

In the latter situation, depending on the scheme chosen, volume or pressure control can be used for mandatory breaths, while pressure control is used for interspersed spontaneous breaths [9, 10]. This is exactly what happens when synchronized IMV (SIMV) is combined with pressure support ventilation (Fig. 3.1b): the mandatory (SIMV) breaths are initiated by time (the rate set on the ventilator) and can be either PC or VC. The pressure support breaths that the patient takes in between the mandatory breaths are initiated by the patient and cycled by the mechanical characteristics of the patient and so are spontaneous. These breaths are delivered in a PC mode [10]. The combinations of what variable the ventilator controls and type and sequence of breaths used are the chief determinants of the various ventilator modes set by clinicians [9–11].

Modes of Mechanical Ventilation

The *mode* chosen for ventilator support refers to how the ventilator interacts with the patient. This includes how each breath is initiated and cycled, the method by which the breath is delivered, and potentially several other conditional or target variables that can modify pressure or flow patterns. Unfortunately, ventilator manufacturers have not embraced a common taxonomy to describe the modes that their products can deliver, leading to a multitude of names for similar modes and confusion or misunderstanding about the type of breaths being delivered on the part of ventilator operators. Clinicians and investigators involved in the study of ventilator function favor the use of a uniform classification system that accurately describes the characteristics of various modes of mechanical ventilation [8–11]. Using that taxonomy, several common modes of ventilation can be analyzed for how the ventilator and patient interact with each other and then indications for when one mode might be preferable over others can be discerned.

Continuous mandatory ventilation (CMV) (Fig. 3.2): this mode of ventilation is commonly referred to as *control ventilation* if there is no opportunity for the patient to initiate any breaths (Fig. 3.2a) or *assist/control* (A/C) *ventilation* if the patient can trigger breaths in between machine-initiated breaths (Fig. 3.2b) [12]. Thus, if the set ventilator rate is below the patient's needs, the patient can trigger the ventilator and receive additional breaths. Whether machine or patient triggered, the delivered tidal volume of each breath will be the same [13]. The breath can be volume or pressure controlled, depending on the operator's preference. In control mode, every breath is time triggered, based on the set respiratory rate of the ventilator. In A/C mode, breaths will be time triggered based on the set rate, or when patient triggered they will be pressure, volume, or flow triggered depending on the characteristics of the ventilator. Every breath is machine cycled based on volume or time. This mode of ventilation reduces respiratory work by providing complete support for every breath while aiming to achieve the desired tidal volume. Control ventilation is used when the patient's respiratory drive is inadequate because of a brainstem lesion, pharmacologic suppression, or in a patient with a high spinal cord lesion who cannot initiate any breathing effort. If the ventilator is set in A/C mode but the set rate is high enough to suppress any spontaneous efforts, the delivered mode is in effect one of control ventilation. If possible, this should be avoided since control ventilation is associated with the development of diaphragm atrophy and loss of function [14].

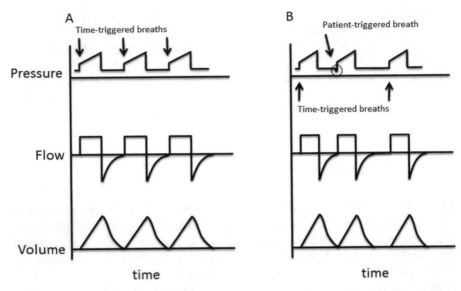

Fig. 3.2 Continuous mandatory ventilation (CMV). (**a**) A patient is receiving VC-CMV. Each breath is machine triggered based on the rate set by the clinician: there is no patient effort to trigger a breath. This type of CMV is also referred to as "control" ventilation. (**b**) A patient is again receiving VC-CMV, but the second breath pictured is triggered by patient effort, before the time interval set by the clinician. In response to patient demand, the ventilator delivers a VC breath that is time cycled and otherwise identical to the breath delivered by machine triggering. This type of CMV has also been referred to as "assist/control" ventilation

Continuous spontaneous ventilation (CSV) (Fig. 3.3a): this type of ventilation pattern refers to modes like pressure support ventilation (PSV) or continuous positive airway pressure (CPAP). Although CPAP does not provide inspiratory positive pressure assistance, it does provide a clinician-set constant pressure while the patient breathes spontaneously [12, 15]. Other modes of CSV like neurally adjusted ventilatory support or proportional assist ventilation are not yet available on portable home ventilators and will not be discussed.

CPAP delivers a baseline elevation of pressure above atmospheric pressure during spontaneous breathing [12, 15]. It is differentiated from positive end-expiratory pressure (PEEP) by virtue of the fact that PEEP is used during mechanical ventilation and refers to control of the baseline pressure during some other mode of mechanical ventilation [12]. It is also conceivable that with a large inspiratory effort, a patient could generate enough negative pressure to cause airway pressure to become subatmospheric during inspiration while still maintaining the set positive expiratory pressure. Such a condition might occur, for instance, if the inspiratory trigger sensitivity of the ventilator were set in such a way that the patient had to exert excessive effort to trigger a breath or if inspiratory flow were inadequate to meet the patient's demand; these represent situations that need to be corrected. CPAP is typically used to maintain functional residual capacity (FRC) in a spontaneously breathing patient. This is especially important in infants and toddlers in

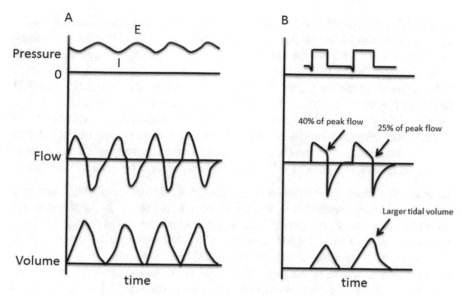

Fig. 3.3 Continuous spontaneous ventilation (CSV). (**a**) A patient is supported by continuous positive airway pressure (CPAP). The baseline pressure is elevated above atmospheric (0) but there is no positive pressure support during inspiration (I). Each breath is patient triggered and cycled. (**b**) This patient is receiving pressure support ventilation (PSV). Each breath is patient triggered. The breath is cycled when inspiratory flow falls below a predetermined threshold. In the first breath, that value is 40 % of the peak flow. Note that the breath is shorter and the resulting tidal volume is smaller than in the second breath, where flow must fall below 25 % of the peak flow to cycle to exhalation

whom the chest wall is more compliant than the lung [16]. Infants actively maintain FRC above resting end-expiratory lung volume by constricting laryngeal adductors and initiating inspiratory muscle contraction during exhalation to retard expiratory flow [17, 18]. Thus, placement of a tracheostomy tube in a newborn with severe upper airway obstruction could impair some infants' ability to maintain FRC; if this were to occur and the function could not be restored with a speaking valve, the infant would require application of CPAP to maintain FRC. CPAP can also be used to raise lung volume above FRC, if that elevated lung volume improves lung mechanics because of the child's underlying condition. In some infants and children with moderate to severe tracheomalacia or bronchomalacia, CPAP is also used to maintain airway patency during exhalation [19].

Pressure support ventilation (PSV) (Fig. 3.3b): is a form of spontaneous breathing in which the breaths are patient triggered and flow cycled, based on the patient's respiratory system impedance: once inspiratory flow falls to a predetermined percentage of the peak inspiratory flow, the ventilator cycles from inspiration to exhalation [20]. The standard flow cycle variable is set to 25 % of peak flow; that is, when the inspiratory flow falls to 25 % of peak flow as the lung fills, the ventilator cycles to exhalation. Some home ventilators, however, (e.g., the LTV® series, CareFusion, Yorba Linda, CA; the Trilogy ventilator, Respironics, Murrysville, PA;

or the HT70, Newport Medical, Costa Mesa, CA) allow the flow cycle level to be adjusted (between 10 and 40 % for the LTV®, between 10 and 90 % for the Trilogy, or between 5 and 85 % for the HT70). Each breath is pressure controlled, and the level of support is adjusted by the clinician based on how much respiratory work is to be assumed by the ventilator [20]. PSV is typically combined either with CPAP to unload respiratory muscles while allowing the patient autonomy with respect to timing of breaths or with intermittent mandatory ventilation to enhance patient comfort and minimize respiratory work. It is also frequently used to assist with weaning from mechanical ventilatory support. Since it involves spontaneous ventilation, the patient's respiratory drive must be intact for it to be a useful modality.

Intermittent mandatory ventilation (IMV) (Fig. 3.4): this mode of ventilation provides a mandatory breath that is time triggered at a rate set by the clinician with a set volume or pressure. In between mandatory breaths, a source of fresh gas is made available to the patient to breathe spontaneously. IMV was actually first described as a feature of a new ventilator for neonates [21], but its use was quickly expanded to adult patients where it was anecdotally hailed as, among other things, a superior mode to Control or A/C ventilation for weaning patients [22]. Other modes of

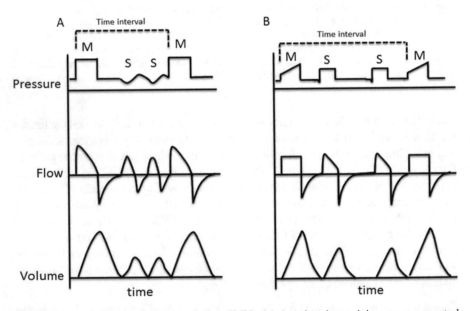

Fig. 3.4 Intermittent mandatory ventilation (IMV). (**a**) A patient is receiving pressure control IMV (PC-IMV). Each mandatory (M) breath is delivered based on the rate set by the clinician. In between mandatory breaths, the patient can breathe spontaneously (S). In this example, there is no positive pressure assistance for spontaneous breaths. This was the original scheme for IMV, and weaning occurred by reducing the set rate and allowing the patient to assume more of the respiratory work by breathing unassisted. (**b**) This patient is receiving volume control IMV (VC-IMV), and pressure support (PSV) has been added to support the patient's spontaneous efforts. The clinician can choose to alter the pressure limit of the PSV breaths, resulting in tidal volumes that match the size of those resulting from mandatory breaths

ventilation have alternately been used to facilitate ventilator weaning, but IMV remains a popular method of ventilator support.

In an effort to avoid unintentional patient-ventilator dyssynchrony and patient discomfort when the mandatory breath would occur during the patient's expiratory phase of the spontaneous breath, *synchronized* intermittent mandatory ventilation (SIMV) was developed [23]. In brief, the ventilator uses a timing window to sense the patient's effort around the time of a scheduled breath and attempts to deliver the mandatory breath in synchrony with the patient's spontaneous breath. In the current generation of mechanical ventilators, mandatory breaths can be delivered in one of three timing scenarios: (1) at the set frequency, (2) only when the patient's spontaneous rate falls below the set frequency, or (3) when the spontaneous minute ventilation (rate x tidal volume/min) falls below a preset threshold [9]. Various home ventilators use schemes based on the first two of these three options, often incorporating a patient-triggered mandatory breath into the scheme in addition to spontaneous breaths (LTV® series, Newport HT50 and HT70). In addition, the Newport HT50 and HT70 ventilators (Newport Medical Instruments, Inc., Costa Mesa, CA) also have a "lockout window" that prohibits additional mandatory breaths for a specified time if the combination of machine- and patient-triggered mandatory breaths exceeds the calculated set rate. Whatever the scheme for synchronization, current home ventilators that offer an SIMV mode also permit the combination of SIMV with PSV so that spontaneous breaths can be partially or completely supported by positive pressure. It is clear that any device that offers either SIMV or PSV must also be able to supply a continuous flow of gas in between mandatory breaths; older generation machines like the LP-10 (Nellcor Puritan Bennett, Inc., Minneapolis, MN) and Respironics® PLV-100 (Respironics, Murrysville, PA) required the patient to open a demand valve for an external supply of air or an H-valve to a reservoir bag for oxygen-enriched air. They permitted the use of an SIMV mode but did not have a PSV option. While these machines are no longer manufactured, there are still patients in the community who use them.

Application of Different Modes of Mechanical Ventilation

Once a child undergoes tracheostomy placement to facilitate mechanical ventilation, there is an implication that the cause of respiratory failure is a chronic one. In an acute setting, efforts are aimed at reducing support with an aim toward liberation from mechanical ventilation as quickly as possible. In contrast, the focus of home mechanical ventilation is not to wean the patient from support: rather, it is to provide adequate support for growth and periods of activity, play, or appropriate developmental interactions [24]. Reduction in ventilator support becomes the natural by-product of improved health, strength, and in some cases resolution of the underlying cause of respiratory failure. The choice of ventilator mode must match the patient's needs, maximize patient comfort, and, when appropriate, allow for the gradual shift of respiratory work from the machine to the patient as the disease improves.

In contrast, there are some children whose disease trajectory can be expected to be static or progressive: these children may actually require increased mechanical ventilatory support over time.

A child who requires assistance to maintain FRC or airway patency may require only CPAP and no other positive pressure assistance. For the child with a normal respiratory drive as well as either an increased respiratory load or reduced respiratory pump function, use of PSV with the required amount of distending end-expiratory pressure (PSV+PEEP/CPAP) is a reasonable way to provide support. Some practitioners prefer to provide a low background mandatory rate to avoid apneas or to simulate a sigh breath to minimize the risk of atelectasis. Here, they set a low SIMV rate (4 or 5 breaths/min) with a targeted tidal volume of 10–15 mL/kg, but allow the infant or child a fair bit of autonomy by providing PSV (SIMV+PSV) to reduce respiratory work and enhance ventilator-patient synchrony. Alternatively, using a higher SIMV rate but lower pressures with PSV breaths is yet another variation that can provide adequate support. Use of PSV is not appropriate for patients with an inadequate respiratory drive: here, mandatory ventilation must be used to assure adequacy of ventilation and to prevent prolonged apneas.

Children with neuromuscular weakness might be able to tolerate PSV alone, but if the child is too weak to trigger a breath, or the respiratory load increases (i.e., with an acute infection, atelectasis or bronchospasm), the modality will provide inadequate support. Additionally, a child with diurnal hypercapnia, who has reset his or her central drive because of chronic hypoventilation, will likely also require mandatory breaths to reestablish eucapnia via modest hyperventilation. Weak patients can do well with A/C ventilation: adequate gas exchange can be guaranteed at rest based on the settings chosen, yet with excitement or exertion the patient's increased demand will be easily met with additional patient-triggered mandatory breaths. As an alternative, SIMV+PSV can be substituted, but to provide the same degree of support as the A/C strategy, the pressure control setting of the PSV breath will have to equal that of the mandatory breath (in PC mode) or be adjusted to provide a similar tidal volume (in VC mode). The use of SIMV+PSV would be expected to be more comfortable for the patient, since the duration of the spontaneous breaths is dictated by the mechanics of the child's respiratory system. Some children will prefer A/C ventilation, however, so that patient feedback and preference should guide the decision of which mode to use whenever possible.

Similarly, there is no universal benefit of choosing to provide mandatory breaths in either volume control or pressure control mode to children with chronic respiratory failure. Fortunately, the current generation of home ventilators can provide mandatory breaths in either mode. For most patients, the choice between modes will be based either on local practice or occasionally on patient preference.

There are, however, situations in which one or the other mode will be preferable. Whenever the situation allows, pediatric practitioners prefer to use the smallest size tracheostomy tube possible to facilitate speech and minimize the risk of damage to the tracheal wall [24, 25]. In a child with a large leak around the tracheostomy tube, the size of delivered tidal volumes in VC ventilation will become highly variable from breath to breath as the leak waxes and wanes. A child can have minimal leak and receive adequate support in VC mode while awake but experience profound hypoventilation when asleep because of excessive leak related to relaxation of pharyngeal musculature [26]. When the leak is large, the volume will be delivered at a low pressure because of the low resistance across the leak and infinite "compliance" of the atmosphere: the mandated volume will escape the respiratory system, and there will be diminished chest wall movement and air entry, resulting in hypoventilation, air hunger, tachypnea, and possibly ventilator-patient asynchrony. An alternative to changing the tracheostomy tube to a larger size or to a cuffed tube is to switch to a PC mode. Here, the ventilator will increase output to provide the level of pressure set by the clinician, even though flow escapes through the mouth and nose. The tidal volume will vary from breath to breath with more or less lost to the atmosphere, but the set peak inspiratory pressure will be maintained, and adequacy of effective ventilation can be preserved [26].

Leaks can affect ventilation in other ways, by exaggerating demand on inspiration or diminishing the signal for cycling of a breath on exhalation. A large leak around the tracheostomy tube can cause problems with ventilator triggering when using a flow-triggered device. Under normal circumstances, the machine monitors flow across the airway opening, and if it is set to deliver a patient-triggered breath (i.e., the mode is assist/control or PSV), it will do so when inspiratory flow falls below the trigger level. If the leak is large, however, the decrease in continuous flow that occurs because of the flow escaping across the leak is interpreted by the ventilator as a patient's inspiratory effort, and the ventilator will deliver the "requested" breath. This can lead to autotriggering of the ventilator, a condition where pressure support or assist/control breaths are delivered almost continuously despite lack of true patient demand. Ventilator autotriggering leads to hyperventilation and metabolic alkalosis and contributes to patient-ventilatory dyssynchrony. If the leak is moderate, some machines have a leak compensation option that can accommodate for the problem, or the trigger sensitivity can be adjusted to compensate manually for the leak and still allow the patient to receive patient-triggered breaths. If the leak is excessive, however, these interventions will be inadequate, and the tracheostomy tube will have to be changed to a larger size or to a cuffed model, or the ventilation mode will have to be changed to one that excludes patient-triggered breaths (e.g., SIMV without PSV or control ventilation).

In PSV mode, a large leak will also cause problems with cycling of a breath (Fig. 3.5). Because the PC breath terminates when flow diminishes to a set percentage of the peak flow based on respiratory system compliance and resistance, a large leak will preclude flow from decreasing as the breath is directed out of the mouth and nose. All ventilators have a backup time limit of 3 s for PSV breaths in case flow does not slow to the cycle threshold. This is too long for most children and leads to patient-ventilator dyssynchrony. Some home machines (e.g., the LTV® series, HT50, HT70) have a backup time termination setting that can be set to limit the duration of the PSV breath in the event of a large leak and failure of the breath to flow cycle.

In addition to situations in which there is a large leak around the tracheostomy tube, pressure control ventilation may also be required for very small infants or those with small lungs as a result of thoracic insufficiency syndrome [27] or pulmonary hypoplasia, since the smallest tidal volume that can be set on current

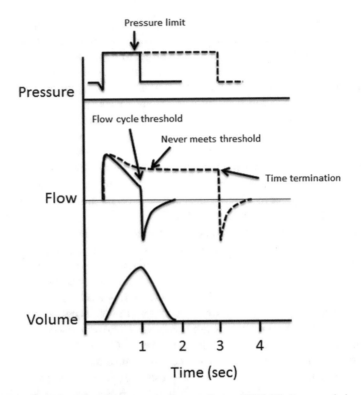

Fig. 3.5 The effect of a leak on pressure support ventilation (PSV). Under normal circumstances (solid tracings), a PSV breath cycles to exhalation when inspiratory flow falls to a preset percentage of peak flow as the lung fills and the pressure difference between airway opening pressure and alveolar pressure approaches 0. When a leak is present (*dashed lines*), however, alveolar and airway opening pressures never equalize, and so flow continues across the airway opening into the atmosphere, never decreasing to the threshold value. Inspiratory time is prolonged: ventilators have an emergency 3 s limit after which the breath will time cycle. During the prolonged inspiration, children will often exhale against the elevated pressure well before the end of the breath. These interactions cause patient-ventilator dyssynchrony and contribute to patient discomfort and inadequate ventilatory support. Several home ventilators allow the cycle threshold to be adjusted to overcome the effect of leaks or have a time termination backup setting that can be adjusted to avoid the prolonged inspiration

home ventilators is 40 mL (iVent, GE Healthcare, Madison, WI) or 50 mL (LTV® series, Puritan Bennett 540, Trilogy, HT70). The HT50 ventilator can be set to deliver a minimum tidal volume of 100 mL. Furthermore, at smaller tidal volumes and high rates, some home ventilators will deliver variable tidal volumes in volume control mode that can be >20 % larger than the intended value [28].

Patients with severe obstructive disease who require a long expiratory time to avoid the development of dynamic hyperinflation might benefit from volume control ventilation with a constant flow pattern. For a given inspiratory time, constant flow can fill the lung faster than flow delivered in a decelerating pattern typical of a pressure control breath: said differently, the inspiratory time for a given tidal volume can be shortened by using constant flow at a higher rate (although the peak inspiratory pressure will also be higher). This will preserve tidal volume but allow for a longer expiratory time and help to prevent breath stacking and dynamic hyperinflation [29].

At present, one home ventilator (iVent 101®) has the capability to provide mandatory breaths in a pressure-regulated volume control (PRVC) mode. This mode represents a method of breath-to-breath dual control, where mandatory breaths are pressure limited and time cycled, and a clinician-set tidal volume is used for feedback to adjust the pressure limit [12]. The ventilator first delivers a "test breath" in volume control mode based on the desired (operator set) tidal volume. The ventilator determines the required pressure and the subsequent breath is delivered in pressure control mode. The ventilator then assesses the size of the resulting tidal volume and adjusts the pressure up or down as necessary in ≤ 3 cmH$_2$O increments until the desired tidal volume is achieved. If the respiratory system compliance or resistance changes, the ventilator will adjust the pressure up or down to maintain the desired tidal volume to a maximum of 5 cm H$_2$O below the preset upper pressure limit. PRVC delivers the desired tidal volume at the lowest pressure necessary and is useful for patients with rapidly changing lung mechanics who would benefit from delivery of a stable tidal volume. As such, its use in a stable home ventilator patient is limited. The mode has been integrated into several bilevel positive pressure generators, but has been found to be unreliable in delivering the set tidal volume in situations where unintended leaks are present [30].

Characteristics of Home Ventilators

The first generation of portable home ventilators were piston-driven, fairly large (weighing about 30–35 lb), delivered breaths in only a volume control mode and did not provide continuous flow [31]. The machines used a single limb circuit with an external PEEP valve. Because there was no continuous flow, however, any leak in the circuit (i.e., around the tracheostomy tube) would result in failure to maintain a set PEEP. Pressure monitoring was used for the inspiratory trigger. Internal battery life was limited, and a lead acid battery (i.e., 12 V car battery) was typically used for portability. Neonates and infants who were too small to be able to use these machines could be supported with small pressure-limited, time-cycled hospital ventilators. These machines required a pneumatic source, and so an electric air compressor had to be used in tandem, making portability impossible. The system provided continuous flow so IMV could be used, making transition from hospital to home easier.

First-generation portable ventilators were generally reliable: a study that reviewed the frequency of home ventilator breakdowns among 150 home ventilator users, of whom 50 were <21 years old, found that equipment malfunction or ventilator failure occurred on average a calculated once every 1.25 years of continuous ventilator use

[32]. Of those requiring ventilator use 24 h/day, however, about 75 % reported at least one equipment problem over the year of observation. Because of the recognized potential for catastrophic outcomes in the event of mechanical ventilator failure, guidelines recommend that ventilator-assisted individuals who require ≥20 h per day of life support [24] or children who cannot maintain adequate gas exchange without mechanical ventilation for ≥2 h [33] have a second (backup) ventilator in the home. These first-generation machines are still in use in the community and can readily fulfill the need of patients who do not breathe spontaneously above a mandatory rate and who do not require a closely maintained level of PEEP to preserve FRC or airway patency.

Most second- and third-generation machines are turbine driven [31]. These machines are smaller and lighter than first-generation machines (most weigh under 15 lb) and have more external battery options, all of which enhance portability. They also offer more options like flow triggering, pressure control (in addition to volume control), SIMV, and PSV. In most models, the PEEP valve is integrated into the ventilator. Some third-generation machines offer graphics for patient monitoring, as well as an ability to download and print reports on patient use and patient-ventilator interaction. Trigger sensitivity varies somewhat between models, but in general is comparable or in some cases superior to that of conventional ICU ventilators [28]. Battery duration also varies widely among different models [28] and is affected by choice of settings: battery life is shortened when using pressure control instead of volume control, when setting higher levels of PEEP, and, depending on the model, when increasing FiO_2 [34]. Battery performance is not just a matter of convenience for portability, but can be lifesaving in the event of a power outage [35–37]. Recently, a ventilator-associated death was reported in an adult with amyotrophic lateral sclerosis because of malfunction of the internal battery, which resulted not only in ventilator malfunction, but also in a reduction of the ventilator alarm volume [38].

As noninvasive mechanical ventilation has gained popularity for the support of children with neuromuscular weakness, restrictive chest wall diseases, and central hypoventilation syndromes, the equipment used to provide that support has become more sophisticated and the distinction between "bi-level pressure generators," also known as "respiratory assist devices," and ventilators has blurred. Sometimes, machines intended for noninvasive use have been used via tracheostomy, and several portable ventilators designed to be used via tracheostomy also have a noninvasive mode. The US Food and Drug Administration (FDA) classifies devices based upon where they are used (facility versus home) and their intended use ("full" or "life" support device versus continuous or noncontinuous, nonlife-supporting device) [39]. Factors including the underlying condition, amount of ventilatory support required, need for alarms or battery backup, local custom, and reimbursement will guide or determine the type of machine that can be used for a given patient.

The improvement in ventilator design of second- and third-generation portable ventilators over first-generation machines is in large part attributable to integration of microprocessor monitoring of ventilator output and patient response. The added complexity of the machines increases the risk for ventilator malfunction, but in the absence of a registry of ventilator-associated individuals, the incidence of serious ventilator-related complications remains unknown. King accessed the FDA Manufacturer and User Facility Device Experience (MAUDE) database and found >150 home mechanical ventilation malfunctions or failures in the United States in 2010 [39]. A recent European review of ventilator-associated problems in the home is more difficult to extrapolate to children requiring home ventilation via tracheostomy, as the number of individuals receiving chronic mechanical ventilation via tracheostomy represented only 1 % of 1211 patients, and only 12 % of the population studied required continuous mechanical ventilation [40]. The authors noted, however, that the likelihood of ventilator malfunction was relatively small (28 % of >3000 calls received over a 6-month period) but increased if the ventilator was >8 years old, if it was a model newly introduced on the market, or if the user required ≥16 h/day of use. The two most common causes of ventilator malfunction included bellows or blower failure or a problem in the circuit board. Ventilator function was also impaired if water entered the pressure lines, a problem that could be circumvented with the use of a filter.

Complications of Invasive Home Mechanical Ventilation

Care of a child who requires chronic mechanical ventilation is complex, and caregivers require specialized training to maximize patient safety and desired outcomes [24]. The presence of a tracheostomy adds complexity to that care and requires that caregivers learn an additional skill set related to care and assessment of the tracheostomy [25]. Potential complications directly related to the tracheostomy include inadvertent displacement or obstruction, swallowing dysfunction and increased risk of aspiration, increased risk of lower respiratory tract infection, creation of a false tract, granuloma formation at the tracheostomy site, acquired tracheal stenosis or suprastomal tracheomalacia, traumatic creation of a tracheo-innominate or tracheoesophageal fistula, and development of a chronic tracheocutaneous fistula following planned decannulation [41–43]. The presence of a tracheostomy necessitates additional equipment, including a heater/humidifier or heat/moisture exchanger (artificial nose) to prevent airway cooling and inspissation of secretions, suction equipment, and additional monitoring. In some regions, the standard practice is to provide skilled nursing care for *at least* 8 h if a child has a tracheostomy and cannot call for help or correct a problem so that parents can sleep but still have their child visually monitored.

Portable ventilators have built-in alarms to detect low pressure or patient disconnection, apnea, low minute ventilation or low tidal volume, high pressure, high tidal volume, high minute ventilation, low battery, and power failure. In the presence of a large leak around the tracheostomy tube, problems with false apnea or low minute ventilation alarms can arise, even when the alarms are adjusted to their lowest settings. Efforts should be made to diminish the leak rather than to turn off these "nuisance" alarms, as they represent important backup systems for identifying inadequate ventilatory support.

Reliance on ventilator alarms alone to detect inadvertent decannulation or other problems, however, could prove disastrous. Using a lung model and simulations of low, medium, and high tidal volume settings, Kun et al. demonstrated that home ventilators failed to alarm if the low-pressure alarm was set 10 cm H_2O below peak inspiratory pressure using tracheostomy tubes with inside diameters ≤ 6.0 mm or with low and medium settings when the tracheostomy tube inside diameter was <4.5 mm, and the low-pressure alarm was set 4 cm H_2O below the peak pressure [44]. Further, the same group subsequently identified several misconceptions that primary caregivers had regarding their ability to rely on alarms to detect either inadvertent decannulation events or episodes of mucous plugging in children receiving positive pressure ventilation via tracheostomy [45]. These findings underline the need for those who care for children reliant on positive pressure ventilation via tracheostomy at home to be vigilant, well trained, and prepared [46].

Outcomes of Children Supported by Positive Pressure Ventilation via Tracheostomy

Survival of children with chronic respiratory failure who require positive pressure ventilation via tracheostomy is generally good. Nineteen single center reports involving a total of 621 children followed for 4.5–25 years describe a survival incidence of 57–100 % and liberation from mechanical ventilation in 0–52 % (see [47] for a table of individual studies). Similarly, the average 5-year cumulative survival calculated from 14 series involving 265 patients was ~85 %, with a mean duration of follow-up of 3.3 years [48].

The presence of a tracheostomy, however, increases the risk for death or catastrophic central nervous system injury, even after a child has been liberated from mechanical ventilation. A comparison of the incidence of tracheostomy-related accidents between hospital and home care in the early 1980s showed that the rate of accidents in home care was eight times greater than the rate in the pediatric ICU (2.3 versus 0.3 accidents per 10,000 patient days, respectively) [49]. In one early report of invasive home mechanical ventilation, Schreiner et al. noted that 30 of 101 patients followed over 18 years died [4]. Six children, including four of eight deaths reported after 24 months of chronic mechanical ventilation, died from airway-related accidents including inadvertent decannulation, unsuspected tube obstruction, or accidental disconnection from the ventilator. Furthermore, three of the five children who died at home had been liberated from mechanical ventilation but were still tracheostomy dependent because of subglottic stenosis. More recently, Edwards et al. reported that 47 (21 %) of 228 ventilator-dependent patients followed over 22 years died: of these, 9 (19 %) deaths were directly attributable to tracheostomy-related accidents [47].

Outcomes of children receiving positive pressure ventilation via tracheostomy are, at least in part, influenced by the child's underlying condition. The wide range of reported survival and liberation percentages in part reflects the characteristics of the center populations being treated: a program that treats a high percentage of children with neuromuscular disease will have a lower proportion of children who are liberated from mechanical ventilation, whereas a center with a large number of

children with chronic lung disease of prematurity will have a much higher proportion of children who can wean completely from mechanical ventilation.

In a retrospective review of children who were ventilator dependent via tracheostomy and discharged from Great Ormond Street Hospital over a 7-year period,
15 (38 %) of 39 children were able to wean from mechanical ventilation whereas
7 (18 %) died [50]. Of those who were able to be liberated from mechanical ventilation, 12 (80 %) had a combination of chronic lung disease and airway disease. In
contrast, those who continued to require ventilatory support were more likely to
have an underlying neuromuscular disorder. Among a population of 35 children
with congenital heart disease who required positive pressure ventilation via tracheostomy followed at Children's Hospital Los Angeles over 15 years, 23 (66 %)
were alive at the time of analysis [51]. Of those, 8 (23 %) had weaned from
mechanical ventilation, 10 (28 %) required continuous mechanical ventilation, and
5 (14 %) used only nocturnal mechanical ventilation. The authors stratified patients
by complexity of their underlying heart disease and surgical repair using the Risk
Adjusted Classification for Congenital Heart Surgery (RACHS-1). Only those
with relatively less complex disease, as reflected by a RACHS-1 score ≤ 3, were
able to wean from ventilation. In contrast, 8/9 (89 %) of those with a RACHS-1
score ≥ 4 died. The 5-year survival for those with a RACHS-1 score ≤ 3 was significantly greater than that of children with a RACHS-1 score ≥ 4 ($p < 0.001$).

To explore how much the characteristics of the underlying disease influenced outcomes, the same group of investigators looked retrospectively at the courses of 228
patients who were supported with positive pressure ventilation via tracheostomy over
22 years (990 patient years) at their institution [47]. Of the group, 41 (18 %) were
liberated from mechanical ventilation and 47 (21 %) died. The cumulative 5-year
incidence of survival for the entire cohort was 80 % (73 %–85 % CI). As previously
noted, a diagnosis of chronic lung disease was significantly positively associated
with likelihood of liberation from mechanical ventilation compared with diagnoses
of respiratory pump weakness or abnormal central drive. Of the 47 patients who died,
the cause of death was ascribed to natural progression of disease in only 16 (34 %);
9 deaths (19 %) were associated with tracheal bleeding, tracheal obstruction, or other
tracheostomy accident, while no death was associated with ventilator malfunction.
There was no relationship between underlying cause of respiratory failure and shortened survival. Approximately 50 % of the deaths were unexpected. The authors speculated that those deaths not related to progression of the underlying disease were
likely associated with non-pulmonary comorbidities that their patients had.

Conclusion

Positive pressure mechanical ventilation via tracheostomy remains an important
component in the armamentarium of therapies for children with chronic respiratory
failure. Improvements in equipment have resulted in more options for the practitioner to enhance patient comfort and portability while maintaining a high degree of
machine reliability. The practitioner must be aware of the effects that the

tracheostomy tube can have on ventilator output and how to compensate for them, especially when leaks around the tracheostomy tube compromise ventilation or patient-ventilator synchrony. Care must be taken to ensure that home caregivers are skilled not only in ventilator management and assessment, but also in the care of the tracheostomy tube and airway. When all of these issues are addressed, outcomes of children with chronic respiratory failure who receive invasive mechanical ventilatory support can be maximized.Acknowledgement The author thanks Julian L. Allen, MD for his critical review of the manuscript.

References

1. Gowans M, Keenan HT, Bratton SL. The population prevalence of children receiving invasive home ventilation in Utah. Pediatr Pulmonol. 2007;42(3):231–6.
2. Graham RJ, Fleegler EW, Robinson WM. Chronic ventilator need in the community: a 2005 pediatric census of Massachusetts. Pediatrics. 2007;119(6):e1280–7.
3. Pilmer SL. Prolonged mechanical ventilation in children. Pediatr Clin North Am. 1994;41(3):473–512.
4. Schreiner MS, Downes JJ, Kettrick RG, Ise C, Voit R. Chronic respiratory failure in infants with prolonged ventilator dependency. JAMA. 1987;258(23):3398–404.
5. Racca F, Berta G, Sequi M, Bignamini E, Capello E, Cutrera R, et al. Long-term home ventilation of children in Italy: a national survey. Pediatr Pulmonol. 2011;46(6):566–72.
6. Wallis C, Paton JY, Beaton S, Jardine E. Children on long-term ventilatory support: 10 years of progress. Arch Dis Child. 2011;96(11):998–1002.
7. Amin RS, Fitton CM. Tracheostomy and home ventilation in children. Semin Neonatol. 2003;8(2):127–35.
8. Mireles-Cabodevila E, Hatipoglu U, Chatburn RL. A rational framework for selecting modes of ventilation. Respir Care. 2013;58(2):348–66.
9. Rabec C, Langevin B, Rodenstein D, Perrin C, Leger P, Pepin JL, et al. Ventilatory modes. What's in a name? Respir Care. 2012;57(12):2138–9. author reply 9–50.
10. Chatburn RL, Volsko TA, Hazy J, Harris LN, Sanders S. Determining the basis for a taxonomy of mechanical ventilation. Respir Care. 2012;57(4):514–24.
11. Chatburn RL, Branson RD. Classification of mechanical ventilators. In: MacIntyre NR, Branson RD, editors. Mechanical ventilation. Philadelphia: W.B. Saunders; 2001. p. 2–50.
12. Branson RD, Campbell RS. Modes of ventilator operation. In: MacIntyre NR, Branson RD, editors. Mechanical ventilation. Philadelphia: W.B. Saunders; 2001. p. 51–84.
13. Singer BD, Corbridge TC. Basic invasive mechanical ventilation. South Med J. 2009;102(12):1238–45.
14. Sassoon CS, Zhu E, Caiozzo VJ. Assist-control mechanical ventilation attenuates ventilator-induced diaphragmatic dysfunction. Am J Respir Crit Care Med. 2004;170(6):626–32.
15. Gregory GA, Kitterman JA, Phibbs RH, Tooley WH, Hamilton WK. Treatment of the idiopathic respiratory-distress syndrome with continuous positive airway pressure. N Engl J Med. 1971;284(24):1333–40.
16. Papastamelos C, Panitch HB, England SE, Allen JL. Developmental changes in chest wall compliance in infancy and early childhood. J Appl Physiol. 1995;78(1):179–84. Epub 1995/01/01. eng.
17. Kosch PC, Hutchinson AA, Wozniak JA, Carlo WA, Stark AR. Posterior cricoarytenoid and diaphragm activities during tidal breathing in neonates. J Appl Physiol. 1988;64(5):1968–78.
18. Mortola JP, Milic-Emili J, Noworaj A, Smith B, Fox G, Weeks S. Muscle pressure and flow during expiration in infants. Am Rev Respir Dis. 1984;129(1):49–53.

19. Panitch HB, Allen JL, Alpert BE, Schidlow DV. Effects of CPAP on lung mechanics in infants with acquired tracheobronchomalacia. Am J Respir Crit Care Med. 1994;150(5 Pt 1):1341–6.
20. Sassoon CS. Positive pressure ventilation. Alternate modes. Chest. 1991;100(5):1421–9.
21. Kirby RR, Robison EJ, Schulz J, DeLemos R. A new pediatric volume ventilator. Anesth Analg. 1971;50(4):533–7.
22. Luce JM, Pierson DJ, Hudson LD. Intermittent mandatory ventilation. Chest. 1981;79(6):678–85.
23. Aoki N, Shimizu H, Kushiyama S, Katsuya H, Isa T. A new device for synchronized intermittent mandatory ventilation. Anesthesiology. 1978;48(1):69–71.
24. Make BJ, Hill NS, Goldberg AI, Bach JR, Criner GJ, Dunne PE, et al. Mechanical ventilation beyond the intensive care unit. Report of a consensus conference of the American College of Chest Physicians. Chest. 1998;113(5 Suppl):289S–344.
25. Sherman JM, Davis S, Albamonte-Petrick S, Chatburn RL, Fitton C, Green C, et al. Care of the child with a chronic tracheostomy. This official statement of the American Thoracic Society was adopted by the ATS Board of Directors, July 1999. Am J Respir Crit Care Med. 2000;161(1):297–308.
26. Gilgoff IS, Peng RC, Keens TG. Hypoventilation and apnea in children during mechanically assisted ventilation. Chest. 1992;101(6):1500–6.
27. Campbell Jr RM, Smith MD, Mayes TC, Mangos JA, Willey-Courand DB, Kose N, et al. The characteristics of thoracic insufficiency syndrome associated with fused ribs and congenital scoliosis. J Bone Joint Surg Am. 2003;85-A(3):399–408.
28. Blakeman TC, Rodriquez Jr D, Hanseman D, Branson RD. Bench evaluation of 7 home-care ventilators. Respir Care. 2011;56(11):1791–8.
29. Kondili E, Prinianakis G, Georgopoulos D. Patient-ventilator interaction. Br J Anaesth. 2003;91(1):106–19.
30. Fauroux B, Leroux K, Pepin JL, Lofaso F, Louis B. Are home ventilators able to guarantee a minimal tidal volume? Intensive Care Med. 2010;36(6):1008–14.
31. King A, McCoy R. Home respiratory care. In: Hess DR, MacIntyre NR, Mishoe SC, Galvin WF, Adams AB, editors. Respiratory care: principles and practice. 2nd ed. Sudbury, MA: Jones & Bartlett Learning; 2012. p. 559–88.
32. Srinivasan S, Doty SM, White TR, Segura VH, Jansen MT, Davidson Ward SL, et al. Frequency, causes, and outcome of home ventilator failure. Chest. 1998;114(5):1363–7.
33. Panitch HB, Downes JJ, Kennedy JS, Kolb SM, Parra MM, Peacock J, et al. Guidelines for home care of children with chronic respiratory insufficiency. Pediatr Pulmonol. 1996;21(1):52–6.
34. Campbell RS, Johannigman JA, Branson RD, Austin PN, Matacia G, Banks GR. Battery duration of portable ventilators: effects of control variable, positive end-expiratory pressure, and inspired oxygen concentration. Respir Care. 2002;47(10):1173–83.
35. Greenwald PW, Rutherford AF, Green RA, Giglio J. Emergency department visits for home medical device failure during the 2003 North America blackout. Acad Emerg Med. 2004;11(7):786–9.
36. Lechtzin N, Weiner CM, Clawson L. A fatal complication of noninvasive ventilation. N Engl J Med. 2001;344(7):533.
37. Shimada S, Funato M. Home mechanical ventilation in the aftermath of the Hanshin-Awaji earthquake disaster. Acta Paediatr Jpn. 1995;37(6):741–4.
38. di Paolo M, Evangelisti L, Ambrosino N. Unexpected death of a ventilator-dependent amyotrophic lateral sclerosis patient. Rev Port Pneumol. 2013;19(4):175–8.
39. King AC. Long-term home mechanical ventilation in the United States. Respir Care. 2012;57(6):921–30; discussion 30–2.
40. Chatwin M, Heather S, Hanak A, Polkey MI, Simonds AK. Analysis of home support and ventilator malfunction in 1,211 ventilator-dependent patients. Eur Respir J. 2010;35(2):310–6.
41. Al-Samri M, Mitchell I, Drummond DS, Bjornson C. Tracheostomy in children: a population-based experience over 17 years. Pediatr Pulmonol. 2010;45(5):487–93. Epub 2010/04/29. eng.
42. Com G, Kuo DZ, Bauer ML, Lenker CV, Melguizo-Castro MM, Nick TG, et al. Outcomes of children treated with tracheostomy and positive-pressure ventilation at home. Clin Pediatr (Phila). 2013;52(1):54–61.

43. Pannunzio TG. Aspiration of oral feedings in patients with tracheostomies. AACN Clin Issues. 1996;7(4):560–9. Epub 1996/11/01. eng.
44. Kun SS, Nakamura CT, Ripka JF, Davidson Ward SL, Keens TG. Home ventilator low-pressure alarms fail to detect accidental decannulation with pediatric tracheostomy tubes. Chest. 2001;119(2):562–4.
45. Kun SS, Davidson-Ward SL, Hulse LM, Keens TG. How much do primary care givers know about tracheostomy and home ventilator emergency care? Pediatr Pulmonol. 2010;45(3):270–4.
46. Boroughs D, Dougherty JA. Decreasing accidental mortality of ventilator-dependent children at home: a call to action. Home Healthc Nurse. 2012;30(2):103–11. quiz 12–3.
47. Edwards JD, Kun SS, Keens TG. Outcomes and causes of death in children on home mechanical ventilation via tracheostomy: an institutional and literature review. J Pediatr. 2010;157(6):955–9. e2. Epub 2010/08/18. eng.
48. Teague WG. Long-term mechanical ventilation in infants and children. In: Hill NS, editor. Long-term mechanical ventilation. Lung biology in health and disease, vol. 154. New York: Marcel Dekker, Inc; 2001. p. 177–213.
49. Downes JJ, Pilmer SL. Chronic respiratory failure—controversies in management. Crit Care Med. 1993;21(9 Suppl):S363–4.
50. Edwards EA, O'Toole M, Wallis C. Sending children home on tracheostomy dependent ventilation: pitfalls and outcomes. Arch Dis Child. 2004;89(3):251–5.
51. Edwards JD, Kun SS, Keens TG, Khemani RG, Moromisato DY. Children with corrected or palliated congenital heart disease on home mechanical ventilation. Pediatr Pulmonol. 2010;45(7):645–9. Epub 2010/06/25. eng.

Chapter 4
Ethical Considerations in Chronic Invasive Mechanical Ventilation in Pediatrics

Walter M. Robinson

Introduction

Placement of a tracheostomy with the intent of chronic ventilation is a momentous decision in a child's life, but it can seem to be a routine clinical decision from the viewpoint of the physician. Physicians and other healthcare providers are used to looking at clinical decisions from the standpoint of damaged physiology and possible technology; we assess whether things are "indicated" by looking at the physical variables such as blood gases, radiograph scans, work of breathing, and so on, and for most clinical decisions, this is the most appropriate way to proceed. But with momentous decisions like the institution of chronic invasive mechanical ventilation, physicians ought to step back and examine the wider context in which their decisions take place, examining their own motivations, institutional pressures, family dynamics, and the influence of their decision on future decisions faced by the child and family.

There is no doubt that the ability to provide chronic ventilation has been a boon to children and families. Dramatic advances in the ability to provide safe, effective, and portable ventilation over the past three decades have increased the number of children who not only survived but thrived outside of institutional environments. Children who would otherwise have died have been saved by advances in care for those with chronic respiratory failure. But as with most technologies which at first seemed miraculous and then became mundane, there are a host of assumptions

W.M. Robinson, M.D., M.P.H. (✉)
Vanderbilt University School of Medicine, Nashville, TN, USA
e-mail: wmacr@mac.com

© Springer Science+Business Media New York 2016
L.M. Sterni, J.L. Carroll (eds.), *Caring for the Ventilator Dependent Child*,
Respiratory Medicine, DOI 10.1007/978-1-4939-3749-3_4

about the institution and maintenance of children dependent on these technologies that ought to be examined. In many cases the institution of chronic mechanical ventilation has begun with high hopes for both the survival and quality of life of the child and for the family's ability to integrate the technology-dependent child into the home. The success stories abound.

But behind this triumphal view of technology lies a more complex set of decisions and influences that ought to be part of the initial consideration of long-term mechanical ventilation. Those of us who are clinicians know the success stories, but we also know the failures. We are well aware of children who were not able to be cared for at home, who did not develop in the manner expected, whose relational ability with their caregivers is minimal, and yet are maintained by chronic ventilator technology, usually in an institutional setting. These children survived, but they did not thrive. The fact that not all decisions to institute chronic ventilation are successful is not a reason to avoid the practice, but it is a reason to examine the set of practices that surround the initiation and maintenance of chronic ventilation. We cannot perfectly predict the future, but we can learn from our experience. We can use our experience to better understand challenges that children and families will face and to change both individual and institutional practices to move toward better outcomes for children and families.

Before Consent

There are three questions with ethical implications to be asked and answered before seeking informed consent to initiation of chronic invasive mechanical ventilation in a child, as shown in Table 4.1.

Table 4.1 Before informed consent: three questions with ethical implications that should be asked and answered *before* seeking informed consent for initiation of chronic invasive mechanical ventilation

1. Is chronic invasive mechanical ventilation for this child a bridge or a destination?
2. What role are institutional factors, such as freeing up an intensive care bed or insurance coverage, playing in the timing of the decision or the rejection of potential clinical alternatives?
3. Have plans for psychosocial, financial, and clinical support been established prior to the decision to begin chronic mechanical ventilation and are such support systems now in place in the community where the family lives?

Bridge or Destination?

There are two broad categories of children who are considered for chronic mechanical ventilation, those for whom ventilation is a *bridge* and those for whom ventilation is a *destination*. In children for whom ventilation is considered a bridge, survival on mechanical support will be temporary, even though it may last for many months or even years, in the expectation that there will be either maturation of lung tissue or healing of an existing pulmonary insult. In children for whom ventilation is considered a destination, there is no expectation that developmental changes or healing will free them from the ventilator; these children have permanent neurological or pulmonary conditions which mean that survival will require mechanical ventilation.

Making this distinction is sometimes easy. Children with neuromuscular conditions resulting in respiratory insufficiency and failure fall clearly into the destination group, while children with lung injury secondary to prematurity are more likely to fall into the bridge group. The distinction is not based solely on the clinical condition of the child at the institution of mechanical ventilation; many factors cited in other chapters of this text should be taken in account when considering the distinction between bridge and destination situations.

Clarity about the distinction is ethically important in order to avoid false promises to the parents. It seems to be part of human nature for most parents to hope for miraculous improvement in their child, but as physicians with experience in the lives of many children, we know otherwise. Children do miraculously improve, but as clinicians we cannot depend on miracles, and part of the skill of managing chronic illness is for the clinician to balance his or her own sense of hope and reality. Parents achieve this balance in different ways, but it is inappropriate for physicians to deceive themselves or parents by encouraging false hope. A better practice is to encourage realistic hopes for connection with their child, for the delight of parenting in spite of the presence of mechanical ventilation, for the mutual joy that parents and children give each other even in the face of serious and debilitating illness.

For some children, making the distinction between *bridge* and *destination* will be difficult. Children who have had a primary lung injury can in many cases show remarkable ability to heal and so progress to independence from mechanical ventilation. Yet the child we expect to heal may not. The vocabulary here is a bit difficult to navigate for both families and clinicians: "temporary chronic" mechanical ventilation may become "permanent chronic" ventilation. Clinicians should be careful not to over-promise healing but instead should emphasize that the path toward removal from mechanical ventilation is a known one, with signposts along the way.

What Is the Role of Nonclinical Factors in the Decision?

Once the distinction between bridge and destination ventilation is clear in the mind of the clinicians—and this includes not just the clinicians in the intensive care unit but those who have expertise in managing long-term ventilation in other settings—then a second set of questions should be addressed before the process of informed consent can begin.

Clinicians must ask themselves in an honest and careful way to what degree factors that are external to the case at hand are influencing the decision to institute mechanical ventilation. Three important factors to address are the understandable need to free up intensive care bed spaces, pressure from third party payers to move the child to a less expensive location for care, and frustration with the pace of improvement of the child in an intensive care setting. Each of these factors can play both legitimate and illegitimate roles in making the decision, and so the issues need to be honestly parsed by those in charge of the care of the child.

First, the need to free up bed space in an intensive care unit is entirely understandable in an environment of restricted resources. Managing scarce resources, such as the time, space, and energy of an intensive care unit, is part of providing ethical care to a community. But pressure to free up a bed space should not be allowed to unduly influence the decision to place a tracheostomy and begin chronic ventilation in a particular child. Part of being an ethical physician is being transparent to oneself and others about the competing goals of clinical care; clinicians have duties to the patient in front of them as well as to other patients, even ones they have not yet met. The worst way to address these competing goals is to do so only on a case by case basis; the best way is to have a flexible but predetermined process for making decisions when the duties to different patients conflict. In any intensive care unit, balancing the needs of various patients is a constant obligation, and rather than making such decisions in a fully ad hoc way, clinicians should develop procedures for addressing these conflicts in a way that involves more than just the clinicians at the bedside. We cannot treat all patients exactly the same, nor would we want to, but we should strive to as much clarity of purpose as can be achieved.

Second, the desire to limit unnecessary expenditure in the American healthcare system often falls to the third party payer system and that system can wield a blunt instrument in individual cases. Pressure may be brought on the bedside clinicians to institute tracheostomy and mechanical ventilation so that the child can be transferred to a less expensive care setting. As with the natural duties to multiple patients, clinicians can manage this conflict best by transparency and planning. Not all pressure to reduce the cost of care is unreasonable, even if that pressure is instituted by those with no connection to an individual patient. But making the decision for tracheostomy and mechanical ventilation solely for financial reason is ethically wrong. Management of resources, including financial resources, is another part of the physician's obligation to the community of patients and that pressure is best managed as a team, with clinician colleagues who are not involved in the care of the individual patient and who can help the individual clinician recognize the pressures to reduce costs for what they are, simply one aspect of many in the appropriate care of the child and family.

Third, clinicians must recognize their own psychological pressures that may play a role in the decision to institute mechanical ventilation. Physicians are asked to bear the psychological burden of the illness of many children, and for many the successes are well worth the hard work. But many of us can fall into a psychological view of our work that valorizes our ability to rescue a child over all other aspects of care. Especially in intensive care, where the rescues can be dramatic, clinicians may become frustrated with children for whom cure is not possible or who make only slow progress. Children who are candidates for chronic mechanical ventilation can be seen from this point of view as failures of the clinician's attempt to rescue a sick child. Unconscious anger at our perceived failures and frustration with the slow progress of the child can lead us to avoid contact with the child and family. Some of this anger and frustration may lead us to suggest chronic mechanical ventilation sooner than we otherwise might. Recognizing and managing these reactions to our work is part of becoming an ethical physician. Just as we best manage our reactions to "difficult patients" by recognizing them and processing them consciously, we ought to examine our own reactions to the child for whom cure is not possible or for whom improvement will be slow. In many cases, those who provide care for chronically ventilated children are self-selected to tolerate this pattern of slow or no improvement, and their input in making decisions about ventilation can be a crucial step in helping the more cure oriented of us make decisions with the best interests of these children and families in mind.

Are Community Supports in Place?

It may seem that the decision to begin chronic invasive mechanical ventilation is a function of the child's clinical status at the time, but success depends on many factors which are independent of the child's clinical condition. The presence in the community of sufficient resources to support the child and family is a necessary precondition for chronic invasive ventilation. Often the funding, function, and existence of these resources lie outside the expertise of the physician making the decision to insert the tracheostomy and begin ventilation. Yet the existence and quality of these resources are part of the responsibility of those who recommend long-term ventilation; the physician is making an explicit and implicit set of promises of how life will go for the child if the plan for ventilation is instituted, and knowledge of the good and bad aspects of the available care outside the hospital is a large part of being able to make such promises in good faith.

A plan for chronic ventilation in the complete absence of community support is an unethical plan for the child and family. We may imagine that a heroic family can manage without such supports, but an honest assessment of our experience would tell us otherwise. This is why the involvement of clinicians with experience in the care of the chronically ventilated child in the community is an essential part of the initial decision. These physicians should know what the benefits and burdens of the existing support for the clinical, psychosocial, financial, and respite care needs of the family are in the community in which the family lives. Providing an accurate picture of the available support is part of avoiding the encouragement of false hope in the family. Knowing that accurate picture may influence the clinical options for the child and family and may increase awareness of hospital-based clinicians of the need to develop community-based resources so that chronic mechanical ventilation is an honest and transparent option that can be offered to parents in good faith.

Table 4.2 The informed consent process: two special aspects of informed consent process for chronic mechanical ventilation

1. Have the clinicians who will provide long-term care to the child and family had sufficient meetings with the parents prior to the decision?

2. Has an experienced clinician had a discussion with the family regarding the constraints that placing the tracheostomy now may place on future decisions to discontinue mechanical ventilation?

The Informed Consent Process

Now that the clinicians have asked and answered the preliminary questions about the decision, the formal process of informed consent can proceed. Questions with special ethical implications that should be asked and answered as part of the informed consent process are listed in Table 4.2.

Parents are expected to provide informed consent to the institution of a tracheostomy and mechanical ventilation, but what does informed consent mean in this context? In some clinical situations, such as the trial of a new medication, parents are asked to approve a treatment which can be reversed, usually without permanent change in the child's health. In other clinical situations, such as surgery for a compound fracture, informed consent means that the parents understand the risks of the surgery and the likely trajectory of the recuperation, but also that the procedure is irreversible.

In chronic mechanical ventilation, informed consent has to include the parents' understanding not only that there are proximate risks of the surgery to place the tracheotomy, but that the recovery of ventilatory independence, if any, has an uncertain trajectory; that there will be an almost certainly heavy burden of caregiving for the child; that there will be a likely considerable financial and emotional toll on them and their family members; that the care of mechanically ventilated child in their home will change the nature of family life; and that the decision to place a tracheostomy now may constrain their decisions about removing the ventilator in the future, should they decide that the burden of mechanical ventilation outweighs the benefits for their child. Because of these complex and uncertain factors, the informed consent process needs to be especially deliberative, transparent, and reflective.

One mistake that is easily avoided is the decision not to discuss these issues, either on grounds that the outcomes are uncertain or that the family cannot stand the emotional or cognitive complexity of the discussion. These issues must be discussed with the family, or informed consent simply has not been obtained.

As to the question of outcomes, it is true that the outcome for this particular child is uncertain: we cannot know the future. But we know what has happened with other similarly situated children and families, and we can make educated assumptions about how things will go with this particular family. We know the past experience of other families, or we ought to, and we have a duty to use this experience to guide families making decisions today.

If we judge that a family cannot withstand the necessary discussion of the possible outcomes, then we ought to take the time and energy necessary to explain it in a manner and setting in which they can understand. In contrast to many medical decisions, this decision is not an emergency. It is a decision about a chronic treatment with long-term implications, and it will take time to explain it. If a family rejects this discussion on the grounds that it is too taxing or emotionally fraught, serious consideration should be made of the family's ability to manage the medical care of this seriously ill child. A family need not have the same moral and spiritual outlook as the physicians for this to be the case. For example, many families may see God or some other divine presence as crucial in their decision, but the clinician should be wary of the family who refuses to understand their own part in the work to come.

Of special importance in the informed consent process is the assessment by the clinicians of the options facing the family. Parents with a child who is a candidate for chronic mechanical ventilation may see no other options, but it is the duty of the clinician to be clear about a particular option, palliative care. The option of palliative care should be made in an earnest and sincere manner, avoiding the description of this option as "giving up" or "doing nothing." Clinicians who are unfamiliar with palliative care should provide access to experts in palliative care for the family. The best option is for those experts to work in concert with the exiting clinical team in order to integrate palliative approaches to care and provide a smooth transition for the family. Again, as with the discussion of the role of rescue above, clinicians must be aware of their own biases and frustrations. Seeing palliative care as "giving up" and transmitting that view in some way to the family inappropriately limits the family's options. The choice not to pursue chronic mechanical ventilation, with the eventual death of the child in comfortable and safe surroundings, should always be discussed. It may take special skill and experience to have this discussion with the family, but there is no excuse for avoiding it altogether. Many families may depend on the skilled clinician to bring up difficult issues which are weighing on their minds, and so it is inappropriate to wait for the family to bring up the option of palliative care. Families may also be waiting for permission to discuss this option, and a clinician avoiding the topic may communicate a moral disapproval of the family's options which is inappropriate and unethical. It is simply a fact that many parents will have consciously or unconsciously wished for their child's suffering to be over, and they may also have been shocked that they even briefly wished for their child to be liberated from a difficult life. Families may express this in spiritual terms by saying that the child "belongs in heaven" or that the child has "suffered enough." Clinicians should be alert to this sort of statement as an opening to discuss the option of palliative care with a compassionate and open frame of mind.

Another essential aspect of the informed consent process is the involvement of the clinical care team that will provide chronic care for the child and family. Not only are these clinicians the most educated specialists about the options for care, but they are especially aware of the benefits and burdens of chronic ventilation as they play out over the life of the child in the months and years to come. A family's faith in this clinical team is an important aspect of the outcome of the decision to pursue ventilation, and their presence and expertise should be sought as early as possible in the informed consent process. These clinicians are likely to have valuable expertise in determining the bridge vs. destination distinction in borderline cases, and they can bring to the informed consent process a wealth of experience-based wisdom and information that can be invaluable to the family. This experienced team, if they are given enough time to do so, can help assess the likely struggles of the individual family with the decision and help the current clinicians individualize the consent process.

Finally, families need to know as part of informed consent that the placement of a tracheostomy and chronic ventilation now may constrain their ability to decide to remove the therapy later. This is a complex topic, and some background information is necessary.

The current ethical consensus in the United States in pediatrics is that families have the right to refuse treatments for their child if the benefits of the treatment are outweighed by the burdens of the treatment, even if that treatment is life sustaining. There are limits on this right, such as the necessity of clinicians to recognize whether the parents' assessment of the benefits and burdens is reasonable and that the parents have the best interests of the child in mind in making the decision. If parents decide that placement of the tracheostomy and chronic ventilation is too excessive a burden given the potential benefits, they will in almost every case have the right to make the decision not to proceed, even if some clinicians disagree. This is in part because the burden of placing the tracheostomy is regarded as sufficiently high, but this is a judgment based in part on the idea of being able to refuse surgery and on the societal view of being dependent on a machine for survival. That societal judgment about the relative burdens of the treatment may change once the tracheostomy has been placed.

Most medical ethicists, especially those with a more philosophical bent, argue that removing a therapy in place is ethically identical to the decision not to institute the therapy; this is the foundation of the assumed lack of ethical distinction between withdrawing a treatment and withholding it. Clinicians are used to withdrawing mechanical ventilation in the intensive care unit, and the boundaries of making the decision to remove the ventilator are fairly well developed. In most cases the decision to treat removing a therapy and withholding it as ethically identical will raise no concerns. But the removal of ventilation from a patient with a tracheostomy who is otherwise medically stable on the grounds of the ventilation being a burden out of proportion to the benefits is a rarer event, and may raise concerns from clinicians.

Part of the issue may arise from the invasive status of the tracheostomy. One reason for placement of the tracheotomy, of course, was to lessen the burden of chronic ventilation. The patient becomes used to the tracheostomy tube, and the physical burden of the tube likely lessens over time. Living on a ventilator with an endotracheal tube either nasally or orally placed is far more burdensome (and far less clinically successful, of course) than being on a ventilator following tracheostomy. After all, the child with a tracheostomy can be on a ventilator at home, whereas the child with a nasal or oral endotracheal tube must remain in an institutional setting.

Over time, we may come to see the burden of being on the ventilator as bearable, but the child is still dependent on and connected to a machine, even though the burden of that machine seems to be easier once the tracheostomy is in place. Additional treatments that would be burdensome for another child might be seen as less burdensome for the ventilated child, who already has endured multiple medical procedures and invasive therapies. We clinicians might thus become more comfortable with aggressive and invasive therapies in a chronically ventilated child than we would in other children. We also might come to believe that the burden of the treatment is zero for the child accustomed to it.

We should pause to consider the implications of this possible desensitization. We have to be careful not to accept a higher degree of suffering for a child simply because the child has undergone burdensome treatment in the past; we should not casually or lightly continue invasive procedures just because the child is used to them. If we adopt that point of view, clinicians are at risk of minimizing the burden of the intervention and so being less likely to allow parents to stop the treatment.

In part this consideration harkens back to the distinction between the use of mechanical ventilation as a bridge or a destination. If we institute ventilation as a bridge, in the expectation of recovery, and that recovery does not occur, then we ought to allow discontinuation of the therapy. If ventilation is considered a bridge, then the methods and pathways to discontinuing it if the outcome is not as expected ought to be discussed with the parents as part of the process of informed consent. This puts chronic mechanical ventilation on the same ethical footing as other invasive therapies with substantial side effects that are put in place for a seriously ill child. Part of the consent process should include a discussion of what will happen if the therapy is unsuccessful.

In children for whom mechanical ventilation is considered a destination, discussion of removal of the ventilator at some time in the future is still important, even though the outcomes of the therapy are viewed in a different way. Parents who agree to life-long mechanical ventilation are not agreeing to the therapy come what may. There may be many instances in the life of the child and the family where circumstances have changed the balance of benefits and burdens, and we must be open to that possibility.

To put it a different way, there appear to be several "natural" moments in the trajectory of a child with life-threatening lung disease; one of these moments is *before* the placement of a tracheotomy. At that "natural moment," it is easier to say no to the treatment than it will be at other moments. Another such natural moment would be the development of additional organ failure, such as the need for a cardiac transplant or for dialysis. These "natural moments" are of course not *natural* at all, that is, they are not functions of human physiology but of the state of technology and medicine. As technology advances, the moments shift; what was once experimental and burdensome becomes routine standard of care.

But parents may not recognize these moments, or they may have other moments, other special times when reassessment of the burden and benefit of care is to them both warranted and necessary. Part of the informed consent process is to tell parents about these moments for the physicians and invite them to share the sort of moments for reassessment that might occur to them. Discussion of these issues is difficult but necessary.

Finally, the informed consent process must involve an explanation of the work that will be expected of the family in caring for the ventilator-dependent child. Other chapters in this text address that burden in detail, but for the purposes of informed consent, it must be part of the discussion. The lives of everyone in the family will be changed in both positive and negative ways, and the informed consent must at least gesture toward a real description of that work. Parents at this stage may be in the mindset of doing everything for their child—they often use the analogy of being willing to "step in front of the bus" to save the child—but the work of caring for a ventilator-dependent child is less heroic and unending. It may be impossible for anyone to know what they are agreeing to, but as clinicians with experience, we ought to explain as best we can.

During Chronic Care of the Child and Family

Ethical issues do not disappear once informed consent has been obtained and the therapy instituted. In addition to all the usual everyday ethical issues that are involved in the care of any chronic illness, chronic ventilation raises four particular issues of an ethical nature, as listed in Table 4.3.

First, for those children for whom ventilation was instituted as a bridge, there is the difficult issue of managing the natural frustration on the part of the family that progress toward decannulation, and respiratory independence has not been faster. No matter how well things are going, families want things to go better and faster. Disagreements about progress or the lack of it can raise substantial trust issues between clinicians and parents, and the accusation of broken promises can be made in anger or frustration. Parents may want to switch physicians, may shop around for the perfect home care company, or may act in other ways that are inadvertently against the best outcome for the child because of the combination of exhaustion and the stress of caring for the child. Clinicians should be alert to the possibility of these events coming and try to head them off. Preparation can forestall disagreements that escalate into ethical struggles.

Second, for children in whom chronic ventilation was instituted as a destination, families and patients may experience some delayed grief at the new limitations on the child's life. The therapy that improved ventilation may have at the same time taken away other important aspects of the child and family's quality of life, such as decreasing the ability to communicate or limiting family travel together. The quality of life

Table 4.3 During chronic care: four questions with ethical implications that should be asked and answered on a regular basis during the care of the child on chronic invasive ventilation

1. For "bridge" children, what are the milestones of progress, if any, toward independence from mechanical ventilation?
2. For "destination" children, how has quality of life changed since the institution of invasive ventilation?
3. What is the impact of the child's chronic ventilation on other family members?
4. What effect, if any, is the lack of progress having on the clinicians' relationship with the family?

may decrease even though the quality of breathing improved. Parents may express this grief in many ways, such as nonadherence to the clinical regimen or isolation from the clinical team. Clinicians should be especially alert to changes in outlook once families and patients have become accustomed to the new normal of life on a ventilator.

Third, as pediatricians and pediatric clinicians, we have an ethical duty to the whole family and not just the one sick child. The impact of a ventilator in the home on the healthy family members is well discussed in Chap. 9, but from an ethical standpoint, it would be wrong not to make some attempt to assess and manage the predictable reactions of family members to the medicalization of the home.

Finally, there is one important ethical issue that is often overlooked in the care of a seriously ill child at home. In many cases, moving the child to a home setting will recast the moral responsibility for the child's progress or lack thereof to the family. Unfortunately, we clinicians can develop an unconscious tendency to attribute setbacks in care to a failure to follow our carefully conceived care plan. In contrast to the hospital setting where our successes are our own and failures are often considered unavoidable, failures at home tend to be seen as the fault of the parents. Clinicians can decide, justified or not, that lack of progress once the child is in a home setting is a function of parental inability or unwillingness to carry out the complex care.

This is simply human nature at work. We want to reward parents who do an excellent job of taking care of their ventilator-dependent child at home, because this is an extremely difficult job. But the flipside of that is that we might blame the parents (subconsciously or not) for setbacks in the child's care once they are at home. In a sense this shifts the moral responsibility for the outcome to the parents, in a way that the physicians and nurses did not bear when the child was in the hospital. To do so is unfair to the parents and can lead to judgmental decisions by the care team when compassion and patience are the better paths to follow. Routine discussion of our affective responses to chronically ill children and their families, in a safe and "backstage" location, can help us reset our expectations and look for solutions to problems that do not involve placing moral blame on parents for the illness of their child. Such routine discussion can also help to identify misunderstandings with parents and is good practice for the promotion of "preventive" ethics.

Special Considerations in Special Populations

Two particular populations bear special mention in consideration of the ethical issues involved in chronic invasive ventilation: the first is teenagers with intact cognition and the second is infants with severely damaged cognition (Table 4.4).

Table 4.4 Two populations with special ethical considerations in the decision to institute mechanical ventilation

Teenagers with intact cognition
Infants with severe cognitive and/or sensory deficits

Teenagers with Intact Cognition

Teenagers make up a small but important subset of patients for whom chronic ventilation is begun during the pediatric years. As discussed in Chap. 14, the primary indication for ventilation in these patients will be neuromuscular conditions, most of which are progressive. From an ethical point of view, this will mean that the teenager will be part of the decision to consider chronic ventilation. The presence of the patient in the discussion means that the process of informed consent must be tailored to address his or her needs for information, privacy, and control. In many cases the discussion may come at a time when the progression of the disease is increasing dependence at exactly the developmental stage when independence is most treasured by adolescents. Many of these teenagers may already have substantially compromised physical independence, and the introduction of the ventilator, with the potential to alter speaking fluency, may remove an important means of asserting individuality. Other teens may have a decreased level of mobility which is further compromised by the addition of the ventilator, necessitating changes in the all important social sphere of life at this developmental stage.

Making a difficult decision with healthy adolescents is challenging enough, but making decisions with dependent and chronically ill adolescents can be especially challenging. Discussion of the care burden for the family may mistakenly give the teen the sense that his existence is a burden rather than his care, and discussion of the option of palliative care may be especially difficult, but all of these discussions are ethically necessary if true informed consent is to be obtained. Some teens may defer certain parts of the decision to their parents; others may want to be in every meeting but not participate; others may want to run every meeting and ask every question. Again, flexibility and patience are the keys to a successful informed consent. Regardless of the teen's approach, they should be involved in the discussion of the options in a manner that suits their wishes. Just as we do not assume that the parents of healthy teenagers understand their child's wishes and desires without asking, we should not assume that the parents of a chronically ill child facing chronic ventilation can speak for their child without asking. It is part of the ethical duty of the clinician to the teenager to insure that the adolescent's questions are answered and wishes are taken into account in any decision regarding invasive ventilation.

Infants with Severely Damaged Cognition or Multiple Sensory Deficits

Infants who are candidates for chronic mechanical ventilation may have other conditions which can seem ethically salient in the decision as to the appropriateness of invasive ventilation. The most common condition which raises ethical issues is a severe cognitive deficit. In these infants, because of their perceived low quality of life, the decision to institute chronic ventilation may be seen as a futile use of resources or as prolonging suffering of the child. Everyone seems to have an opinion about the use of chronic ventilation for these infants, and few hesitate to express it; to some it is the unacceptable use of scarce resources for those who cannot benefit, while to others to withhold such treatment based on assumptions about quality of life is misguided and discriminatory.

It is beyond the scope of this chapter to settle the issue. However, there are several issues that the clinician facing such decisions ought to keep in mind. First, the decision is not really up for a public vote; it is the concern of the parents, the clinicians (*all* the clinicians, including those who will be involved only temporarily), and the hospital. Second, the decision is not truly irreversible, although as stated above, it may be harder to reverse than was previously expected. Third, we are currently in a difficult era with regard to the infant brain and its capacity for improvement: while there are new instances of neural plasticity unexpected in previous decades, there are also some injuries from which no brain can be expected to recover. Knowing which is which may take time, wisdom, and judgment; we should reserve room to make different decisions in similar cases during this time of flux in our understanding.

Conclusion

Most aspects of the practice of medicine are suffused with ethical considerations, and chronic invasive mechanical ventilation is no exception. Patience, foresight, and teamwork are essential in addressing clinicians' ethical obligations to children and families facing chronic ventilation; attention to these concerns before, during, and after the institution of mechanical ventilation is the best ethical practice.

Chapter 5
Palliative Care and End-of-Life Considerations in Children on Chronic Ventilation

Jeffrey D. Edwards

Alleviating illness and suffering and preventing premature death are fundamental duties embraced by professional medical caregivers. However, despite our best efforts, not all conditions are curable, and premature death is sometimes the result. Unfortunately, this is also true for some conditions affecting children. Nevertheless, when caring for children confronted with life-limiting conditions, professional caregivers are challenged to strive to alleviate the child's and family's suffering and to fulfill life goals when possible. This often involves implementing palliative care paradigms in the context of the family and their various needs.

Chronic respiratory failure is one such condition or manifestation of numerous conditions that often cannot be cured. Instead, portable, high-efficiency respiratory devices for both noninvasive and transtracheal support have evolved to assist or replace this vital function. These technological advancements have meant more options, more decisions, and often more care responsibilities for patients and families.

"Family" and "familial caregiver" are used here to mainly refer to those nonprofessionals who have a long-standing relationship with the patient and devote themselves to his or her care and are surrogate decision-makers for them. In most cases, this implies parents. However, biological mothers and fathers are not always the functional parents or primary caregivers of children with intensive healthcare needs. "Family" also refers to other nuclear and extended relatives who are impacted by the child's substantial, ongoing care needs. It may also include non-related caregivers—friends, home health aides, and private duty nurses—who have become an integral part of the child's life and vice versa. These extended family members should not be overlooked and should be supported in the course of palliative care. In addition, despite the language in this

J.D. Edwards, M.D., M.A., M.A.S. (✉)
Division of Pediatric Critical Care Medicine, Columbia University College of Physicians and Surgeons, 3959 Broadway, CHN 10-24, New York, NY 10032, USA
e-mail: jde2134@columbia.edu

© Springer Science+Business Media New York 2016
L.M. Sterni, J.L. Carroll (eds.), *Caring for the Ventilator Dependent Child*,
Respiratory Medicine, DOI 10.1007/978-1-4939-3749-3_5

chapter, it should not be presumed that all children on chronic ventilation are incapable of participating in goals and values assessments or decision-making. The age and intellectual ability of each child should be considered, and each child should be allowed to participate and assent to the extent of her own capacity.

Chronic ventilation has been shown to be a relatively safe and effective means to assist children with chronic respiratory failure [1, 2]. Nevertheless, given that interruption of assisted ventilation can be life-threatening for those with continuous dependence and/or an artificial airway, it remains a risky technology [3]. Even those with some intrinsic respiratory function risk acceleration of serious cardiopulmonary complications if they are noncompliant with assisted ventilation. Some children on chronic ventilation have underlying conditions that have a known terminal trajectory with variable life expectancies (e.g., spinal muscle atrophy type 1, Duchenne muscular dystrophy) [4, 5]. Others have conditions (e.g., cerebral palsy, trisomy 21) that, while not terminal, will result in shortened life spans, compared to children without these conditions [6, 7]. Many children on chronic ventilation live with complex chronic conditions, other than chronic respiratory failure, that put them at risk for acute, critical deterioration that can be life-threatening [8–11]. Often, children with life-limiting or complex chronic conditions can have fluctuations in health over time that vary from slow or rapid progressive declines in health to a pattern of relative stability interspersed with acute illnesses sometimes followed by new lower plateaus [12]. Thus, while deterioration and premature death are real risks for many children on chronic ventilation, prognostication of their timing is usually difficult to impossible, as there are many factors in play, only some of which are modifiable.

It is important to recognize that chronic ventilation is relatively safe and effective for children primarily because of the diligent, meticulous daily care provided by familial and professional caregivers. Often their care needs are substantial and ongoing. Thus, chronic ventilation and the child's underlying conditions have a profound impact on the family, as well [13–22].

For these reasons, professional caregivers of children on chronic ventilation are charged with addressing these patients' and families' multiple and various needs beyond effective ventilation. These needs can take many forms, from symptom management to developmental issues. It also involves caring for these children and families as their conditions worsen and they approach the end of their lives. Preparing for and providing such care to any patient and family can be challenging. Because the premature death of a child violates our sense of the "natural" order, preparing children and families has additional challenges. Even more potential obstacles arise in this cohort because the child is already dependent on an extraordinary, life-assisting technology. Attentive care, in general, and palliative care, specifically, offer the means and paradigms to address these diverse needs and challenges.

The purpose of this chapter is to address how and why palliative care is relevant to children on chronic ventilation and their families. It also seeks to explore potential challenges to palliative and end-of-life care in the context of caring for children on chronic ventilation, as well as possible approaches to avoid or minimize them.

What Children on Chronic Ventilation and Their Families Want and Need

Several studies of patients with life-limiting or complex chronic conditions and their families have sought to elucidate their needs when cure or prolongation of life is not possible. Few specifically studied children on chronic ventilation. Also, it should be noted that much of this family-centered research is potentially limited by small sample sizes, relatively low response rates, and, thus, selection bias. So while there is likely much that can be gleaned from this body of research and our anecdotal experience, the best resource to learn the wishes and needs of patients and families are the patients and families themselves.

A simplified synopsis of most families' wishes for their children is for them to be as healthy, functional, and free of suffering as possible for as long as possible. This wish was undoubtedly a motivation for choosing chronic ventilation and understandably remains a goal after it is initiated. Other related wishes of families with children with life-limiting or complex chronic conditions include:

- Symptom management, including pain, dyspnea, depression [23, 24]
- Access to quality, compassionate medical care and a medical home with coordination of providers/services [11, 25]
- Adequate, competent home health services and respite services [25, 26]
- Prevention of further deterioration to new, lower plateaus of health and function
- A reduction in life disruptions and maintenance of normality for the child and family [12, 15, 21, 27]
- Opportunity to discuss medical and nonmedical issues, have their concerns and wishes heard, and make decisions (sometimes sharing this decision-making with professional caregivers)
- Preparation and advanced planning for the future [11, 25, 28–32]. Most professional and some familial caregivers are aware that this includes the end of life, in order to avoid unnecessary suffering with interventions that may add more burden than benefit
- Respect and affirmation of the child as a whole person and member of the family. Patients with complex chronic conditions and disabilities and their families often feel stigmatized and thus misunderstood or disrespected [23, 25, 31]
- Hope in the face of crises [33–35]
- Family members sometimes need to feel that there is always something they can do to improve their child's suffering (i.e., that they are "fighting" for the child) [27]

Some of these needs may fall out of the usual province of subspecialty care that might be focused on one organ system or prolonging life, but within the scope of palliative care.

What Is Palliative Care and Why It Is Applicable to Children on Chronic Ventilation and Their Families

Palliative care evolved with the recognition of patients' suffering and unmet needs at the end of life. Instead of focusing on disease-specific cures, it aims to treat the whole individual and integrate medical (both physical and psychological), emotional, and spiritual support. Although best begun at diagnosis, palliative care is appropriate at any stage of a serious, chronic, or life-limiting illness. In other words, it is not mutually exclusive from or an afterthought to curative/life-prolonging goals and treatments [36–38]. There should not be a discrete, divergent switch from life-prolonging therapy to palliative care. Rather palliative, chronic, and life-prolonging care should be integrated and complementary within total care [39, 40]. Palliative care commonly does and should play an increasingly more prominent role as life-limiting conditions progress and death becomes more probable. As such, palliative care eventually also involves a transition from hope for a cure or prolongation of life to hope for other things of importance [41]. Given that the patient is a member of a family, palliative care also seeks to support the family, both while the patient is alive and with bereavement support after their death.

The relevance of palliative care for the majority of children on chronic ventilation is evident given they have chronic respiratory failure, other life-limiting conditions, and/or substantial medical and nonmedical needs. Even those children with regressive causes of chronic respiratory failure (e.g., bronchopulmonary dysplasia) sometimes have concurrent comorbidities that are chronic and carry risks for acute deterioration (e.g., severe intraventricular hemorrhage requiring cerebral spinal fluid shunt, feeding intolerance requiring gastrostomy). Perhaps even more commonly, children on chronic ventilation have static or progressive causes of chronic respiratory failure. Furthermore, while underlying conditions may be static (e.g., cerebral palsy), their associated complications can be progressive (e.g., contractures, neuropathic scoliosis). Thus, palliative care is indicated for most children on chronic ventilation and should not be thought of as mutually exclusive of it, as a technological life-assisting intervention. Given the goal of chronic ventilation is not just to prolong but also to improve life, chronic ventilation itself can be thought of as palliative in these children.

Given their numerous, various, and complex needs, palliative care for children on chronic ventilation is an ongoing, demanding task. How to address all its elements is beyond the scope of this chapter. Similarly, comprehensive provision of palliative care is beyond the scope of one provider. Recognition of its importance and that it is tantamount to "good" medical care in general are important starting points. Professional caregivers wishing to provide palliative care should pursue an interdisciplinary approach and avail themselves of other professionals (e.g., palliative care experts/teams, other subspecialists, generalists who care for medically fragile children, psychologists, social workers, case managers, dieticians, and respiratory, physical, and occupational therapists, as well as community resources such as clergy and respite providers).

One core element of palliative care for children on chronic ventilation and their families that deserves attention is preparing them for the future. As part of good care, professional caregivers are obliged to help children and families anticipate and prepare for the range of probable events that they may encounter. This sort of preparation requires two interrelated approaches: anticipatory guidance and advance care planning. Anticipatory guidance is simply providing information and preventive advice to families about the child's expected future. It is usually generalizable to all children but can be specific to the individual, and it is considered integral to well-child care. Parents have reported increased healthcare satisfaction when anticipatory guidance is provided [42]. Advance care planning is a proactive, incremental, four-stage process of guiding patients and surrogates (1) to an understanding of their diagnosis and, if possible, their prognosis; (2) to an understanding of their core values and goals that will help them prioritize future care options; (3) to then consider the potential options and decisions they will face in the future; and finally (4) to make anticipatory choices based upon their values and goals and before crises occur that force and strain decision-making. Studies have shown that parents of children with life-limiting conditions and special healthcare needs found advance care planning helpful and desirable [28–30]. In one study, parents reported such planning helped communicate and ensure desired care, provided time and information to make decisions, and offered peace of mind [29].

Specific anticipatory guidance for children on chronic ventilation should focus on the limitations and risks of these technologies and prevention of complications. Appropriate topics to be raised with patients and families are highlighted in Table 5.1. For many children, the probability of some of these events is relatively low. However, because they do occur unpredictably and their impact and sequelae are significant, they deserve addressing with families. Much of this anticipatory guidance is best introduced before chronic ventilation is initiated in order to help ensure that expectations are realistic and that an informed decision is made when considering whether to initiate ventilatory support. Professional caregivers should periodically reinforce and expand pertinent points during longitudinal care.

Given that many children on chronic ventilation have life-limiting illnesses and/ or are at risk for acute, critical deterioration, end-of-life advance care planning is appropriate and necessary for this group. The goal of this planning is for children and families to understand the possible circumstances under which death might occur, the potential decisions they may face, and their overall goals, values, and best interests of the child and family that should guide their decision-making. A secondary goal is to avoid unnecessarily subjecting the child to interventions that may prolong or increase the child's suffering with little relative benefit. Advance care planning should be initiated early once the life-limiting or complex illness is diagnosed and should be continued throughout the course of that illness [30].

Admittedly, it is difficult to address all potential end-of-life scenarios; the choice of which ones depends on the individual child. At minimum, cardiopulmonary resuscitation (CPR) should be discussed. Families must understand that chest compressions with possible defibrillation and cardiac medications are the indiscriminate

Table 5.1 Topics appropriate for anticipatory guidance for children on chronic ventilation

- Chronic ventilation is only an assistive, never a curative, technology for respiration; it cannot alter static or progressive conditions or the risks and burdens of comorbidities
- Weaning from chronic ventilation is possible for some children, depending on their underlying conditions and other factors
- The child's goals of care will likely need to be readdressed when the child's condition worsens, which can happen without warning
- A perceived state of improved health can sometimes occur after initiation of chronic ventilation; this new plateau is sometimes temporary [59, 80]
- Acute illness sometimes precedes or leads to a new and more fragile state of chronic health [12]
- Common respiratory illnesses that are usually of little consequence to other children can result in severe illness in children on chronic ventilation
- Home ventilators are often inadequate for assisting respiration during acute illness
- Rehospitalization is often necessary for children with acute illness
- Noninvasive ventilation, even when administered in a hospital, may be inadequate to support respiration during acute illness, necessitating consideration of tracheal intubation
- In some cases, tracheal intubation is needed to support children normally sustained on noninvasive ventilation (e.g., acute illness, surgery). In some of these instances, tracheal extubation and return to noninvasive support are not possible and consideration of tracheostomy is necessary
- Children initiated on noninvasive ventilation can sometimes not be optimally sustained on it, and tracheostomy and transtracheal ventilation must be considered
- Tracheostomy complications and accidents—such as airway obstruction, decannulation, ventilator disconnection, false track replacement, aspiration, and tracheal bleeding—are potentially life-threatening [3, 8]. Similarly, for some patients on noninvasive ventilation, airway obstruction, ventilator disconnection, and ineffective mask fit can be potentially life-threatening. Caregiver competence in tracheostomy care, airway suctioning, bag-tracheostomy ventilation, bag-mask ventilation, and cardiopulmonary resuscitation can be lifesaving
- Even in children who are only partially dependent on assisted ventilation, noncompliance can accelerate life-threatening cardiopulmonary complications of their chronic respiratory failure

default medical response in the face of cardiac arrest. In order for informed families to assent to or forgo these measures, families should also understand that CPR is usually only successful when the arrest is triggered by an acute reversible cause and that nonfatal arrests can lead to new neurologic morbidity [43–46]. Because the causes of acute deterioration can be initially unclear and may be reversible, CPR is appropriate when deterioration is unexpected, even for children with life-limiting conditions. Thus, familial caregivers learn basic life support and airway management, and professional caregivers are obliged to attempt resuscitation. However, as the child's illness progresses or deteriorations become more frequent, severe, or irreversible, the burden of aggressive CPR may outweigh any benefits. Thus, preemptive decisions on CPR and other interventions may change over time.

However, simply addressing advance directives such as Do Not Resuscitation (DNR) orders or Physician Orders for Life-Sustaining Treatment (POLST) forms are often insufficient. Decisions faced during critical illness and at the end of life are more complex than the narrow topics addressed by these directives. Other decisions that may warrant advance care planning include utilization of hospice services, place of death, the use of other treatments (e.g., antibiotics, artificial nutrition), and organ donation. For patients on chronic noninvasive ventilation, why and when tracheal intubation might be indicated should be discussed before it becomes a life or death decision. Often it is appropriate to transcribe advance decisions into a signed written care plan that indicates what medical care is (and is not) desired for the child and why [29]. This care plan can be given to professional caregivers who are unfamiliar with the child in emergencies or when family is not present.

Hospice care should also be considered and discussed as viable options when appropriate and available. Commentators have argued that hospice care can be concurrent with disease-directed curative or life-assisting interventions [36, 47], which would include chronic ventilation.

Understandably, clinicians may first think of end-of-life preparation when considering advance care planning for children with life-limiting or complex chronic conditions. While this may be appropriate, a single-minded focus on end-of-life issues may become an obstacle to dealing with this and other issues. The future for children on chronic ventilation is as varied and complex as the children themselves. It can range from independent living as young adults (e.g., for those with congenital central hypoventilation syndrome) to progressive loss of functionality that requires escalating intervention. As part of caring for the whole person and their family, future non-end-of-life issues also deserve advance care planning. These often include progressive mobility and feeding difficulties, but can also include many other care issues, some of which can be controversial (e.g., growth attenuation [48]). In addition, when possible and appropriate, transition to adult healthcare providers should be strategized for any adolescent on chronic ventilation expected to survive into adulthood. Importantly, issues relevant to supporting the family also deserve attention, such as respite, emotional/psychological/financial distress, relationship strain, social isolation, and sibling psychosocial development.

The Challenges of Palliative Care and Advance Care Planning

It can be challenging to help any patient and family come to terms with their life-limiting condition and to participate in end-of-life palliative care and advance care planning. This challenge is both personal and cultural, as death has become something unfamiliar and to be avoided in Western culture [49]. Our healthcare system also has systems barriers to providing this sort of care, including a relative lack of expertise and training and insufficient resources/reimbursement [50]. Different and perhaps even greater challenges arise when the patient is a child, as the death of a child is seen as an injustice to the natural order of life [51]. Similarly, there are unique challenges to palliative care and advance care planning for children with complex chronic conditions and those on chronic ventilation. These unique challenges are often interrelated and can be linked to the idiosyncrasies of the child's underlying conditions, chronic ventilation itself, families, and even professional caregivers. These challenges can culminate and contribute to palliative care not being optimized and advance care planning not being done.

One of the most common and fundamental challenges is the difficulty of prognosticating disease trajectory and death for a particular patient [12, 52, 53]. Professional caregivers and usually families are aware that children with complex chronic conditions and chronic respiratory failure can die prematurely from progression of their underlying disease or acute critical illness related to their comorbidities [12, 54, 55]. In a large, single-institutional cohort study of children on chronic transtracheal ventilation, the 5- and 10-year cumulative incidences of death were 20% and 37%, respectively [8]. Strikingly, progression of an underlying condition accounted for only a third of the deaths, and half of the deaths were unexpected. So while shortened life expectancies can be anticipated, the timing and cause of these patients' deaths can often not be accurately predicted [40]. This inability to prognosticate can result in both professional and familial caregivers being hesitant to initiate palliative care. Both may choose to focus only on life-prolonging treatments until professional caregivers are "sure" of the child's imminent demise [11, 52]. In addition, arbitrary and spurious estimates of when death will occur can hinder attempts to address end-of-life issues. Erroneous guesses can lead to mistrust and misplaced focus. As Brook and Hain put it, "Numbers are always memorable; the concept they illustrate less so" [56].

While professional caregivers tend to view uncertain prognoses as a simmering "threat" to the child and want families to acknowledge the possible negative outcomes, families may view them as a possibility for a good outcome or for an extended period of not worrying about bad ones [35]. Despite this disconnect, uncertain prognosis should be a sign that palliative care is needed, even when it is not yet appropriate to focus on end-of-life care [52]. Importantly, it is not just the timing and cause of death that can be difficult to prognosticate. Other events/processes such as deteriorations of functionality or failure of noninvasive ventilation and the need to consider transtracheal ventilation can also be impossible to predict but substantially impact child and family.

Second and related to the inability to prognosticate death, it is not uncommon that children on chronic ventilation have survived previous "near-death" illness, sometimes more than once [11, 12, 40, 54, 57]. Scenarios where professional caregivers erroneously pronounce or speculate that the child will die can lead to a variety of familial responses from desensitization to the gravity of future deteriorations to mistrust or doubt in professional caregivers. Families may become increasingly reluctant to limit future interventions [40] or rely on their own intuition on these grave matters and thus move away from shared decision-making with professionals [58]. One way of looking at this is families are doing nothing different than what professionals do—they interpret and project the prior benefit of interventions onto future scenarios. Professional caregivers may become unwilling to share ominous predictions in the future even when their probabilities are higher and the need to address end-of-life issues greater.

Third, while chronic ventilation may be "palliative," in some cases, it can become a barrier to the provision of other palliative care. Commentators have reported their anecdotal experience that families of children on chronic ventilation can adopt an unrealistically positive view of the life-prolonging capabilities of these technologies [44, 59]. This view can hinder participation in palliative care and advance care planning for the end of life, especially when the child is clinically stable. In addition, it is likely that this extraordinary intervention becomes "ordinary" for the child and family. It is rare that families of children on chronic ventilation are offered or request that assisted ventilation be withdrawn at the end of life [44]. The choice for chronic ventilation can implicitly and explicitly be a sign that other extraordinary, life-prolonging interventions will be favored in the future. Reconciling the acclimation to and preference for extraordinary interventions can become a challenge when the child's underlying condition worsens more significantly or the care team concludes that the child's critical illness is likely not reversible. Thus, this preference, while initially appropriate, often needs to be gently recalibrated as circumstances and family readiness change [60]. Other familial and professional challenges to palliative care and advance care planning for children on chronic ventilation are listed in Table 5.2.

Table 5.2 Familial and professional challenges to palliative care for children on chronic ventilation

Familial challenges
• Familial caregivers can assume (sometimes divergent) roles of primary and medical provider [19]
• A mutually dependent relationship can develop between the child and familial caregivers who have devoted so much energy to their child's care [40, 68]
• Familial caregivers and patients can adopt a "live for the moment" attitude [11, 52]
• Familial caregivers can understand their child's life-limiting diagnosis on an "intellectual" level, but not believe it on an "emotional" level, making them not ready to participate in advance care planning [52, 81]
• After choosing chronic ventilation, the family presumes that they cannot or should not discontinue assisted ventilation or forgo subsequent interventions when the child's condition deteriorates
• Familial caregivers consciously or unconsciously withdraw from a mutually respectful patient-family-provider relationship when the child's condition worsens and there are disagreements with providers over the relative benefits and burdens of interventions, potentially feeling that providers are "giving up" on their child [67]
• There can be conflict among familial caregivers on goals of care
• Some children on chronic ventilation live outside of a home and are wards of the state. Who can make decisions about limiting life-sustaining interventions can vary by state. Detached surrogate decision-makers can potentially be the result
• Some children on chronic ventilation live outside of a home, and, rarely, families are not as involved in their child's care as would be ideal [54, 82]. Detached surrogate decision-makers can potentially be the result
Professional challenges
• With chronic ventilation, the child's medical home can shift from generalist to potentially intervention-oriented specialist [40]
• Professional caregivers have difficulty integrating life-prolonging-oriented care and palliative care [40]
• Professional caregivers erroneously presume that because a family has chosen chronic ventilation, they will always choose extraordinary measures to prolong their child's life

(continued)

Table 5.2 (continued)

• Professional caregivers erroneously interpret a family's difficulty in discussing grave issues as an implicit rejection of palliative care and advance care planning [11]
• Professional caregivers avoid raising sensitive, difficult issues with family members and project their own lack of readiness to discuss these issues onto them
• Professional caregivers may have little experience caring for or providing palliative care to children with such complex needs
• Professional caregivers' time may be constrained and feel as though they cannot adequately address all relevant topics [52]
• Professional caregivers can sometimes make assumptions (and thus recommendations/ decisions) based on brief or intermittent interactions with a patient during crises, which may not reflect the child's usual health state [12]
• Professional caregivers can sometimes make assumptions (and thus recommendations/decisions) about the child's quality of life and the family's burden of care based on their own values and biases, which may not reflect those of the child or family [83, 84]. Professional caregivers may make conscious or unconscious attempts to impose their own values on the family
• Professional caregivers consciously or unconsciously withdraw from a mutually respectful patient-family-provider relationship when the child's condition worsens and there are disagreements with families over the relative benefits and burdens of interventions, worrying that the family has "false hopes" [35, 40]
• Professional caregivers may be unwilling to accept their patient's fate
• Professional caregivers can sometimes use confusing language when discussing complex issues [27]
• Different professional caregivers can sometimes provide noncomplementary or contradictory information or recommendations [85]

Addressing These Challenges and Talking About End-of-Life Topics

While there is no point-by-point framework to address these challenges, they usually can be avoided or minimized. Awareness of them is the first and most important step. Next, using patience, sincerity, compassion, and candor is imperative when dealing with patients and families. Similarly, other broad, important strategies include good communication, avoiding abandonment, and propitious timing.

- Good communication

    Listening, understanding, exploring, explaining, and teaching are the platforms on which to build the patient-family-provider relationship [61]. Doing these things effectively and thoughtfully with patients and families is vital for facilitating palliative care. In one study of children with life-limiting oncologic or cardiac conditions and their parents, five domains of physician communication were identified as salient and influential to quality palliative care—relationship building, demonstration of effort and competence, information exchange, availability, and appropriate level of child and parent involvement [62]. Physician characteristics that were reported as harmful to palliative care included disrespectful or arrogant attitudes, not establishing a relationship with the family, breaking bad news in an insensitive manner, withholding information from parents and losing their trust, and changing a treatment course without preparing the patient and family. Other adult studies found significant associations between more empathic or emotionally supportive physician statements and higher family satisfaction with communication during deliberations about limiting life support [63]. Strategies and their corresponding mnemonics have arisen to aide professional caregivers empathically communicate difficult topics and explore patient and family experience, understanding, and concerns [64]. Importantly, good communication is not one-sided. Active listening and families having more time to talk have been shown to increase family satisfaction in the care of their critically ill family member [65, 66]. Professional caregivers must balance being compassionate with the need to always be forthright. Even before crises arise, they should explain this intention. They should inform families that it would be inappropriate to keep their concerns from them, that they are obliged to sometimes discuss difficult, sensitive topics, and that these topics will increasingly need to be addressed if and when the child's condition declines.

- Avoid any suggestion of abandonment

   Families who feel that their professional caregivers are "giving up" on their child can be resistant to engaging in important discussions related to end-of-life care [67]. In addition, families who demand what is considered "futile" treatment by their providers may be struggling with fears of abandonment [39]. Children and families should and need to be promised and feel that, no matter the circumstances, there will be an overriding commitment to addressing their needs and improving their situation. When families feel their providers are working diligently for their child in all cases, doubt, mistrust, and other threats to the patient-family-provider relationship may be avoided or minimized. This promise and corresponding action permits for hope that things can get better. Parents of dying children often retain an emotional component of hope for a "good" outcome while still intellectually understanding the inevitability of their child's condition. They do not see these states in competition with each other [35, 57]. At the end of life, this frame of mind should be channeled into a hope for their child's suffering to end through a peaceful death [39]. It also helps families to feel that they too are doing all they can for their child, when life-prolongation is no longer possible.

- Timing is everything

   Occasionally, the family themselves introduce the topic of end of life [29]. When this is not the case, appreciating when patients and families are ready to discuss end-of-life issues is an important step in facilitating advance care planning. As mentioned, the most appropriate timing for initiating end-of-life discussions is early in the patient's illness and before crises [68]. Early introduction of palliative and end-of-life options can give patients and families more time to hear, question, reflect on, and understand the difficult choices they may be forced to face [52].

Ideally, advance care planning would be introduced when chronic respiratory insufficiency is diagnosed (i.e., before chronic respiratory failure and before initiation of chronic ventilation). End-of-life issues are undoubtedly touched upon or inferred during early conversations about whether to initiate chronic ventilation. However, the expectation may not be realistic that families will connect pre-initiation conversations that include how not initiating chronic ventilation will allow the child's chronic respiratory failure or other underlying conditions to take their natural terminal course and advance care planning conversations after initiation. For many children with recognized and unrecognized chronic respiratory insufficiency, chronic ventilation is not discussed until after an acute illness pushes the at-risk child into failure [11, 69–73]. So, while end-of-life issues may have been introduced before initiation of chronic ventilation, it would be rare for advance care planning to not be modified by this new life-assisting intervention. It needs to be reintroduced early after initiation and before new crises, meaning that family readiness for such conversations needs to be reassessed early and often. Furthermore, if their child has never had a "near-death" illness or a visible decline in health from their long-standing baseline or if initiation of chronic ventilation resulted in an improved plateau of chronic health, asking families to make end-of-life decisions can be disorienting and without context [57].

While it is important for families to become partners in palliative care and advance care planning at their own pace, professional caregivers should continuously gauge family readiness and even create an environment that families recognize their benefit [52]. Facilitating families' acceptance of end-of-life palliative care can be augmented by first integrating life goals and non-end-of-life palliative care goals into the usual chronic care management [40, 74]. Similarly, a period of stability after initiation of chronic ventilation and other non-end-of-life palliative care is a good time to reintroduce end-of-life advance care planning. Other potential opportunities include development of a new comorbidity, the child approaching the upper range of the anticipated lifespan, prior to major surgical procedures, when the child starts to be left in the care of others, the death of another child the family knows, and other transition points [44, 75] Less ideal, but common, is reintroducing end-of-life topics after or during acute or chronic deteriorations of health [44]. Given that palliative care and advance care planning are inclusive with life-prolonging options, there should not be an abrupt switch to end-of-life issues. Just as patients' clinical condition can fluctuate, where the emphasis of advance care planning should be placed can fluctuate. Similarly, "all or nothing" paradigms, such as only focusing on DNR orders, should be avoided.

Although they may stem from a wish to provide compassionate care, suggestions to abruptly redirect goals of care can be negatively received. When families are not ready to discuss end-of-life issues and the child is clinically stable, overemphasizing this topic can make families believe that they are "on different pages" with providers and obstruct the patient-family-provider relationship. Constantly reminding families of their child's serious diagnosis or overwhelming them with negative anticipatory guidance risks quelling hope and sabotaging the relationship. Ill-timed discussions also risk families feeling that their child's presumed poor quality of life or other unintended reason prompted the discussion, as opposed to the anticipated trajectory of his conditions. However, by communicating belatedly or in a manner that is not forthright, physicians risk under-informing families.

If the child is clinically stable, it is not necessary for families to preemptively articulate their preferences for future scenarios. Rather, it is sufficient for them to gain a realistic understanding of their child's condition and risks and think through the values and goals that will likely shape their decisions. To help with the latter, one approach is to regularly recommend that families contemplate what they want for their child when he is in a period of relative health and what they want when he is threatened with serious acute illness or progression of an underlying condition. Likely, the values and goals that surface when contemplating "positive" scenarios can inform those that will be drawn upon to handle difficult ones. This approach encourages families to reflect on the inevitability or the serious risks of their child's condition while still focusing on their positive and hopeful goals. It also permits the professional caregiver to understand the family's life goals and the opportunity to show that she will work to help achieve them. Finally, it allows assessments of the family's readiness for end-of-life advance care planning. Regular encouragement to contemplate and possibly discuss these goals would ideally be offered during regular outpatient visits, but it could also be provided during hospitalizations.

The amount of time and effort professional caregivers should expend discussing scenarios of relative health versus illness depends on the child's condition and trajectory. As a child's condition worsens, ensuring that families are contemplating end-of-life goals and eliciting more specific preferences become more crucial. During periods of instability, the situation's gravity trumps family readiness, and the professional caregiver must alert the family of significant concerns related to morbidity or death.

Just like any advance directive, advance care plans can be modified at any point. The reasons for the desired change should be explored with the same sensitivity and focus on overall goals and values that facilitated the initial plan. Professional caregivers should ensure that the desired change is not prompted by confusion, doubt, new stressor, or outside coercion. Otherwise, advance care plans should be reviewed regularly with patients and families to ensure all are still in agreement.

When conflict over what is in the best interest for the child arises between professional and familial caregivers, the family's role as surrogate decision-maker should be respected. The family's love and commitment to their child's welfare should rarely be questioned. Finally, families are usually the ones who will have to deal with the consequences of whatever decisions are made [76, 77]. Sometimes, while shared decision-making is the goal, it is sometimes appropriate for professional caregivers to take the weight of the difficult decisions onto their own shoulders in order to help ameliorate the family's suffering [78]. Sometimes professional caregivers should compromise and agree to a plan that leads to a greater level of intervention than they believe is ideal in order to maintain a partnership with the family. Over time and as the child's condition deteriorates, a less invasive plan can usually be agreed upon [75]. Rarely, professional caregivers will feel obligated to involve outside parties, such as ethic committees or the legal system, in conflicts.

Discussions around palliative care and advance care planning should be documented in the patient's medical record, even when no decision has been reached.

Such documentation can help future caregivers know what has been discussed and where families are in terms of readiness, respond to allegations that important topics were not discussed, and support reimbursement claims related to counseling [79]. While the points above are predominately for the longitudinal caregiver, even those professionals who only sporadically interact with these children and families must be aware that their interactions can impact patients and families and help or hinder family readiness for advance care planning.

Palliative care is a necessary part of the total care for children on chronic ventilation and their families. It complements life-prolonging or cure-oriented therapies by providing other medical, psychological, emotional, and spiritual care. Through advance care planning, it also offers families the chance to preemptively think through future scenarios that their child will face because of his medical conditions and think through the values and goals that will inform their ultimate decisions. Importantly, while end-of-life palliative care and advance care planning should be a focus, end of life should not be the sole focus. Rather, helping children and families achieve life goals at all its stages is an overarching imperative, one that should not be derailed by any combination of challenges.

Acknowledgments Special thanks to Drs. Gloria Chiang and Robert Graham for their reading portions of the manuscript and for their suggestions.

References

1. Srinivasan S, Doty SM, White TR, Segura VH, Jansen MT, Davidson Ward SL, Keens TG. Frequency, causes, and outcome of home ventilator failure. Chest. 1998;114(5):1363–7.
2. Chatwin M, Heather S, Hanak A, Polkey MI, Simonds AK. Analysis of home support and ventilator malfunction in 1,211 ventilator-dependent patients. Eur Respir J. 2010;35(2):310–6.
3. Boroughs D, Dougherty JA. Decreasing accidental mortality of ventilator-dependent children at home: a call to action. Home Healthc Nurse. 2012;30(2):103–11.
4. Gregoretti C, Ottonello G, Chiarini Testa MB, Mastella C, Ravà L, Bignamini E, Veljkovic A, Cutrera R. Survival of patients with spinal muscular Atrophy type 1. Pediatrics. 2013;131(5):e1509–14. doi:10.1542/peds.2012-2278.
5. Ishikawa Y, Miura T, Ishikawa Y, Aoyagi T, Ogata H, Hamada S, Minami R. Duchenne muscular dystrophy: survival by cardio-respiratory interventions. Neuromuscul Disord. 2011;21(1):47–51.
6. Brooks JC, Strauss DJ, Shavelle RM, Tran LM, Rosenbloom L, Wu YW. Recent trends in cerebral palsy survival. Part II: individual survival prognosis. Dev Med Child Neurol. 2014;56(11):1065–71.
7. Bittles AH, Glasson EJ. Clinical, social, and ethical implications of changing life expectancy in Down syndrome. Dev Med Child Neurol. 2004;46(4):282–6.
8. Edwards JD, Kun SS, Keens TG. Outcomes and causes of death in children on home mechanical ventilation via tracheostomy: an institutional and literature review. J Pediatr. 2010;157(6):955–9.
9. Edwards JD, Kun SS, Keens TG, Khemani RG, Moromisato DY. Children with corrected or palliated congenital heart disease on home mechanical ventilation. Pediatr Pulmonol. 2010;45(7):645–9.

10. Jernigan SC, Berry JG, Graham DA, Bauer SB, Karlin LI, Hobbs NM, Scott RM, Warf BC. Risk factors of sudden death in young adult patients with myelomeningocele. J Neurosurg Pediatr. 2012;9(2):149–55.

11. Parker D, Maddocks I, Stern LM. The role of palliative care in advanced muscular dystrophy and spinal muscular atrophy. J Paediatr Child Health. 1999;35(3):245–50.

12. Steele RG. Trajectory of certain death at an unknown time: children with neurodegenerative life-threatening illnesses. Can J Nurs Res. 2000;32(3):49–67.

13. Carnevale FA, Alexander E, Davis M, Rennick J, Troini R. Daily living with distress and enrichment: the moral experience of families with ventilator-assisted children at home. Pediatrics. 2006;117:e48–60.

14. Blucker RT, Elliott TR, Warren RH, Warren AM. Psychological adjustment of family caregivers of children who have severe neurodisabilities that require chronic respiratory management. Fam Syst Health. 2011;29(3):215–31.

15. Toly VB, Musil CM, Carl JC. A longitudinal study of families with technology-dependent children. Res Nurs Health. 2012;35(1):40–54.

16. Noyes J, Hartmann H, Samuels M, Southall D. The experiences and views of parents who care for ventilator-dependent children. J Clin Nurs. 1999;8(4):440–50.

17. Heaton J, Noyes J, Sloper P, Shah R. Families' experiences of caring for technology-dependent children: a temporal perspective. Health Soc Care Community. 2005;13:441–50.

18. O'Brien ME, Wegner CB. Rearing the child who is technology dependent: perceptions of parents and home care nurses. J Spec Pediatr Nurs. 2002;7:7–15.

19. Kirk S, Glendinning C, Callery P. Parent or nurse? The experience of being the parent of a technology dependent child. J Adv Nurs. 2005;51:456–64.

20. Alexander E, Rennick JE, Carnevale F, Davis M. Daily struggles: living with long-term childhood technology dependence. Can J Nurs Res. 2002;34:7–14.

21. Toly VB, Musil CM, Carl JC. Families with children who are technology dependent: normalization and family functioning. West J Nurs Res. 2012;34(1):52–71.

22. Thyen U, Kuhlthau K, Perrin JM. Employment, child care, and mental health of mothers caring for children assisted by technology. Pediatrics. 1999;103(6 Pt 1):1235–42.

23. Donnelly JP, Huff SM, Lindsey ML, McMahon KA, Schumacher JD. The needs of children with life-limiting conditions: a healthcare-provider-based model. Am J Hosp Palliat Care. 2005;22(4):259–67.

24. American Academy of Pediatrics Policy Statement. Pediatric palliative care and hospice care commitments, guidelines, and recommendations. Pediatrics. 2013;132:966–72.

25. Dawson S, Kristjanson LJ. Mapping the journey: family carers' perceptions of issues related to end-stage care of individuals with muscular dystrophy or motor neurone disease. J Palliat Care. 2003;19(1):36–42.

26. Cockett A. Developing a long-term ventilation service in a children's hospice: an illustrative case study. Int J Palliat Nurs. 2012;18(6):301–6.

27. Carroll KW, Mollen CJ, Aldridge S, Hexem KR, Feudtner C. Influences of decision making identified by parents of children receiving pediatric palliative care. Am J Bioeth Prim Res. 2012;3(1):1–7.

28. Friedman SL. Parent resuscitation preferences for young people with severe developmental disabilities. J Am Med Dir Assoc. 2006;7(2):67–72.

29. Hammes BJ, Klevan J, Kempf M, Williams MS. Pediatric advance care planning. J Palliat Med. 2005;8(4):766–73.

30. Wharton RH, Levine KR, Buka S, Emanuel L. Advance care planning for children with special health care needs: a survey of parental attitudes. Pediatrics. 1996;97(5):682–7.

31. Steinhauser KE, Clipp EC, McNeilly M, Christakis NA, McIntyre LM, Tulsky JA. In search of a good death: observations of patients, families and providers. Ann Intern Med. 2000;132:825–32.

32. Liberman DB, Pham PK, Nager AL. Pediatric advance directives: Parents' knowledge, experience, and preferences. Pediatrics. 2014;134(2):e436–43.

33. Hill DL, Miller VA, Hexem KR, Carroll KW, Faerber JA, Kang T, Feudtner C. Problems and hopes perceived by mothers, fathers and physicians of children receiving palliative care. Health Expect. 2013;18(5):1052–62. doi:10.1111/hex.12078.
34. Feudtner C. Hope and the prospects of healing at the end of life. J Altern Complement Med. 2005;11 Suppl 1:S23–30.
35. Reder EA, Serwint JR. Until the last breath: exploring the concept of hope for parents and health care professionals during a child's serious illness. Arch Pediatr Adolesc Med. 2009;163(7):653–7.
36. Miller EG, Laragione G, Kang TI, Feudtner C. Concurrent care for the medically complex child: lessons of implementation. J Palliat Med. 2012;15(11):1281–3.
37. American Academy of Pediatrics, Committee on Bioethics and Committee on Hospital Care. Palliative care for children. Pediatrics. 2000;106(2 Pt 1):351–7.
38. Viallard ML. Some general considerations of a human-based medicine's palliative approach to the vulnerability of the multiply disabled child before the end of life. Cult Med Psychiatry. 2014;38(1):28–34.
39. Gillis J. We want everything done. Arch Dis Child. 2008;93(3):192–3.
40. Graham RJ, Robinson WM. Integrating palliative care into chronic care for children with severe neurodevelopmental disabilities. J Dev Behav Pediatr. 2005;26(5):361–5.
41. Kane JR, Barber RG, Jordan M, Tichenor KT, Camp K. Supportive/palliative care of children suffering from life-threatening and terminal illness. Am J Hosp Palliat Care. 2000;17(3):165–72.
42. Schuster MA, Duan N, Regalado M, Klein DJ. Anticipatory guidance: what information do parents receive? What information do they want? Arch Pediatr Adolesc Med. 2000;154(12):1191–8.
43. Haque IU, Udassi JP, Zaritsky AL. Outcome following cardiopulmonary arrest. Pediatr Clin N Am. 2008;55(4):969–87.
44. Edwards JD, Kun SS, Graham RJ, Keens TG. End-of-life discussions and advance care planning for children on long-term assisted ventilation with life-limiting conditions. J Palliat Care. 2012;28(1):21–7.
45. Matos RI, Watson RS, Nadkarni VM, Huang HH, Berg RA, Meaney PA, Carroll CL, Berens RJ, Praestgaard A, Weissfeld L, Spinella PC, American Heart Association's Get With The Guidelines–Resuscitation (Formerly the National Registry of Cardiopulmonary Resuscitation) Investigators. Duration of cardiopulmonary resuscitation and illness category impact survival and neurologic outcomes for in-hospital pediatric cardiac arrests. Circulation. 2013;127(4):442–51.
46. Girotra S, Spertus JA, Li Y, Berg RA, Nadkarni VM, Chan PS, American Heart Association Get With the Guidelines–Resuscitation Investigators. Survival trends in pediatric in-hospital cardiac arrests: an analysis from get with the Guidelines-Resuscitation. Circ Cardiovasc Qual Outcomes. 2013;6(1):42–9.
47. United States, et al. Compilation of Patient Protection and Affordable Care Act (PPACA) as amended through November 1, 2010, including PPACA health-related portions of the Health Care and Education Reconciliation Act (HCERA) of 2010. Washington, DC: U.S. Government Printing Office; 2010.
48. Wilfond BS, Miller PS, Korfiatis C, Diekema DS, Dudzinski DM, Goering S, Seattle Growth Attenuation and Ethics Working Group. Navigating growth attenuation in children with profound disabilities. Children's interests, family decision-making, and community concerns. Hastings Cent Rep. 2010;40(6):27–40.
49. Callahan M, Kelley P. Final gifts: understanding the special awareness, needs, and communications of the dying. New York: Bantam; 1997.
50. Himelstein BP, Hilden JM, Boldt AM, Weissman D. Pediatric palliative care. N Engl J Med. 2004;350(17):1752–62.
51. Jecker NS, Schneiderman LJ. Is dying young worse than dying old? Gerontologist. 1994;34(1):66–72.
52. Davies B, Sehring SA, Partridge JC, Cooper BA, Hughes A, Philp JC, Amidi-Nouri A, Kramer RF. Barriers to palliative care for children: perceptions of pediatric health care providers. Pediatrics. 2008;121(2):282–8.

53. Hynson JL, Gillis J, Collins JJ, Irving H, Trethewie SJ. The dying child: how is care different? Med J Aust. 2003;179(6 Suppl):S20–2.
54. Grossberg RI, Blackford M, Friebert S, Benore E, Reed MD. Direct care staff and parents'/legal guardians' perspectives on end-of-life care in a long-term care facility for medically fragile and intellectually disabled pediatric and young adult residents. Palliat Support Care. 2012;10:1–8.
55. Serwint JR, Nellis ME. Deaths of pediatric patients: relevance to their medical home, an urban primary care clinic. Pediatrics. 2005;115:57–63.
56. Brook L, Hain R. Predicting death in children. Arch Dis Child. 2008;93(12):1067–70.
57. Hauer J. Medical treatment and management at the end of life. In: Friedman SL, Helm DT, editors. End-of-life care for children and adults with intellectual and developmental disabilities. Washington, DC: American Association on Intellectual and Developmental Disabilities; 2010. p. 93–120.
58. Michelson KN, Koogler T, Sullivan C, Ortega Mdel P, Hall E, Frader J. Parental views on withdrawing life-sustaining therapies in critically ill children. Arch Pediatr Adolesc Med. 2009;163(11):986–92.
59. Birnkrant DJ, Noritz GH. Is there a role for palliative care in progressive pediatric neuromuscular diseases? The answer is "Yes! J Palliat Care. 2008;24(4):265–9.
60. Hill DL, Miller V, Walter JK, Carroll KW, Morrison WE, Munson DA, Kang TI, Hinds PS, Feudtner C. Regoaling: a conceptual model of how parents of children with serious illness change medical care goals. BMC Palliat Care. 2014;13(1):9.
61. Singer GR, Koch KA. Communicating with our patients: the goal of bioethics. J Fla Med Assoc. 1997;84(8):486–7.
62. Hsiao JL, Evan EE, Zeltzer LK. Parent and child perspectives on physician communication in pediatric palliative care. Palliat Support Care. 2007;5(4):355–65.
63. Selph RB, Shiang J, Engelberg R, Curtis JR, White DB. Empathy and life support decisions in intensive care units. J Gen Intern Med. 2008;23(9):1311–7.
64. Coyle N, Peereboom K. Facilitating goals-of-care discussions for patients with life-limiting disease—communication strategies for nurses. J Hosp Palliat Nurs. 2012;14(4):251–8.
65. McDonagh JR, Elliott TB, Engelberg RA, Treece PD, Shannon SE, Rubenfeld GD, Patrick DL, Curtis JR. Family satisfaction with family conferences about end-of-life care in the intensive care unit: increased proportion of family speech is associated with increased satisfaction. Crit Care Med. 2004;32(7):1484–8.
66. Thornton JD, Pham K, Engelberg RA, Jackson JC, Curtis JR. Families with limited English proficiency receive less information and support in interpreted intensive care unit family conferences. Crit Care Med. 2009;37(1):89–95.
67. Hinds PS, Schum L, Baker JN, Wolfe J. Key factors affecting dying children and their families. J Palliat Med. 2005;8 Suppl 1:S70–8.
68. Durall A, Zurakowski D, Wolfe J. Barriers to conducting advance care discussions for children with life-threatening conditions. Pediatrics. 2012;129(4):e975–82.
69. Shneerson JM. Home mechanical ventilation in children: techniques, outcomes and ethics. Monaldi Arch Chest Dis. 1996;51(5):426–30.
70. Simonds AK. Respiratory support for the severely handicapped child with neuromuscular disease: ethics and practicality. Semin Respir Crit Care Med. 2007;28(3):342–54.
71. Fraser J, Henrichsen T, Mok Q, et al. Prolonged mechanical ventilation as a consequence of acute illness. Arch Dis Child. 1998;78(3):253–6.
72. Sritippayawan S, Kun SS, Keens TG, Davidson Ward SL. Initiation of home mechanical ventilation in children with neuromuscular diseases. J Pediatr. 2003;142:481–5.
73. Gillis J, Tibballs J, McEniery J, Heavens J, Hutchins P, Kilham HA, Henning R. Ventilator-dependent children. Med J Aust. 1989;150:10–4.
74. Nelson JE, Hope AA. Integration of palliative care in chronic critical illness management. Respir Care. 2012;57(6):1004–12.
75. Wolff A, Browne J, Whitehouse WP. Personal resuscitation plans and end of life planning for children with disability and life-limiting/life-threatening conditions. Arch Dis Child Educ Pract Ed. 2011;96(2):42–8.

76. American Academy of Pediatrics Committee on Bioethics. Ethics and the care of critically ill infants and children. Pediatrics. 1996;98(1):149–52.
77. Burns JP, Mitchell C. Do-not-resuscitate orders and redirection of treatment. In: Friedman SL, Helm DT, editors. End-of-life care for children and adults with intellectual and developmental disabilities. Washington, DC: American Association on Intellectual and Developmental Disabilities; 2010. p. 147–59.
78. Clark JD, Dudzinski DM. The culture of dysthanasia: attempting CPR in terminally Ill children. Pediatrics. 2013;131(3):572–80. doi:10.1542/peds.2012-0393.
79. Lustbader DR, Nelson JE, Weissman DE, Hays RM, Mosenthal AC, Mulkerin C, Puntillo KA, Ray DE, Bassett R, Boss RD, Brasel KJ, Campbell ML, Cortez TB, Curtis JR, IPAL-ICU Project. Physician reimbursement for critical care services integrating palliative care for patients who are critically ill. Chest. 2012;141(3):787–92.
80. Simonds AK, Muntoni F, Heather S, et al. Impact of nasal ventilation on survival in hypercapnic Duchenne muscular dystrophy. Thorax. 1998;53(11):949–52.
81. Feudtner C, Carroll KW, Hexem KR, Silberman J, Kang TI, Kazak AE. Parental hopeful patterns of thinking, emotions, and pediatric palliative care decision making: a prospective cohort study. Arch Pediatr Adolesc Med. 2010;164(9):831–9.
82. Stein GL. Providing palliative care to people with intellectual disabilities: services, staff knowledge, and challenges. J Palliat Med. 2008;11(9):1241–8.
83. Freed MM. Academy presidential address. Quality of life: the physician's dilemma. Arch Phys Med Rehabil. 1984;65(3):109–11.
84. Levy J, van Stone M. Ethical foundations and legal issues. In: Friedman SL, Helm DT, editors. End-of-life care for children and adults with intellectual and developmental disabilities. Washington, DC: American Association on Intellectual and Developmental Disabilities; 2010. p. 31–49.
85. Meert KL, Eggly S, Pollack M, Anand KJ, Zimmerman J, Carcillo J, Newth CJ, Dean JM, Willson DF, Nicholson C, National Institute of Child Health and Human Development Collaborative Pediatric Critical Care Research Network. Parents' perspectives on physician-parent communication near the time of a child's death in the pediatric intensive care unit. Pediatr Crit Care Med. 2008;9(1):2–7.

Chapter 6
Transition from Hospital to Home

Sherry L. Barnhart and April Carpenter

Introduction

With clinical and technological advancements in neonatal and pediatric care, more children are surviving critical illnesses. Survival however is often accompanied by respiratory failure and other complex conditions that remain unresolved at hospital discharge [1]. The result is a population of technology-dependent children who require either permanent or temporary mechanical ventilator assistance. With portable mechanical ventilators and nursing care available in the home, these children are no longer remaining hospitalized. Today they are discharged home with oxygen, tracheostomy tubes, positive pressure ventilators, airway clearance devices, and other medical interventions that formerly would have only been available in a hospital [2].

Transitioning the ventilator-dependent child from the hospital to home requires a coordinated effort between the child's family and a multidisciplinary healthcare team. The ultimate goal throughout the discharge process is to move the child into a home where the family can safely and independently provide daily care that will result in a healthy and optimum quality of life with a minimum of recurrent hospitalizations.

S.L. Barnhart, R.R.T-.N.P.S., F.A.A.R.C. (✉)
Respiratory Care Discharge Planner, Respiratory Care Services, Arkansas Children's Hospital, 1 Children's Way, Little Rock, AR 72202, USA
e-mail: barnhartsl@archildrens.org

A. Carpenter, A.P.R.N.
Arkansas Children's Hospital, University of Arkansas for Medical Sciences, Little Rock, AR, USA

© Springer Science+Business Media New York 2016
L.M. Sterni, J.L. Carroll (eds.), *Caring for the Ventilator Dependent Child*, Respiratory Medicine, DOI 10.1007/978-1-4939-3749-3_6

Benefits of Going Home

Along with the high cost of care, there are multiple developmental and psychological disadvantages to caring for a medically stable ventilator-dependent child in the
hospital. Most caregivers prefer their child be at home because this causes less
disruption in family activities. Moving care into the home can improve the quality
of life of not only the child but the entire family.

Enhanced Psychosocial Development and Quality of Life

Ventilation at home has long been considered as the respiratory technology-dependent
child's best option for optimum psychosocial development, social integration, and
quality of life [3]. Families can provide far more love and dedication while caring for
their child at home than a nurse has time to give in an inpatient facility. Children tend
to thrive in the home environment and master developmental milestones at an increasingly faster pace than while hospitalized. They are found to excel in the home environment with improved activities of daily living (ADLs). Additional benefits are
improvement in skin integrity and musculoskeletal alignment, functional mobility,
communication skills and ability to use sign language, and overall independence [4].
    Although few in number, studies have shown that participation in recreation and
leisure activity improves the quality of life in children dependent on long-term
mechanical ventilation. These activities include watching television, listening to
music, playing computer and board games, eating at restaurants, and attending movies
and sporting events [4]. Improvement in psychosocial outcomes are also noted when
these children are no longer separated from their families and are able to participate in
age appropriate peer activities. Many of them take pleasure in hobbies and everyday
activities and view their dependence on technology as a very small part of their lives.

Reduced Cost

The financial burden of caring for a child who is ventilator-dependent includes
medical equipment and supplies, hospital stays, ambulance transport, medication,
and other primary medical services [4]. Although reports indicate that 24-h nursing
care at home is more expensive than a standard children's hospital ward, it is far less
expensive than care in a long-term ventilation unit or an intensive care unit [4].
Caring for the child at home has been found to be less costly by as much as 70 %
when compared to the cost of staying in an intensive care unit or step-down unit [5].
Savings in providing care at home can in some part be attributed to family members
bearing the cost of housing and providing a portion of the nursing care. Cost is
further reduced when home care minimizes the number of hospital readmissions.

Risks of Providing Care at Home

As is often the case, with many benefits there are also risks. In a recent study of parents whose children attended a pediatric home ventilator clinic, one quarter of the families reported financial struggles and over half reported unmet needs for care [6]. This included therapeutic services and skilled nursing care, with inadequate staffing being the major barrier to nursing care. Probable caregiver depressive disorder was also associated with an unmet need for care. However, transferring a respiratory technology-dependent child from an inpatient facility to home carries considerable risk even when 24-h nursing is provided in the home.

Risk of Mortality

Despite the technological advances in home monitoring of mechanically ventilated patients, the preventable death rate among children has not changed significantly during the last two decades [7]. The primary causes for preventable death in this population are inadequate caregiver training, improper caregiver response to monitor and ventilator alarms, improper response to the child's clinical symptoms, and lack of appropriately trained caregivers [7]. To reduce the risk of mortality the American Thoracic Society (ATS) has developed guidelines for the home care of children of children with tracheostomy [8]. These guidelines are based on research and expert opinion and have been adopted by most children's hospitals as the standard of care to successfully transition children receiving mechanical ventilation from hospital to home. However, published standards for the care of children on long-term invasive and noninvasive ventilation are still needed.

Inadequate Home Nursing Care

The lack of available home nursing along with an increasing number of inadequately trained nurses has hugely impacted the ability of families to care for their ventilator-dependent child at home. Besides noting that there is a decrease in the number of nurses willing to work in pediatric home care, literature also shows that most nurses employed in the home have little to no prior experience providing tracheostomy or ventilator care to a child in a hospital setting. For many, their competency is based on simulation and online teaching methods [7]. Despite the advantages of learning through simulation with mannequins, the value of experiential learning with humans cannot be replaced. Simulation, whether online or in a classroom setting, often does not adequately prepare nurses for the unique needs of children and the unpredictability of real-life circumstances [7].

Caregiver Stress, Fatigue, and Financial Loss

The needs of a technology-dependent child can change family dynamics and affect the caregivers' coping mechanisms. As family caregivers are responsible for a large amount of their child's medical care, the resulting stress impacts their marriage, siblings, and extended family. A recent review reported that the demands of caring for a chronically ill child created greater stress for the caregivers than the severity or length of the child's illness [9].

Due to the nursing shortage and cuts by the payer source, children requiring chronic mechanical ventilation often receive only 12–16 h of skilled home nursing per day or even less. Because nursing hours approved by insurance or Medicaid are often grossly insufficient to meet the child's needs at home, family caregivers are now expected to become experts in the care of their medically complex child [10]. Being an expert includes providing their child with physical, occupational, and speech therapies at home. It also requires that they manage highly technical equipment including ventilators, cardiopulmonary monitors, oxygen, and feeding pumps, as well as provide tracheostomy and gastrostomy tube care. The 24-hours-per-day responsibility of assessing and monitoring their child and responding to ventilator and monitor alarms can lead to a sense of isolation. These caregivers desperately need respite time, a temporary break from the pressures of caring for their child in which they can rest and replenish their energy. Unfortunately respite care is often difficult if not impossible to acquire.

The care that their child requires can place considerable time demands on the entire family. This often negatively impacts the caregivers' employment, social life, and ability to participate in the activities of their other children [11]. Although employment outside of the home may provide a form of respite, many caregivers experience missed days of work and disruption in their schedules which can lead to reduced productivity and lower household income. Because of the added workload, caregivers often suffer from sleep disruption, which causes fatigue and burnout and puts them at high risk for physical illness and poor mental health outcomes [4]. Financial loss, chronic lack of sleep, feelings of guilt and resentment in not being able to meet all of the needs of the rest of the family, and the around-the-clock vigilance required often results in an enormous amount of emotional stress and isolation [12]. This alone places these children at risk for re-hospitalization.

Lack of Community and Financial Resources

Often times caring for ventilator-dependent children at home can become a financial burden to the family as their community resources and government aide runs thin [3]. Families must constantly stay abreast of reimbursement and medical coverage issues to avoid the aggravation of denials and the challenges of obtaining necessary equipment and community assistance [13].

Children dependent on medical technology have unique healthcare needs and it has become increasingly difficult to find clinicians who are qualified to care for them at home. More hospitals are training physicians to be primary caregivers who unfortunately often lack the ability to care for tracheostomy and ventilator-dependent children. Traditional care doesn't work for these children; they require an educated clinician who can collaborate with the family and other medical team members to make decisions that will benefit their care [10].

Alternative Sites of Care

The commitment to provide a child with chronic mechanical ventilation requires determining the eventual site at which long-term care will be provided. Major factors impacting this decision are the assessment of the family, the adequacy of the home environment, and the medical needs of the child. Despite the benefits of discharging a mechanically ventilated child home there are circumstances that prevent this outcome. In the event that the child cannot be discharged safely to a home setting with trained caregivers, it is recommended that transfer be made to an alternative site of care. This may be an extended specialty hospital, a foster home, or a pediatric skilled nursing facility where optimal nursing care can be continued [2]. Alternative sites of care may serve three possible purposes: transitional care, respite care, or long-term care.

Transitional care may consist of moving the child to an alternative site just until the family caregivers are better prepared to bring the child home. During transitional care emphasis is placed on the caregivers continuing training while gradually increasing the care they provide to their child. Respite care may be provided in an institution or medical foster home. Transitional care and respite care are also utilized by families when there is an emergency or the home becomes an inappropriate setting of care for a short period of time. Long-term care is for children whose caregivers are either unable or unwilling to have them cared for at home. Some states do not have facilities that provide such care for infants or children. In those situations the care is provided in a subacute or step-down transitional unit within an acute-care hospital setting. In most cases, the care in alternative sites is temporary and the ultimate goal is for the child to be reunited with the family.

Multidisciplinary Team Approach to Discharge

Discharging technology-dependent children from the hospital is a complex and challenging process. Planning for the discharge of any patient should ideally start before or at admission. However in many cases it is not known at admission that a child will be ventilator-dependent upon discharge. Deciding that a child is medically appropriate for home mechanical ventilation and caregivers' committing to provide it usually occurs later in the hospital course. For these children, it is when that decision is made that discussion of discharge needs should begin. Effective discharge planning for them involves a skilled multidisciplinary team approach with each healthcare professional having a clearly defined role [13].

Team Composition

The multidisciplinary discharge planning team should include, but not be limited to, hospital and community healthcare workers who can provide expertise and empower families as they prepare to independently care for their child. Although team composition will vary per hospital, Table 6.1 lists those who may be represented on the team. At the center of this team are the caregivers and their child; family-centered care is widely embraced as an essential component of the medical home and is a core-objective of the Maternal Child Health Bureau's goals for the care of children with special healthcare needs [14] (See Chap. 7).

Table 6.1 Composition of multidisciplinary discharge team

- Patient and Caregivers
- Physician
- Advanced nurse practitioner
- Specialty nurse
- RN case manager/discharge planner
- Respiratory case manager/discharge planner
- Social worker
- Nutritionist
- Child life specialist
- Respiratory therapist
- Occupational therapist
- Physical therapist
- Speech therapist
- Pharmacist
- Chaplain
- Home medical equipment provider
- Home nursing agency representative
- Insurance case manager
- School nurse
- Alternative site (e.g., subacute specialty hospital, foster home, pediatric skilled nursing facility) representative

Responsibilities of the Team

The discharge planning team's goal is to provide the caregivers and the ventilator-dependent child with a successful transition from the hospital. This is done by (1) establishing a target length of stay, (2) identifying issues that must be resolved prior to discharge, and (3) developing a discharge plan unique for each individual child and family. Together the team should make decisions and agree upon the discharge process and the appropriate time for discharge. Because of the number of members involved in this multidisciplinary collaboration, it is essential that communication remain effective. This can be accomplished through team rounding within the hospital units, discharge planning team meetings, designated liaisons for the medical equipment company and the nursing agency, progress notes and team meeting summaries accessible by both hospital and home care staff through the electronic medical record, caregiver competency documentation, and personal contact with the caregivers by phone or at the bedside [15].

Communication with Caregivers

Efficient lines of communication are essential during the ventilator-dependent child's transition to home. Information is an invaluable means of enhancing the caregiver's sense of control. Regularly scheduled meetings with the caregivers and the multidisciplinary team provide a time for every one present to ask questions and voice their concerns. It is helpful to have one team member responsible for scheduling the meetings and communicating these dates and times with the caregivers.

Keeping the caregivers informed about their child's medical progress and discussing their understanding of the condition and prognosis provides an opportunity to address any misconceptions. It is important to determine what caregivers expect to occur prior to and following discharge home. They also need a clear understanding of the roles of the various healthcare providers. There is often a wide difference between the caregivers' expectations of the community healthcare services that will be provided at home and what actually occurs.

It is vital that the family caregivers meet the team as soon as it is determined that their child will require long-term mechanical ventilation. The initial meeting may have only the family, physician, nurse practitioner or specialty nurse, and social worker in attendance. The primary purpose of this meeting is to inform the caregivers of the process that is followed when discharging a ventilator-dependent child to home and the options available to them. The caregivers should be provided with educational material explaining the discharge process for their child. This should include information about what their child will need at home, what skills the caregivers are expected to learn, and the steps that must be followed in preparing for their child's discharge.

Members of the multidisciplinary team should meet often with the caregivers to identify and work through any barriers relating to discharge. These meetings provide an opportunity to set goals and priorities for the family and review the level of responsibility expected of them. Figure 6.1 provides an example of a handout that may be given to the team members for use at a meeting. Caregiver meetings should occur at least every 2–4 weeks, depending upon how close it is to the expected discharge date. As discharge day nears for a child, the team may choose to meet more frequently. Scheduling a final meeting within a week of discharge is often helpful in making sure that everything is in place with the caregivers, the home, the medical

CAREGIVER/FAMILY MEETING -- PREPARING TO GO HOME

Date: _____

Tentative Date for Discharge Home is _____

CAREGIVERS

Name & phone # of caregivers who will complete the training to take your child home:

1 _____ Phone # _____
2 _____ Phone # _____
3 _____ Phone # _____

You need to complete the following training before beginning the 24-hour in-hospital stay with your child:
_____
_____
_____

You need to have the following before your child will be discharged:
___ car seat   ___ crib or bed   ___ stroller or wheelchair
___ smoke alarms   ___ fire extinguishers   ___ home/electrical repairs completed

Other things you need before discharge: _____
_____
_____

Your 24-hour in-hospital stay is tentatively scheduled to occur on: _____

If you have questions about your training or what you need at home, contact your child's nurse or social worker.

HOME NURSING AGENCY

Name of agency that will provide nursing care in your home: _____

   Location: _____ Phone # _____
   Supervisor: _____ Phone # _____

Home visit from nursing agency will occur on: _____

If you have questions about home nursing, contact: _____

Fig. 6.1 Caregiver handout for use during family meetings

HOME RESPIRATORY EQUIPMENT COMPANY

Name of company providing the ventilator and respiratory equipment:

_____

    Location: _____   Phone # _____
    Manager: _____   Phone # _____

The home visit from the respiratory equipment company will occur on: _____

Dates you will receive ventilator and respiratory equipment training: _____

Your training will be held at ___ your home, ___ the hospital, ___ the equipment company.

The respiratory equipment/supplies will be delivered to your home on: _____

If you have questions about your home equipment, contact: _____

FEEDS/ENTERAL SUPPLIES COMPANY

Name of company providing feeds and enteral supplies: _____

    Location: _____   Phone # _____
    Manager: _____   Phone # _____

Dates you will receive feeds/enteral supplies training: _____

Your training will be held at ___ your home, ___ the hospital, ___ the equipment company.

The feeds/enteral supplies will be delivered to your home on _____

If you have questions about your feeds/enteral supplies, contact: _____

IMPORTANT DATES TO REMEMBER:

Home Visit from Nursing Agency: _____
Home Visit from Respiratory Equipment Company: _____

Ventilator & respiratory equipment training: _____
Feeds & enteral equipment/supplies training: _____

24-hour in-hospital stay (tentative date): _____
Discharge date (tentative date): _____

Fig. 6.1 (continued)

equipment company, and the nursing agency. Barriers to communication include extensive distance from the hospital, limited transportation options, and limited caregiver education level. For those caregivers who have a language barrier, it is essential that interpreters are provided during all training sessions and caregiver meetings with the discharge planning team. It is also helpful to identify intermediaries within an ethnic community and establish linkages with community-based services.

Pre-discharge Criteria

Specific criteria must be met before the ventilator-dependent child can be considered for discharge. Following these criteria has been found to result in a reduction in hospital length of stay, unplanned readmissions, and post-discharge medical costs. Table 6.2 lists criteria that should be met before discharge is considered.

Medical Stability of Child

Each child must be evaluated and medically stable prior to hospital discharge. If the child has a condition that may require readmission to the hospital within 1 month following discharge, then that child is not considered medically stable [5]. The tracheostomy must be secured and stabilized to reduce the risk of obstruction or inadvertent decannulation. Children who are receiving noninvasive ventilation must be tolerating well the airway interface (e.g., mask, nasal pillows) and accompanying headgear. A stable oxygenation and ventilatory status is present if the FiO_2 requirement is less than 0.40 and blood gas CO_2 levels are considered appropriate for that child's diagnosis [16]. When a ventilator-dependent child is discharged home for the first time, the same model of ventilator that will be used at home should be used for at least a 1–2 week period before going home. For at least 1 week prior to discharge there should be no changes made in the medical plan of care including no changes in the ventilator settings or supplemental oxygen. Making changes in the medical plan in the week prior to discharge is an important predictor of unplanned readmissions to the hospital within 3 months of discharge [17].

Table 6.2 Pre-discharge criteria for home mechanical ventilation

• Medically stable child
• Secure and stable airway
• Stable oxygenation with FiO_2 requirement at an acceptable level for home use
• Stable ventilatory status with appropriate CO_2 level
• Two supportive and skilled caregivers who have completed training and met competency requirements
• Safe and stable home environment
• Available home equipment and supplies
• Adequate home nursing care
• Adequate funding of home equipment and nursing
• Available community resources
• Provisions for emergency care

Identification and Assessment of Caregivers

Caregivers are fundamental in ensuring the survival and quality of life of their ventilator-dependent child. Most hospital policies require two adult caregivers in the home—a primary caregiver and a secondary caregiver. They must be willing and able to commit to the ongoing training required prior to discharge home and be capable of successfully completing all competency assessments. This commitment to provide complex care must continue into the home. For that reason it is essential to determine the extent of the caregivers' desire to invest their time and energies into the care of their child [2].

Identifying appropriate caregivers for the child is critically important and often fraught with problems. No matter how strong and sincere the commitment to care for the child may be, other factors may become barriers to a successful discharge home. Assessment of the maturity level, emotional stability, and mental status of caregivers is a necessary component of anticipating their ability to provide safe care for their child. How well they understand the child's medical condition, reasons for hospitalization, and expectations for progress may well be indicative of their maturity level and/or cognitive abilities. Problems in accessing transportation may become apparent when caregivers are unable to visit their child while in the hospital. There are also sociocultural and religious practices that may need to be addressed.

Evaluation of Home Environment

Evaluating the family's home is one of the most critical steps in determining if the child can be discharged into the care of their family. It doesn't matter how well equipped and competent the family is in caring for their child or that equipment and nursing staff are available, if the home environment is not safe or accessible for the child, then discharge home is not feasible.

The medical equipment company performs a home safety assessment. Electrical capacity and outlets are inspected to determine if they will support the ventilator and other medical equipment. Outlets must be grounded and have a dedicated circuit for the ventilator and other medical equipment. Functional smoke detectors, carbon monoxide monitors, and fire extinguishers are required. The child's room must have adequate lighting and be large enough to house the respiratory equipment and still allow rapid exit in case of an emergency. The evaluation also includes identification of an area where supplies may be stored as well as an area where reusable equipment can be cleaned and dried. A bathroom connected to the child's room is helpful although not mandatory. Should the company find problems within the home during the initial assessment, the family is responsible for correcting the inadequacies. A follow-up assessment must be performed by the company and if all corrections have been made then the company will proceed with providing equipment and training.

Figure 6.2 is an example of a home safety assessment form that may be used by a home medical equipment company.

The nursing agency also inspects the home for cleanliness and fire safety. Evaluation includes ensuring that there is a crib or bed for the child and a bedside chair and table available for the nurse to use. There must be no infestation of bugs or rodents. Some agencies require a landline phone, even if the family has mobile phone service. Architectural barriers and the home's ability to accommodate large equipment, such as lift systems and hospital beds, must also be considered [2].

HOME MEDICAL EQUIPMENT COMPANY

HOME ASSESSMENT FORM

Patient Name: _____

Home Address: _____

Date of Assessment:_____

Individual Completing Assessment: _____

Wiring – Electrical   **Main Service is _____ amps.**

Home is equipped with circuit breakers. ___ Yes ___ No

Electrical outlets are 3-prong and grounded. ___ Yes ___ No

Heating – Cooling

Source of home heating: _____. Heating source is adequate. ___ Yes ___ No

Source of home cooling: _____. Cooling source is adequate. ___ Yes ___ No

Physical Space   **Patient's room is approximately ___ x ___ ft.**

Room has adequate space for equipment and supplies. ___ Yes ___ No

Accommodations are adequate for cleaning equipment and storing supplies. ___ Yes ___ No

Source of room lighting is ___ lamp(s) _ceiling light. Lighting is adequate. ___ Yes_ No

Communication and Safety

Home has a land-line phone. ___Yes (phone #___ - ___ - _____) ___ No

Home has 9-1-1 service. ___ Yes ___ No

Home has smoke detectors. ___ Yes (number of detectors: ___) No

Home has fire extinguishers. ___ Yes (number of extinguishers: ___)   ___ No

Summary & Recommendations

_____
_____
_____

Fig. 6.2 Home safety assessment form

Children with a tracheostomy and those who require noninvasive mechanical ventilation are very sensitive to all forms of smoke. This includes secondhand tobacco smoke in the house and car as well as on clothing. A ventilator-dependent child's environment must be smoke-free at all times. Caregivers and family members should be encouraged to stop smoking and provided with information on smoking cessation assistance. If they continue to smoke they should be advised to smoke outside of the home and to remove clothing that smells of smoke before they hold or care for their child.

Assessment of Available Financial Resources

Adequate financial resources must be available to provide equipment, supplies, medication, therapies, and nursing care in the home. Healthcare funding coverage (e.g., private insurance, Medicaid) must be verified and it must be determined if there is a limit or if there are alternate payment sources. Alternative coverage is sometimes obtained through state Medicaid waiver programs, state-funded respite programs, or private payment through an agency or charitable organization.

The family's ability to finance healthcare costs after discharge should also be assessed. It is critical that they have the financial resources to maintain the daily cost of living, including food, housing and utilities, and transportation to clinic visits.

Availability of Home Equipment and Nursing Care

Providing appropriate equipment for the home requires selection of a home medical equipment company. The company must be able to provide the required equipment and capable of servicing the geographic area in which the child resides. Qualified staff that are available 24 h per day is essential in providing home equipment for a ventilator-dependent child.

Although there are currently no universal standards stating the required hours per day of nursing care in the home of a ventilator-dependent child, it is understood that it must be in place before a child can be discharged from the hospital. The period immediately following discharge is a difficult transition for most families. It is during this time that 24 h per day skilled home nursing care is recommended to prevent caregiver stress and disruption in the child's care. The additional support provided by skilled nurses is directly related to a better quality of life [20].

Primary Care Provider and Pulmonologist

A primary care provider (PCP) must be identified prior to hospital discharge. This physician must be willing to provide care for a medically complex child who requires chronic mechanical ventilation and be knowledgeable about the child's diagnosis, treatment, and long-term goals. Prior to discharge from the hospital, the

PCP should be informed of the discharge date. The PCP should also receive a detailed summary of the child's hospital course, information about the ventilator and the settings, a list of medications and therapies, the dates and frequency of subspecialty clinic visits, and community services that will be provided [2]. In addition, a child on long-term mechanical ventilation should have an identified Pediatric Pulmonologist or other qualified practitioner skilled in ventilator management and specialized pulmonary care (e.g., Pediatric Critical Care or Anesthesia specialists in some areas). As discussed in detail in Chap. 7, the primary medical home provider should be identified and the respective roles of the primary and all subspecialty providers should be clearly delineated.

Home Medical Equipment and Supplies

Respiratory equipment and supplies for the home are obtained through a home medical equipment company that, in the United States, is certified by the federal agency Centers for Medicare and Medicaid Services (CMS), within the US Department of Health and Human Services. The home medical equipment company may or may not be hospital based. This company is responsible for obtaining a home assessment, delivering and maintaining the equipment and supplies, providing caregiver education on the equipment provided, coordinating preventable maintenance, and replacing equipment as needed. The family should be provided with a list of available equipment providers. Selection of this company is usually through caregiver preference, although this may not always be possible as choices can be limited due to equipment availability, in-network healthcare financing status, and geographic location.

Determining which company to use depends upon several factors. The company must be located within the service area where the child will reside following discharge. It is best to be in-network with the healthcare funding source and it should provide 24 h a day, 7 days a week staffing availability for response to equipment failure or malfunction. If more than one company is available, then the child's caregivers should be given the choice of which company will provide the equipment.

Identification of the equipment provider should be done as soon as possible to reduce the risk of delaying discharge. Since most companies will not agree to provide equipment or caregiver training until an acceptable home evaluation has been obtained, a referral to the company should be made as soon as the need for home mechanical ventilation is determined. Scheduling the home evaluation as early as possible allows more time to make any needed changes to the home, such as providing grounded electrical outlets, adding wheelchair ramps, or widening doors. Early planning also gives the company plenty of time to order equipment and supplies and schedule training sessions for the caregivers [2].

Respiratory therapists or nurses from the home medical equipment company are usually responsible for providing caregivers with instruction sessions regarding care and operation of the ventilator and respiratory equipment provided. This training may occur at the company's office, in the child's home, or at the bedside in the hospital. Sessions should be scheduled in advance of discharge so that caregivers

Table 6.3 Home equipment
and supplies for the
respiratory technology-
dependent child

- Oxygen - portable tank or liquid canister
- Oxygen - stationary concentrator or liquid base unit
- Suction machine - stationary and portable
- Pulse oximeter
- Apnea monitor
- Heated humidifier
- Mechanical ventilator + circuit
- Airway clearance devices
- Air compressor
- Resuscitation bag
- Suction catheters
- Tracheostomy tubes
  Tracheostomy ties
  Tracheostomy care kits
  Trach Go Bag
  Emergency home power generator

have ample opportunity to become familiar with the equipment and become skilled in its use prior to the in-hospital stays and discharge home.

The equipment required varies depending upon the child's individual needs. For each piece of equipment selected for the home it is important to consider its portability and durability, alternative devices for use in case of malfunction, available power sources for travel, and ease of use. Table 6.3 lists medical equipment that may be used in the home. Depending upon the location of the home and the equipment required during the transport home, medical equipment and supplies may be delivered to the hospital, to the home, or to both. A ventilator-dependent child cannot be cared for in the home without the necessary equipment and supplies. Any problem that prevents the child from obtaining the equipment will also prevent the child from being discharged home.

All equipment that will be provided in the home must have a physician order. Orders must include the brand and model of mechanical ventilator and ventilator settings, type of oxygen devices and flow rates, pulse oximetry and/or apnea monitor alarm settings, and airway clearance devices. State Medicaid and insurance providers require proof of medical need for the equipment. This may be provided in the form of letters of medical necessity, sleep studies, lab values, or through documentation in the history and physical, progress notes, and flow sheets within the child's medical record.

Home Nursing

A ventilator-dependent child requires complex and time-consuming care which is usually unfeasible for the family alone to provide. This often results in parents experiencing sleep deprivation, emotional and physical stress, and financial loss [21]. Professional nursing support in the home may improve the health and well-being of caregivers [22]. It gives the caregivers an opportunity to be away from their child, either outside of the home or just a break from being a medical caregiver. Full-time private duty nursing by an LPN or RN provides care with procedures that cannot be legally provided during brief and periodic visits by home health aides. Nursing services are generally funded through insurance or Medicaid and payers must approve coverage before care can begin.

The level of nursing support required varies with each child and family. Parents need time to sleep, work at jobs outside their home, and care for other siblings. A child may initially receive approval from the healthcare funding source for 24 h per day nursing care. However coverage is very likely to decrease to as low as 8–12 h per day after the child has been home for a period of time. Caregivers must also be made aware that there will be times when even though nursing staff is scheduled to be in the home, they will not work because of illness, family issues, an emergency occurs, or they just fail to show up. Contingency plans should be in place for families to follow in case nurses are unavailable [2]. Clinical issues that can affect the support needed include changes in the child's medical condition, the child's ability to breathe spontaneously, the amount of time mechanical ventilation is required per day, frequency and duration of therapies, and nutrition requirements. There are also family and caregiver issues that can impact home nursing need, especially those placing greater demands on a family's time. Examples are loss of the primary or secondary caregiver, siblings with medical conditions, additional children, and changes in job commitments. Other factors that may result in a decrease in nursing coverage are changes in healthcare funding, a lack of available nurses, and the family's inability to cope with the child's needs.

Although nursing care supports the family, it may also intrude on their privacy and cause the family to prefer to have less nursing care or none at all [12]. Parents who work outside the home may choose to have nursing coverage only during the hours that they work or only when they sleep. Nursing professionals must have a high-level of skills in airway management that includes tracheostomy care, ventilator management, troubleshooting alarms, airway clearance therapies, and CPR with tracheostomy emergency protocols [7]. Professional nursing care is for many families a critical factor in the quality of care at home. However, nursing care is not always available. Due to the shortage of skilled pediatric nurses in some communities, it may be difficult to obtain adequate staffing for a patient and result in discharge being delayed. There are also situations in which families report that care has been disrupted by a nursing staff with inadequate levels of skill [23].

Preparing the Caregivers

In most situations constant home nursing care cannot be guaranteed and parents or other adult family members must be responsible for part or all of the day to day medical care [24]. In order for care at home to be effective, it is paramount that the caregivers are dedicated to caring for their child and are available and willing to learn how to provide all medical interventions. They must develop the skills to competently and independently perform routine and emergency tracheostomy tube changes, operate and troubleshoot the ventilator and other equipment, administer medications and feedings, and provide airway clearance therapies. They must also be able to recognize signs and symptoms of respiratory distress and understand the technological supports their child requires. As a result the caregivers must be provided with a structured training program which covers all aspects of the knowledge necessary to provide a safe home environment and allows opportunities for supervised practice and skills to be developed.

Establish Expectations

The burden of caring for a ventilator-dependent child at home is often underestimated. The transition from a parent or family member to the caregiver role is a dynamic process with consequences that impact the entire family [25]. Caregivers must assume a role for which they have little or no experience and which they never expected to take. They may feel shocked and overwhelmed by the uncertainty of assuming all aspects of their child's medical care at home. To work successfully with family members who are designated caregivers, it is important to have a shared understanding of what their role entails and to establish realistic expectations of their level of involvement and the education required. For adult caregivers to achieve educational goals, the goals should be clearly defined [24]. Prior to discharge, in order to better understand the skills and the care required, it may be helpful for them to meet with other caregivers who have a ventilator-dependent child at home.

Caregiver Education

Effective educational programs begin early in the discharge plan and incorporate a variety of progressive learning activities including bedside teaching, computer modules, videos, educational manuals, and simulation models with interactive sessions [26, 27]. Consistent and thorough training is provided by designated nursing staff, therapists, and nutritionists. Allowing caregivers multiple opportunities to observe techniques and actually perform the interventions builds their confidence and competence in caring for their child.

Caregivers should be provided instruction in the technical aspects of operating equipment and alarms, identifying equipment problems, and administration of therapies, medications, and feedings [28]. They should also receive training in emergency preparedness including their response to an obstructed airway, cardiac arrest, weather emergencies, and equipment malfunction [29]. CPR instruction must include resuscitation of a child with a tracheostomy [7]. Using simulation educational models may be the most effective way to train caregivers and to check proficiency in response to emergency scenarios. Caregivers can benefit from a manual that provides information

Table 6.4 Content of manual for caregivers of ventilator-dependent children	• Understanding medical terms
	• Caregiver's role at the hospital
	• Required classes and training sessions
	• Procedures for equipment operation and therapies
	• In-hospital stays
	• Preparing the home
	• Medical equipment in the home
	• Home nursing care
	• Discharge day
	• Clinic visits
	• Preparing for emergencies at home
	• Troubleshooting equipment problems

about caring for their child. The manual may discuss what the caregivers can expect during the discharge process, including caregiver responsibilities and information detailing operating medical equipment as well as steps to take in performing procedures. Table 6.4 lists content that may be helpful to include in a caregiver manual. Table 6.5 lists those educational items that caregivers are typically required to show proficiency in before discharge to home. It may take several weeks of training before caregivers have acquired the skills needed to care for their child at home, with some caregivers progressing through the training at a faster or slower rate than others. Assessment of skills should include return demonstration of medical interventions, successful activity during a simulation, and verbal responses to scenarios. Training is considered complete when caregivers can demonstrate competency in all of the required tasks and correctly respond to verbal or simulated emergency scenarios. Figure 6.3 is an example of a proficiency checklist that may be used to document a caregiver's competency level. An ongoing evaluation of the caregiver training process should be in place to identify opportunities for improvement [24].

Caregiver In-hospital Stays

Before the child is discharged home it is common practice that the caregivers are scheduled to stay overnight in the hospital room with their child where they are responsible for independently providing most if not all of the care [2]. Hospitals have various terms for this in-hospital stay including "family care stay," "family care session," and "rooming-in." During in-hospital stays the caregivers take turns sleeping or leaving the room, with at least one caregiver in the room and awake at all times. Both must be in the room during any procedure that requires two people, such as changing tracheostomy ties or changing a tracheostomy tube. It is important to document any difficulties the caregivers have or unexpected issues that

Table 6.5 Required skills of caregivers of ventilator-dependent children

Demonstrate Proper Operation (as applicable)
• Portable oxygen—tank, liquid canister
• Stationary oxygen—concentrator, liquid base unit
• Pulse oximeter—apply probe, respond to alarms
• Resuscitation bag—demonstrate manual ventilation
• Suction machine—stationary, portable
• Mechanical ventilator—check/change settings, respond to alarms
• Heated humidifier with ventilator
• External ventilator battery and charger
• Heated humidifier with tracheostomy collar
• Air compressor with tracheostomy collar
• Enteral feeding pump
Demonstrate Proper Technique
• Hand washing and infection control
• Bathing
• Mouth care
• Assessing respiratory status
• Changing oxygen flow
• Tracheostomy tube change
• Tracheostomy ties change
• Tracheostomy cleaning
• Suctioning a tracheostomy
• Suctioning using sterile suction technique
• Suctioning using clean suction technique
• Suctioning using a mucus trap
• Response to tracheostomy tube obstruction
• Response to accidental tracheal decannulation
• Chest physiotherapy
• Use of airway clearance devices
• CPR with modification for tracheostomy
• Administering medications
• Providing feedings

arise during the stays. Although hospital policy may require a minimum number of stays, caregivers should be encouraged to continue performing as many aspects of their child's medical care while still in the hospital, even after successfully completing the required minimum in-hospital stays.

Using a Portable Oxygen Tank

Caregiver: _____   **Date:** _____

Nurse/Therapist: _____

	S	U	NP	Comments
Attach Regulator and Set Oxygen Flow				
1. Collect the oxygen tank, regulator, and oxygen tubing				
2. Wash hands				
3. Attach the regulator to the tank				
4. Use wrench to open the tank				
5. Check the pressure gauge				
6. Connect the oxygen tubing				
7. Turn on the oxygen flow				
8. Secure the tank or canister so it does not tip over				
8. Wash hands				

Fig. 6.3 Sample of proficiency check for caregiver of ventilator-dependent children

Disconnect Regulator				
1. Bleed the regulator				
2. Remove the regulator from tank				
3. Wash hands				
S=Satisfactory U=Unsatisfactory NP=Not performed				

Fig. 6.3 (continued)

Some institutions have two levels of family care stay or "rooming in." The initial stay is often scheduled early in the child's hospitalization and may occur before all training has been completed. It usually lasts only 24 h. During this stay, caregivers may be responsible for bathing and feeding their child, administering medications, suctioning and using the resuscitation bag, and providing tracheostomy cleaning care. The purpose of this stay is to focus on the caregivers becoming familiar with their child's needs. They do not have to be functioning independently at this time because the nurses and therapists are still actively helping them learn about their child's care. This initial stay provides an opportunity to see how well the caregivers are coping, if the caregivers are well prepared, or if more training is needed.

The next level of in-hospital family care stay should occur only after successful completion of all required training, including the ventilator, respiratory-related equipment, and feeding pumps. This stay usually lasts 24–48 h, although some caregivers require longer periods. As with the initial stay, caregivers stay together in the room with their child. However during this stay, in addition to the responsibilities covered during the initial stay, they will also check the ventilator settings, respond to all alarms, administer medications and all forms of therapy, and perform tracheostomy tube changes. Nursing staff and therapists should be available as a resource to answer questions but are not expected to assist with the child's care. Unlike the initial in-hospital stay, this is not a time for continued teaching or for competency checks to be completed. The main purpose of this stay is to provide the caregivers with a simulation of being responsible for total care at home without any nursing assistance. Having the caregivers repeat this stay may be necessary if the child's condition changes or if the prior stay reveals that they are not prepared to care for their child alone, in which case additional training should be provided. In some cases it becomes apparent that the caregivers may never be able to safely care for their child alone at home. When this occurs other discharge options must be considered, including medical foster care or alternative sites of care.

Transportation Plan

Prior to discharge, caregivers must be prepared to transport and provide care for their child outside of the home. A safe and predictable means of transportation should be discussed with the caregivers. They should be given a checklist of all the supplies and equipment that are needed for travel and advised to carry a mobile phone with them when their child is outside the home. For oxygen or for devices that require electrical or battery power, caregivers should ensure that they have enough for at least double the expected time they anticipate they will be away.

If traveling in a car, the back seat is the safest place for the child to ride. When the child has a tracheostomy in place or is requiring a mechanical ventilator, one adult must ride in the back seat of the vehicle with the child. The family should be encouraged to make frequent stops if traveling long distances. It may be helpful for the family to apply for a parking permit for handicapped or disabled individuals if they must carry multiple pieces of equipment when they are outside their home. An emergency plan should be developed for the family to use if their child has a medical emergency while traveling and advise the family to keep a copy of this plan inside the car.

Some facilities require the caregivers to take their child in a stroller on a small trip inside or outside the hospital, such as to the cafeteria, gift shop, or garden prior to discharge. It is also helpful for them to load equipment into their family vehicle and properly secure the equipment to prevent it from rolling or hitting other pieces. This helps prepare them for assembling the needed equipment and familiarizes them with the steps necessary to safely transport their child outside the home.

Emergency Plan for Home

Prior to discharge, the family should be given an emergency plan to follow at home. This includes a checklist of all items that should be kept in the "Trach Go Bag" which contains supplies for tracheostomy related emergencies inside and outside of the home. A telephone list that includes the phone numbers of emergency providers, physicians, medical equipment providers, and the home nursing agency should also be provided. Emergency medical services in the child's local community should be notified that a ventilator-dependent child is a resident at that particular address. The local electric company is also notified that the home has a child who requires an electrically powered ventilator. Figure 6.4 is an example of a telephone contact list that could be used in the home of a ventilator-dependent child. Written plans on managing an acute pulmonary exacerbation, an airway obstruction, or cardiac emergency should be established and reviewed prior to discharge.

TELEPHONE CONTACT LIST

COMMUNITY CONTACTS	PHONE NUMBER
Ambulance – Police – Fire	**9-1-1**
Hospital Emergency Department	_____
Electric Company	_____
Gas Company	_____
Water Company	_____
Phone Company	_____
Pharmacy: _____	_____
Home Nursing Agency: _____	_____
Respiratory Equipment Company: _____	_____
Feeds/Enteral Company: _____	_____
Insurance Case Manager: _____	_____

HOSPITAL– CLINIC CONTACTS	PHONE NUMBER
Pediatrician: Dr. _____	_____
Pulmonologist: Dr. _____	_____
Specialist: Dr. _____	_____
Nurse Practitioner: _____	_____
Social Worker: _____	_____
Respiratory Therapist: _____	_____
Speech Therapist: _____	_____
Physical Therapist: _____	_____
Occupational Therapist: _____	_____

Fig. 6.4 Telephone contact list for home

Preparing the Home

In addition to correcting any issues that were found during the home safety assessment and the evaluation by the nursing agency, the healthcare team should assist the family in preparing the home for the child's return. Occasionally there are changes or home modifications to be made that will take several days or weeks to complete, such as building a wheelchair ramp, widening doorways, or providing grounded electrical outlets. In some cases the home environment is so unacceptable that the family must move to another location before their child can be discharged. To prevent delaying the discharge, it is wise to get an early start in preparing the home.

The ventilator-dependent child should have a private room and bed that is not shared with caregivers or siblings. This is necessary so that nursing staff can stay in the room with the child during sleep hours. The room must be large enough to accommodate a crib or bed and all medical equipment. As the equipment generates heat, a small room may become uncomfortably warm. Space must be available around the bed so that respiratory treatments and other therapies can be provided. An area where supplies and medications can be stored must be available, organizing the supplies with those used daily in one area and the monthly supplies in another area can be useful. Rolling carts and cabinets with multiple drawers are helpful in keeping equipment and supplies organized and readily available. Placing labels on the drawers assists nursing staff in finding items and in putting supplies away. Provide an easily reached area near the bed where emergency equipment, such as the Trach Go Bag and the suction machine, can be placed. While in the home, even during the hours of sleep, nurses are expected to stay awake and closely monitor the child. A comfortable chair is needed near the bed for the nurse to use. Designate an area in the home where reusable equipment can be cleaned and dried. This is often in a kitchen or bath where a sink is available.

Preparing for Outpatient Care

When the child is meeting the criteria for discharge from hospital to home the medical team begins working with the family on community integration. According to Boroughs and Dougherty, "Successful discharge of ventilator-dependent children from hospital to home can be traced to a smooth, collaborative effort by a skilled team of physicians, nurses, social workers, therapists, and family members." [30] The same need for coordination of care, advocacy, and communication that the families experience in a hospital setting is equally important in the community.

Child Life Education Specialists

Child life educators use creative play and educational materials about procedures and treatments to help alleviate children's stress and address psychological concerns. They also coordinate events and facilitate interaction between patients and staff. Child life educators work closely with parents and siblings to educate them about the healthcare process. This may be in the form of providing information about surgeries and other medical procedures, leading hospital tours, and assisting with communication between the family and healthcare providers.

Child life educators play a key role in the child's ability to adapt to surroundings outside of the hospital setting. During the hospitalization the child life educator coordinates and assists with taking the child on activities outside of the hospital room. These may include trips to hospital playrooms, outside play areas, and other places within the hospital that are unfamiliar to the child. Including the parents and other family members on these trips is an essential part of preparing them for living at home. These outings allow the child to become familiar with and slowly adjust to unknown environments that may initially feel threatening. Child life educators also strive to help families adjust to taking their child to places outside of the hospital. This can include trips to malls, parks, restaurants, and church. The goal is to provide the family with the necessary tools that allow their child to feel comfortable in normal everyday socialization outside of a hospital setting.

Preparation for School-Based Education

Many ventilator-dependent children will attend school once they are discharged home. Nurses or other caregivers can function as aides to these children while in the school setting. As previously discussed, these children are often discharged home with 24 h coverage of home nursing. Once they reach elementary school age the tendency is for nursing coverage to be reduced significantly. The role of the school nurse becomes vital for the integration of technology-dependent children into the school setting. Meeting their educational needs is a challenge for parents, educators, and the medical team. Prior to discharge it is often helpful to discuss the needs of the child with the school staff, including the teachers and school nurse. In some cases, especially for children with a tracheostomy or enteral feedings, the school personnel should be provided with training that is specific to that child's equipment and needs [2].

The Individuals with Disabilities Education Act (IDEA) ensures educational and related services for students with special needs. However the polices set forth from this act fail to address the entire scope of education and health-related requirements of children who are chronically ill or technology-dependent [31, 32]. School systems rely heavily on guidelines and policy mandates for this patient population. In the absence of guidelines specifically for respiratory technology-dependent children, some schools will not serve their needs appropriately or, even worse, refuse to admit them into the school system [31]. Education placement for these children continues to be highly dependent on the available resources, which are often affected by a child's geographic location and state and federal funding for such programs. Due to the vast number of diagnoses that can result in a child being ventilator-dependent there is little to support what is the best educational placement for these children. There continues to be a small population of ventilator-dependent children who receive home-based services either because they are not of school age or because their disability classification makes it challenging for them to attend public or private schools.

Researchers from the University of Kansas looked at the types of educational placement and services these children received within the school system. The study showed that school-based students spent from 7.5 to 40 h per week in school, while home-based students received 1–20 h per week of educational service, with the average equaling 7.9 h per week. The study also reported that the most important issues affecting placement were academic needs, socialization needs, healthcare needs, psychological/emotional needs, and therapy needs for the child. Educational placement was found to be determined by not any one factor but a multitude of factors that when considered by educators and parents in collaboration can increase the likelihood of years of satisfaction in this student population within the school setting [31]. Many parents feel that some form of school program is essential because it helps normalize the childhood experience.

Outpatient Medical Team and Clinic Visits

Once a ventilator-dependent child is discharged home, the child will require a regular follow-up by the outpatient medical team responsible for their pulmonary care. Children with tracheostomies require follow-up with Otolaryngology and most medically complex, ventilator-dependent children require outpatient follow-up by other specialty services (e.g., Cardiology, Neurology, etc.). The outpatient pulmonary healthcare team may be different from that in the hospital. There may be some individuals in the outpatient setting that were also involved with the transition from the hospital to home. However in most cases the majority of the outpatient staff will be unfamiliar faces to the family and the child. In many hospitals this is the team who the family will contact for questions and concerns once their child is home. Therefore, if possible, it is helpful for the family and child to meet the members of this team prior to discharge home. Models of outpatient care for medically complex children are discussed in detail in Chap. 7.

Prior to discharge family and caregivers should be provided with information concerning their outpatient clinic visits, detailed office-hours and after-hours contact information and clear instructions concerning indications for calling and whom to call for specific issues (e.g., equipment issues, illness, non-respiratory medical questions or illness, etc.). This should include the location of the outpatient clinics, how to prepare for and schedule a clinic visit, and what to expect during the visits. Table 6.6 is a list of what the family may be required to bring to a clinic visit.

Count Down to Discharge Day

Although caregivers may have been anxiously looking forward to the day they can take their child home, they tend to become more anxious the closer it gets to that date. Discharge day can become emotional and quite intense for some families. It is best to arrange discharge for a day that benefits the family and guarantees adequate staffing from the nursing agency and the home medical equipment company.

Table 6.6 Items the ventilator-dependent child brings to clinic visits

• Actual medications or list of medications and dosages
• Name and contact phone numbers for the home equipment company and home nursing agency
• Ventilator, circuit, electrical adaptor, battery (bring even if child only uses at night)
• Trach Go Bag—Containing all disposable supplies required for managing tracheostomy-related emergencies (e.g., extra tracheostomy tube and obturator, a size smaller tracheostomy tube, tracheostomy ties, suction catheters, lubricant)
• Face mask (if using noninvasive ventilation)
• Portable oxygen (if using)
• Portable suction machine
• Extra feeds, diapers, medications (to use if visit takes longer than expected)

Communicate Expectations

Planning a meeting with the caregivers and the multidisciplinary discharge team within 1–2 weeks of discharge is helpful in keeping the family and the healthcare team on schedule. A representative from the home medical equipment company, nursing agency, and school may be invited to the meeting. The purpose of the meeting is to communicate expectations to the caregivers about activities that will take place on the days leading up to discharge as well as what will occur on discharge day. This meeting also provides the caregivers with an opportunity to ask questions and a chance for the entire team to review the plan of care with the family.

Advise the family on what specific pieces of home equipment must be brought to the hospital to use during the transport home. Many hospitals and home medical equipment companies have policies requiring the child to be maintained, prior to hospital discharge, on the actual mechanical ventilator that will be used in the home. This often has a specified time period of 24–72 h prior to discharge. In addition to the ventilator and circuit, the family should be reminded to have a car seat available for the ride home. This is required if the child is transporting home in an ambulance or in the family vehicle. The family should also meet with hospital financial counselors if there are any issues concerning insurance or Medicaid.

Transportation and Arrival Home

Transportation home from the hospital following initiation of chronic mechanical ventilation may be either in an ambulance or in the child's family vehicle. Whichever one is utilized tends to be determined by several factors including hospital policy, insurance or Medicaid reimbursement, proximity of the home and hospital, parental preference, and the child's medical diagnosis. In most situations discharge is planned to occur as early in the day as possible. This allows for more time to transition the child inside the home and for the home medical equipment company and nursing agency staff to attend to the child.

The healthcare staff from the medical equipment company and the nurse should be at the home upon the child's arrival. They should assist the family in moving the child and all equipment into the home.

Barriers to Discharge

In spite of beginning early, having a comprehensive discharge plan in place, and working with a skilled multidisciplinary team, significant delays in discharge from the hospital to home still exist. The most common barriers to discharge revolve around (1) instability in the child's medical condition, (2) the inability of family/caregivers to provide safe care in

Table 6.7 Barriers to discharge of the ventilator-dependent child

Unstable Medical Condition of the Child
• Unstable airway
• Respiratory support needs exceed appropriate levels for home
• Unable to transition to home-type ventilator
Family Barriers
• Inability/unwilling to learn and participate in care
• Failure to complete required training
• Unable to meet requirement of two caregivers
• Unreliable transportation
• Not adhering to medical regimen
• Unstable financial status
• Failure to cooperate with home medical equipment company
• Failure to cooperate with home nursing agency
Equipment Barriers
• Inadequate funding for equipment
• Unavailable equipment
• Unsafe home environment
• Lack of equipment providers that accept ventilator-dependent children
Home Nursing Barriers
• Insufficient nursing staff
• Unqualified nursing staff
• Incomplete or delayed funding
• Unsuitable home environment

the home, (3) unqualified or insufficient home nursing staff, (4) incomplete or delayed funding of home care, (5) an unsuitable home environment, and (6) lack of or delays in obtaining home medical equipment [4]. Early identification of the barriers and open communication between the family and the medical team are the best ways to minimize the risk of a discharge being delayed. Table 6.7 lists barriers to discharge [33].

Future Needs

Transitioning a ventilator-dependent child from the hospital to home requires a complex, coordinated interaction of multiple care and equipment providers, both inside and outside of the hospital, and there are numerous opportunities for pitfalls and delays. The key components to a smooth and successful transition may well be to employ a multidisciplinary team approach and begin the process as early as possible. It is also important to consider the medical and social needs of the child and caregivers and to check often for their understanding of the discharge plans. Allow caregivers and the child as much self-determination as possible in planning for care and needs. Ensuring that the home and community services are adequate following discharge is also an essential component to maintaining safe and competent care at home.

As we continue to have more children discharged home dependent on long-term mechanical ventilation, additional clinical research is needed to better understand the needs of this diverse patient population. There is currently little research examining patterns of discharge planning for specific clinical subgroups [34]. Also needed are recognized standards of practice in the discharge process and a better understanding of reimbursement and coverage [13]. This includes standardized criteria for caregiver competence and how to best demonstrate accomplished skills [2]. Further research is also needed to develop and implement pre-discharge interventions that will promote the physical and mental well-being of caregivers. Additional research topics may include the impact of involving the home nursing staff in the child's care prior to discharge—whether this would affect the high turnover rate among skilled home pediatric nurses—and the use of simulation educational modules for caregiver and home nursing staff.

References

1. Simon TD, Berry J, Feudtner C, et al. Children with complex chronic conditions in inpatient hospital settings in the United States. Pediatrics. 2010;126:647–55.
2. Elias ER, Murphy NA, Council on Children with Disabilities. From the American Academy of Pediatrics Clinical Report: home care of children and youth with complex health care needs and technology dependencies. Pediatrics. 2012;129:996–1005.
3. Hammer J. Home mechanical ventilation in children: indications and practical aspects. Schweiz Med Wochenschr. 2000;130:1894–902.
4. Dumas HM. Rehabilitation considerations for children dependent on long-term mechanical ventilation. ISRN Rehabilitation. 2012;2012:756103.
5. Kohorst J. Transitioning the ventilator-dependent patient from the hospital to home. Medscape. 2005.

6. Hefner JL, Tsai WC. Ventilator-dependent children and the health services system. Unmet needs and coordination of care. Ann Am Thorac Soc. 2013;10:482–9.
7. Boroughs DS, Dougherty JA. Decreasing accidental mortality of ventilator-dependent children at home: a call to action. Home Healthc Nurse. 2012;30:103–11.
8. Sherman JM, Davis S, Albamonte-Petrick S, et al. Care of the child with a chronic tracheostomy. This official statement of the American Thoracic Society was adopted by the ATS Board of Directors, July 1999. Am J Respir Crit Care Med. 2000;161(1):297–308.
9. Cousino MK, Hazen RA. Parenting stress among caregivers of children with chronic illness: a systematic review. J Pediatr Psychol. 2013;38:809–28.
10. Capen CL, Dedlow ER. Discharging ventilator-dependent children: a continuing challenge. J Pediatr Nurs. 1998;3:175–84.
11. Heaton J, Noyes J, Sloper P, et al. Families' experiences of caring for technology-dependent children: a temporal perspective. Health Soc Care Community. 2005;13:441–50.
12. Aday LA, Wegener DH. Home care for ventilator-assisted children: implications for the children, their families, and health policy. Child Health Care. 1988;17:112–20.
13. Lewarski BS, Gay P. Current issues in home mechanical ventilation. Chest. 2007;132:671–6.
14. Kuo DZ, Houtrow AJ, Arango P, et al. Family-centered care: current applications and future directions in pediatric health care. Matern Child Health J. 2012;16(2):297–305.
15. Tamasitis J, Shesser L. A hospital-to-home program for ventilator-dependent children sets the standard of care. AARC Times. 2012;33(6):44–52.
16. American Thoracic Society Document. Statement on home care for patients with respiratory disorders. Am J Respir Crit Care Med. 2005;171:1443–74.
17. Kun SS, Edwards JD, Ward SLD, Keens TG. Hospital readmissions for newly discharged pediatric home mechanical ventilation patients. Pediatr Pulmonol. 2012;47(4):409–14.
18. Gershon RRM, Pogorselska M, Qureshi KA, et al. Home health care patients and safety hazards in the home: preliminary findings. In: Henrcksen K, Battles JB, Keyes MA, Grady ML, editors. Advances in patient safety: new directions and alternative approaches, assessment. 1st ed. Rockville, MD: Agency for Health Care Research and Quality; 2008. AHRQ Publication No. 08-0034-1.
19. Markkanen P, Quinn M, Galligan C, et al. There's no place like home: a qualitative study of the working conditions of home health care providers. J Occup Environ Med. 2007;49:327–37.
20. Abresch RT, Seyden NK, Wineinger MA. Quality of life. Issues for persons with neuromuscular diseases. Phys Med Rehabil Clin N Am. 1998;9:233–48.
21. Carnevale FA, Alexander E, Davis M, et al. Daily living with distress and enrichment: the moral experience of families with ventilator-assisted children at home. Pediatrics. 2006;117:e48–60.
22. Meltzer LJ, Boroughs DS, Downes JJ. The relationship between home nursing coverage, sleep, and day-time functioning in parents of ventilator-assisted children. J Pediatr Nurs. 2010;25:250–7.
23. Reeves E, Timmons S, Dampier S. Parents' experiences of negotiating care for their technology-dependent child. J Child Health Care. 2006;10:228–39.
24. Tearl DK, Hertzog JH. Home discharge of technology-dependent children: evaluation of a respiratory therapist driven family education program. Respir Care. 2007;52:171–6.
25. Huang TT, Peng JM. Role adaptation of family caregivers for ventilator-dependent patients: transition from respiratory care ward to home. J Clin Nurs. 2010;19:1686–94.
26. Bakewell-Sachs S, Porth S. Discharge planning and home care of the technology-dependent infant. J Obstet Gynecol Neonatal Nurs. 1995;24:77–83. doi:10.1111/j.1552-6909.1995.tb02382.x.
27. Hill DS. Coordinating a multidisciplinary discharge for the technology-dependent child based on parental needs. Issues Compr Pediatr Nurs. 1993;16:229–37.
28. Simonds AK. Risk management of the home ventilator dependent patient. Thorax. 2006;61:369–71.
29. Graf JM, Montagnino BA, Hueckel R, McPherson ML. Children with new tracheostomies: planning for education and common impediments to discharge. Pediatr Pulmonol. 2008;43:788–94.
30. Boroughs DS, Dougherty J. A multidisciplinary approach to the care of the ventilator-dependent child at home. A case study. Home Healthc Nurse. 2010;28:24–8.

31. Jones DE, Clatterbuck C, Marquis JG, et al. Educational placements for children who are ventilator assisted. Except Child. 1996;63:47–57.
32. Walker DK, Jacobs FH. Chronically ill children in school. Peabody J Educ. 1984;61:28–74.
33. Noyes J. Barriers that delay children and young people who are dependent on mechanical ventilators from being discharged from hospital. J Clin Nurs. 2002;11:2–11.
34. Benneyworth BD, Gebremariam A, Clark SJ, et al. Inpatient health care utilization for children dependent on long-term mechanical ventilation. Pediatrics. 2011;27:e1533–41.

Chapter 7
The Model of Care for the Ventilator-Dependent Child

Dennis Z. Kuo and John L. Carroll

Chapter Objectives

- Learn the importance of the Medical Home and family-centered care for the ventilator-dependent child
- Learn how to best coordinate care between tertiary and primary care settings

Sean is a five-month-old child who was born at 25 weeks gestation. Due to surfactant deficiency and tracheomalacia, he received a tracheostomy and receives 24/7 ventilation. He is also dependent on a gastrostomy tube for feedings. He has 16 h of nursing and lives 75 miles from the children's hospital where long-term ventilator support was initiated. The second night Sean is home, he vomits his gastrostomy tube feeds. The third night home his parents notice that Sean needed to be suctioned every 2 h and his oxygen needs rose from 0.5 to 2 L. They turn the oxygen up because they don't want to bother anyone. The oxygen saturation monitor alarms every 30 min. The next day his mother goes to work, concerned that she is going to lose her job because of the time off. She takes the car. Home nursing arrives, but Sean has developed a low-grade fever and they seem to be running out of suction catheters. His father calls the primary care doctor, a friend they've known for 4 years because of Sean's older sister. The doctor has never seen Sean and hasn't received the discharge summary yet, and suggests calling the pulmonologist instead. Meanwhile, Sean's oxygen saturations are now 91 %. His father calls 911.

D.Z. Kuo, M.D., M.H.S.
Center for Applied Research and Evaluation, Arkansas Children's Hospital, 1 Children's Way, Little Rock, AR 72202, USA

J.L. Carroll, M.D. (✉)
Division of Pediatric Pulmonary and Sleep Medicine, University of Arkansas for Medical Sciences, Little Rock, AR, USA
e-mail: CarrollJohnL@uams.edu

© Springer Science+Business Media New York 2016
L.M. Sterni, J.L. Carroll (eds.), *Caring for the Ventilator Dependent Child*,
Respiratory Medicine, DOI 10.1007/978-1-4939-3749-3_7

Why Is This Chapter Important?

Sean's first medical crisis at home appears to require early involvement of a pulmonary care specialist to prevent being rehospitalized. Could his vomiting have caused aspiration pneumonia? Whose responsibility is it to monitor changes in his symptoms, change his formula, or titrate his enterally administered medications? Might his medical event be avoided if his feeds were run continuously or if his feeds were run more slowly through a feeding pump? Finally, could Sean's impending hospitalization been prevented had the parents reached a pulmonologist the night before?

This chapter discusses how to ensure that the ventilator-dependent child effectively receives the best possible healthcare while residing in the home setting. Medical technology has allowed increasing numbers of children with ventilator dependence to reside at home, achieving what was unthinkable even just a few years ago. There is little doubt that, all else being equal, that home is the best place for the ventilator-dependent child and the family. However, the home setting is full of unpredictable challenges, not the least of which is the ability of the family to manage what can accurately be referred to, in Sean's case, as continuous life support!

The number of children who are discharged to home while on long-term ventilator support is increasing [1], along with the indications for initiating home ventilation. Indications for home ventilator dependence include primary lung disease, chest wall disorders, muscle weakness, respiratory control disorders, or a combination of the above. Many such children also have accompanying non-pulmonary medical disorders. Some of these disorders may impact the overall health and functioning of the child, such as seizure disorders and severe neurologic impairment; feeding intolerance; and cardiac disorders. The prognosis of the ventilator dependence thus depends not only on the underlying respiratory system disease, but also the severity of the accompanying medical concerns. Some children improve and are able to discontinue use of the ventilator in a short period of time; others with degenerative disorders continue to worsen. Many children are in between the two extremes.

Regardless, all ventilator-dependent children share some of the highest levels of medical fragility, requiring a very high learning curve by families for home management. These family caregivers assume a tremendous caregiving burden, due to the time, technical expertise, and financial commitment needed to care for a ventilator-dependent child [2, 3]. The caregiving burden often comes at the expense of their personal health, employment, and family time, and ultimately can impact the ability of the best-laid care plans to be effectively carried out.

Ventilator-dependent children at home require a potentially mind-boggling array of services and surveillance in order to grow and thrive happily. The pulmonologist or intensivist is responsible for the initiation of the ventilator assistance, and the role of the pulmonary care specialist certainly is crucial to the long-term health and survival of the child. The pulmonary team will develop deep and longstanding relationships with the family because of the frequency and intensity of the required services. However, a typical ventilator-dependent child will require caregiving services from his parents, siblings, neighbors and friends; primary care physician, nurses, respiratory therapists, medical equipment companies, pharmacists, social worker, and other specialists; a tertiary care facility and a place to receive acute care; teachers and therapists; transportation; legal and financial support; adequate insurance; and community services. **Individually, all these services are important, but within the context of a child's life, each individual service is just one player out of many.** All of these services must work competently and in coordination with each other for a child and family to reach their maximum potential. The experience of all of these services with a ventilator-dependent child may vary considerably.

Practically speaking, the family must learn how to be proactive and recognize problems before they happen or get worse; they must know who to call, when to call, where to call, how to call, and understand the instructions they are provided. Similarly, all services that participate in caring for a ventilator-dependent child must be comfortable and competent with a high level of medical fragility.

How do we put all of these care components together so families know what they need to do in a situation like Sean's?

Introduction to Care Models for Ventilator-Dependent Children

Home ventilation is a relatively recent development. However, care models for children with disabilities and special healthcare needs have been evolving over the last 50 years. The experience and lessons learned from these care models can be applied to ventilator-dependent children.

In 1998, the Maternal and Child Health Bureau, Health Resources and Services Administration, defined children and youth with special healthcare needs (CYSHCN) as:

Children with special healthcare needs are those who have or are at increased risk for a chronic physical, developmental, behavioral, or emotional condition and who also require health and related services of a type or amount beyond that required by children generally [4].

This definition of CYSHCN is thus **not** dependent on any particular diagnosis. Rather, the definition spans a spectrum of diagnoses and disabilities, from asthma to spina bifida to autism and undiagnosed conditions. Ventilator-dependent children are at the extreme end of service need and intensity. However, models of care developed for CYSHCN can—and should—be applied to ventilator-dependent children.

In the past, many CYSHCN lived in institutional settings. Deinstitutionalization of children with disabilities through the 1950s and 1960s led to families advocating for greater support services at home. Family advocacy led to a number of legislative victories, attention from the Surgeon General's office, and national recognition in 1987 for a "family-centered, community-based system of care." [5] Since then, the need for a family-centered, community-based, system of care for children with disabilities and special healthcare needs has been affirmed as a national priority, as evidenced by *Healthy People 2010* and *2020* and the Department of Health and Human Services. This has led to legislation, funding, and initiatives earmarked for family support groups, electronic medical records, education, payment reform, and other supportive initiatives. Families of children with special healthcare needs, however, report that the care system continues to be fragmented and is difficult to navigate [6, 7].

The medical care of the ventilator-dependent child is initiated within the tertiary care center. After discharge, the pulmonary team is essential for home management but must be integrated smoothly with other support services to achieve effective care delivery. It is essential that healthcare providers who care for the ventilator-dependent child understand the historical context, current understanding, and future directions on the optimal care model for the child with disabilities and special healthcare needs. **No one model of care is optimal for all situations**, but the theoretical framework is the same. Executing the model of care depends greatly on the family involvement, knowledge of the providers involved, and communication among each other in a co-management model of care.

The pulmonary team is in a particularly influential position to partner with the family to navigate the healthcare system. Initially, the pulmonary team will work closely with families to teach and support home medical management of life-supporting technology. The pulmonary team is also in a position to learn about the psychosocial challenges families face and counsel about available services, including services that are outside the scope of care for the pulmonary team. It is important that the pulmonary team is aware of the care components of the ideal care model that families will need, and how to implement this care model. *In many cases, an ideal integrated care service model may not locally exist,* leaving the pulmonary team to coordinate the multiple components of care.

The Medical Home for the Ventilator-Dependent Child

Macy is a two-year-old child with spinal muscular atrophy and is ventilator-dependent. She presents for her routine pulmonary follow-up and her mother says all is well and her shots are up to date. The alert pulmonary fellow pulls her vaccine records from the state registry and discovered she never received any of her one year vaccines, even though she has received influenza vaccines at the pulmonary clinic. Her mother appears bewildered and says she cannot remember the last time she saw her primary care physician because she has so many visits to the children's hospital. You further discover that her ranitidine dose hasn't been adjusted for weight since she was six months old. Macy's mother admits that she has trouble making appointments because she works and she has two older children, and she has no other support.

Macy's care has fallen through the cracks, so to speak. Who was responsible for making sure that Macy received her immunizations? What about adjusting her ranitidine dose? Did anyone screen Macy's mother for financial needs? What about maternal depression?

The most well-known of comprehensive care models for CYSHCN is the Medical Home. The Medical Home care concept was first mentioned in 1967 by the American Academy of Pediatrics (AAP) as a central place for medical records for children with special healthcare needs and disabilities [8]. The subsequent two decades found a number of community-based initiatives dedicated to improving the medical care delivery for CYSHCN, generally wrapped around the primary care-based Medical Home. This led to development and refinement of the Medical Home concept towards applying to all children. By 1992, the AAP declared that the Medical Home should be the standard of care for all children and that all children should have a medical home.

Today, the Medical Home is defined by the AAP as a concept of care delivery, rather than an actual locus of care or a building or specific provider. The Medical Home describes care that is: [9]

- Accessible
- Comprehensive
- Compassionate
- Continuous
- Coordinated
- Culturally Competent
- Family-Centered

It is critical to emphasize that the Medical Home concept, as originally envisioned by the AAP, is not synonymous with the primary care setting. The AAP does not specifically state that the Medical Home should be located in the primary care setting, nor is the care concept localized to one specific setting. **Rather, the Medical Home is the concept of care delivery that encompasses all medical care sites.** However, the AAP states that the Medical Home "should be delivered or directed by well-trained physicians who provide primary care and help to manage and facilitate essentially all aspects of pediatric care." [9] The statement directly implies that the continuity, relationships, and community that the primary care setting provides are essential to providing the Medical Home. Thus, the Medical Home MUST have a strong primary care involvement.

The specific steps necessary to provide care consistent with the Medical Home are not always consistently defined and may likely vary between practices and settings. The AAP concept of the Medical Home also leaves the question open as to whether a specialty service can be responsible for directing the Medical Home for a particular child, although the AAP definition does emphasize that the primary care physician must be involved at some level. The Medical Home Index (MHI) [10–12] is an example of a tool designed for practices to assess their level of delivering Medical Home services consistent with the AAP concept. Practices that had higher MHI scores demonstrated lower emergency department use [10]. In addition, a review by Homer [13] found broad applicability of the Medical Home concept associated with improved child and family outcomes specifically for children with special healthcare needs [13]. Many studies to date have been tempered by weak designs and inconsistent conceptualizations of the Medical Home.

Nonetheless, the Medical Home concept—sometimes referred to as the Patient-Centered Medical Home—has found its way into national and legislative priorities, and subsequently tied to healthcare reform activities. *Healthy People 2020 Objective MICH-30.2* is to "increase the proportion of children with special healthcare needs who have access to a medical home." [14] The Joint Principles of the Patient-Centered Medical Home, published in 2007 and signed by multiple medical societies, acknowledged the importance of the Medical Home for adults for the first time [15]. However, the Joint Principles specifically state that the PCMH is an approach to providing "comprehensive primary care," and while it does not specify where the primary care should be located, the stipulation is clear about the director role of the primary care physician. From here, further discussion about the Medical Home has focused on the role of the primary care physician, including in the 2009 Affordable Care Act legislation, primary care practice transformation efforts by groups such as TransforMED, and standards for operationalizing the National Committee for Quality Assurance (NCQA), with implications for tying higher Medical Home assessment scores to payments for primary care services.

Given the importance of the Medical Home to the national dialogue on healthcare reform, research, and legislation, **it is clear that primary care services should be active participants within all care models for children and adults alike**. For the ventilator-dependent child, however, the medical and technical expertise of the pulmonologist is crucial to the health and well-being of the child. Implementing a Medical Home thus leads to these specific questions:

- What services should the primary care setting provide for the ventilator-dependent child?
- What services should the pulmonologist provide for the ventilator-dependent child?
- Who is responsible for ensuring that the primary care setting is capable and willing to provide appropriate services for the ventilator-dependent child?
- Who is responsible for ensuring that the Medical Home model of care is provided for the ventilator-dependent child?

The Medical Home specific to the ventilator-dependent child must be able to deliver:

- Community-based primary care
- Specialty care and close involvement by the pulmonologist
- Technical support for tracheostomy and ventilator
- 24/7 access to care
- A central provider that is responsible for comprehensively assessing and managing all aspects of the child's care

Finally, it is important to remember that children are not "little adults." Stille [16] and the Academic Pediatric Association (APA) delineated five specific characteristics on how the pediatric Medical Home need to be considered in a different light from adult Medical Homes [16]. The five "D" characteristics are:

- Developmental Change—children grow, develop, and require habilitation, not *re*habilitation
- Dependency—children are dependent on adults, and thus parents are essential partners in ensuring care delivery
- Differential Epidemiology—children have a relatively large number of rare chronic conditions, thus no "one size fits all"; moreover, pediatric subspecialists tend to be located in academic medical centers, which may be far from where the child lives.
- Demographic Patterns—children have disproportionate rates of poverty and have disproportionate racial and ethnic diversity
- Dollars—overall costs of child healthcare are low but frequently have a long-term investment over a life course

Specific to ventilator-dependent children, the 5 "Ds" are a reminder that the medical needs of children vary over the life course of the child; parents are essential partners; and the pulmonary team, critical for effective care delivery, may be located far away from the residence of the child. Even if the pulmonary team is located near the residence of the child, the team members may not be familiar with the numerous community support services that the family engages with. In that scenario, the community-based primary care physician may be more familiar with such services. These issues are highly relevant when considering how to effectively deliver healthcare for the ventilator-dependent child at home.

How the System of Healthcare Appears to the Ventilator-Dependent Child

Josiah is eight years old and ventilator-dependent due to thoracic dystrophy. He is home schooled and acting out because of his frustrations with difficulty communicating. His mother wants to know if there is a way to help him because she believes "he's much smarter than people think." He gets speech therapy but his mother says that they have only been working on his oral motor skills.

Clinical experience and emerging literature documents what families of ventilator-dependent children have long known: the health and welfare of the child depends highly on the quality of pulmonary care, primary care, and the community-based services that reach far beyond the medical home setting. In fact, the Medical Home is only one key component of the system of services that are needed to

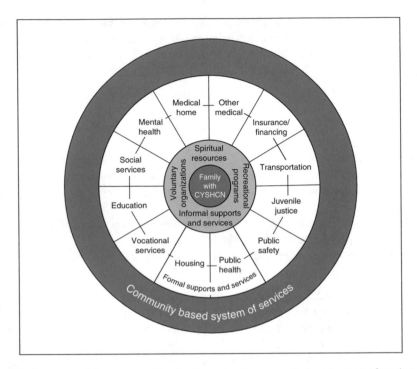

Fig. 7.1 A conceptual framework of the family-centered, community-based system of services for children and youth with special healthcare needs. Reproduced with permission from Archives of Pediatrics & Adolescent Medicine. 2007. 161(10):933-936. Copyright© 2007 American Medical Association. All rights reserved

support the health and welfare of a child. Wagner's Chronic Care Model, for example, demonstrates that the Medical Home must exist within the context of a supportive community of services and healthcare policies.

Figure 7.1 provided a conceptual framework of the "family-centered, community-based system of services" for CYSHCN generally [17]. The center of the framework is the family with CYSHCN, surrounded by informal supports and services. Beyond that informal network of support services are the formal support services, which includes the Medical Home—but also includes social services, education, vocational services, housing, transportation, and insurance/financing, to name a few.

No framework of care has been derived directly for the ventilator-dependent child up to this point. However, a framework developed by Cohen [18, 19] of the child with medical complexity is instructive in understanding the care needs of the ventilator-dependent child (Fig. 7.2) [18]. The Cohen framework defines medical complexity as the presence of the following four domains of need:

- Chronic conditions
- Healthcare use
- High level of family-identified needs
- Functional limitations: technology dependence

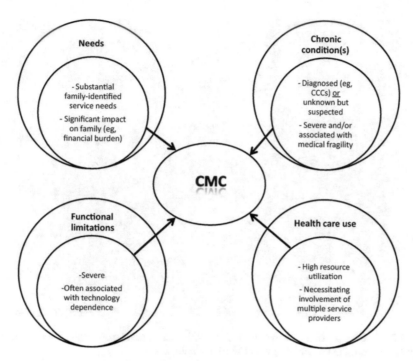

Fig. 7.2 A framework of medical complexity. Reproduced with permission from *Pediatrics,* Vol. 127(3), Pages 529-538. Copyright © 2011 by the AAP

The framework applies well to the ventilator-dependent child, who will have a chronic condition with technology dependence and high healthcare use. If anything, the ventilator-dependent child epitomizes medical complexity due to the fragility of having airway complications and a risk of sudden death. The ventilator-dependent child has home nursing needs, high equipment needs, the need (often) for 24/7 monitoring, and in some cases, the stigma of needing equipment that may limit the child's ability to enjoy a normal routine. All of these medical needs typically drives a high level of family-identified needs, and the longer the duration of ventilation, the greater the needs [2].

However, it is family-identified needs—whether financial, psychosocial, transportation—that rounds out the level of medical complexity. "Care mapping" is a process in which families provide a diagram of all of the services that a child with special healthcare needs. Figure 7.3 shows one example of the care map of a child with special needs. A child's care map provides the most complete illustration of the level of healthcare utilization and family challenges.

The extreme level of family need—medical, financial, psychosocial—demands the highest level of comprehensive care that successfully integrates all services that the child may need. Primary care practices, by themselves, are typically not set up to be able to provide the necessary level of comprehensive care services for the ventilator-dependent child. We have already discussed how tertiary care centers may not always provide Medical Home level services, as the scope of practice of the

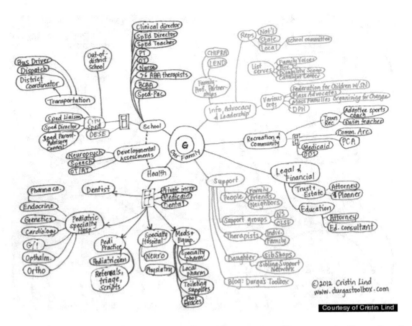

Fig. 7.3 An example of a care map for a child with special healthcare needs. Reproduced with permission from Cristin Lind. Copyright © 2012 Cristin Lind

individual specialty service is narrowly drawn. The pulmonologist, with rare exception, is not delivering well child care or anticipatory guidance consistent with primary care services, and many are not able to identify and coordinate the community-level services needed for the care of the ventilator-dependent child. *Who is thus responsible for ensuring that the ventilator-dependent child receives the comprehensive care that he or she needs?*

Unfortunately, the family frequently becomes the responsible entity by default. Many families are not well-prepared to handle every aspect of the child's care, due to the myriad needs, stresses, and financial burden [7, 20]. It is also important to recognize that the nature of family support typically changes over time, from informal supports during infancy to increasing levels of formal support by school age [21]. The family also experiences "chronic sorrow" due to the perceived loss of a healthy child, which may lead to outright depression of the parent caregiver [22]. Nevertheless, the family is ultimately responsible for the effective delivery of healthcare. It becomes paramount, therefore, for providers to understand how to meet the needs of families when considering how to deliver effective healthcare. Meeting the needs of family, and providing family-centered care, is the key link to being able to translate medical recommendations into effective care.

Ensuring Family-Centered Care for the Ventilator-Dependent Child

Gladys is a 3-year-old child who is dependent on a ventilator due to severe broncho-pulmonary dysplasia. Her parents speak little English and sometimes arrive with their own interpreter, but sometimes they do not. She has missed multiple appointments and has had difficulty growing. There has been suspicion that she is not getting her feedings and that her mother has been feeding her by mouth against medical advice. You obtain a trained Spanish interpreter and cultural broker and her mother is able to tell you that Gladys vomits her formula regularly and pulls out her gastrostomy tube, but the doctors keep increasing the amount of formula because she does not grow. In addition, she has not had a good swallowing evaluation and her mother thinks she is ready to eat more by mouth.

For Gladys, the pulmonary management has been compromised by a number of issues that the family readily identifies. Centering the care approach on the family-needs is the essence of family-centered care (FCC). Although frequently misunderstood, FCC is increasingly recognized as key to providing effective care for the ventilator-dependent child. It is important to understand the principles of FCC in order to ensure family-centered care for the ventilator-dependent child.

FCC has been described, at its core, as a partnership approach to healthcare decision-making. In recent years, FCC—and a related term, patient-centered care—has received increasing attention as not only the standard of care for all persons but also crucial to patient health, satisfaction, and healthcare quality. Kuo et al. [23] examined and compiled general principles of FCC in the literature, which includes: [23]

- Information sharing
- Respecting and honoring differences
- Partnership and collaboration
- Negotiation
- Care in context of family and community

Like the Medical Home concept, the FCC principles were developed through consensus, but do not necessarily translate into specific clinical practices. Kuhlthau [24] reviewed practices that were consistent with FCC principles as related to care of the child with special needs, finding improvement on health literacy and self-management; other reviews similarly suggest improved child health and behaviors [24]. Empowered families are considered *essential* to delivering chronic care; family knowledge and empowerment are suggested as the mediating factors towards improved health outcomes [25] and the key mediating outcomes in Wagner's Chronic Care Model [26].

FCC is especially important for effectively caring for the ventilator-dependent child because of the enhanced caregiving role that parents must play for the child. The caregiving role is 24/7. The airway and the life-supporting ventilation must be managed by the family and the risks of a tracheostomy and the technology dependence are assumed by the family. There are always sets of physician and nursing instructions that need to be understood, accepted, and implemented by the family. With everything to manage, undoubtedly every family will encounter a stage where they may not comprehend medical advice, prioritize other needs, or simply disagree with the recommendations. Sometimes this family is labeled a "bad" or "noncompliant" family. We urge avoiding such labels.

With medical fragility depending so heavily on family home care management, it is critical to create any care plan through meeting the family's caregiving needs and working in partnership with family. The FCC approach would not inherently judge the family as "noncompliant." Rather, the FCC approach emphasizes a *partnership* approach to healthcare. The very term "partnership" emphasizes that the family and provider bring their mutual strengths to decision-making. This is a frequently misunderstood concept! A common misconception is that FCC means families make the final decision. Rather, respecting mutual strength acknowledges that the physician has the medical expertise while acknowledging that the family usually knows the home situation, the child's behavior, the caregivers' abilities and the caregiving needs better. These factors all need to be taken into account when jointly making a care plan. There are very few medical care plans that should be made unilaterally. In Gladys's case, unilateral recommendations for feeding did not consider the impact on the family. As a consequence, Gladys was not able to receive the total volume. A negotiated plan for feeding frequency could have improved the outcome.

Ensuring FCC for the ventilator-dependent child is achieved through everyday actions, not by implementing a specific intervention or tool. For example, "person-first" language and respectfully discussing the family's needs among team members is critical. This approach is particularly crucial for the leader of the medical team, as the leader sets the tone for the remainder of the team. Examples include respectful language, joint consideration of care plans, family presence during procedures when feasible, and integration of families at all levels of care between bedside, institution and community. Care teams should involve family input, potentially in a formal advisory capacity, and leadership should actively support the involvement of families at an administrative level. Physicians and families frequently have differing understanding of the needs of the child [27], thus ensuring FCC is critical to proper assessment, consideration, and addressing of family-needs that ensures good care.

National Priorities: The Maternal and Child Health Bureau Six Core Outcomes for CYSHCN

As previously noted, families of children with disabilities and special healthcare needs report that fragmentation of care and healthcare system navigation are the biggest challenges to implementing effective healthcare delivery. It is reasonable to assume that the families of ventilator-dependent children are similar in their needs. Families actually report that the direct medical care can actually be one of the *easier* aspects of caregiving for the child with special healthcare needs [21]. The system navigation is the toughest aspect to meet. **The pulmonologist needs to recognize that meeting the needs of families of ventilator-dependent children MUST address the system navigation and care fragmentation issues.**

National oversight for implementation of a broad system of care is under the jurisdiction of the Maternal and Child Health Bureau (MCHB), Health Resources and Services Administration, Department of Health and Human Services. MCHB is the federal-level agency responsible for maternal and child health programming, and funds are authorized through Title V of the Social Security Act of 1935.

Since 1989, the Maternal and Child Health Bureau (MCHB) has been authorized through the Omnibus Budget Reconciliation Act (P.L. 101-239) to address the core elements of community-based systems of care for CYSHCN. In response, state Title V CYSHCN groups work with family advocates, providers, and other partners to implement six Core Outcomes of a system of services based on evidence-based practices for CYSHCN. The six MCHB Core Outcomes, developed through family and professional consensus, are: [28]

- Family–professional partnerships at all levels of decision-making
- Access to coordinated, ongoing, comprehensive care within a medical home
- Adequate private and/or public insurance to pay for needed services
- Early and continuous screening for special healthcare needs
- Organization of community-based service systems for easy use
- Youth transition to adult healthcare, work, and independence.

States report on meeting the MCHB Core Outcomes through the National Survey of Children with Special Healthcare Needs. As such, the Core Outcomes reflect a general synopsis of how well the system of care is operating broadly for children with special healthcare needs. State Title V agencies are also responsible for a broad array of services and infrastructure designed to support healthcare access for children with special healthcare needs. In addition, many Title V agencies have worked closely with provider and community partners to ensure access to comprehensive services, funded through the Title V Block Grants. Ventilator-dependent children can take advantage of such supportive services, which vary by state, and pulmonologists can work with Title V agencies to be aware of the available services.

Overall, families continue to report widespread deficiencies in having their needs met. The 2009–2010 National Survey of Children with Special Healthcare Needs is the latest in a series of national telephone surveys that examine how well states are meeting the Core Outcomes. The results of the survey found that only 17.6 % of CYSHCN are served by healthcare systems that met all age-relevant Core Outcomes. Data specifically on ventilator-dependent children are not found in the National Survey, but children with medical complexity have worse findings on the National Survey [29].

The findings of the National Survey simply reflect the ongoing stress that families endure and the inability of the healthcare system to meet their needs that continues despite over 25 years of state- and national-level programs, funding, and initiatives designed to integrate systems. More recently, the Affordable Care Act has encouraged states and systems, particularly through the Center for Medicare & Medicaid

Innovation, to design novel healthcare delivery systems as well as the payment structure that supports the integrated care that ventilator-dependent children require. Examples of payment reform may include accountable care organizations, integrated healthcare systems, paying for care coordination through a continued fee-for-service structure, and integrating support services through Health Homes. State Title V agencies and the MCHB have some oversight of developing comprehensive systems of services for ventilator-dependent children.

As changes in healthcare payment reform continue to develop, it will be up to the individual healthcare providers to implement changes in their own practices that take advantage of payment incentives and system changes. For example, increased payments for care coordination would enable a provider office to hire additional care coordinators who would be responsible for ensuring that families are connected to the services that they require—specialty care, medications, and therapies—ideally in a proactive manner. It is important to realize that many of these reforms may be directed towards the primary care setting or separate community-based or state agencies under Health Home activities, which, in essence, defaults to the pulmonologist in a supportive role when it comes to managing the ventilator-dependent child. Put another way, the coming years may very well see additional financial support for healthcare providers to coordinate care and promote family-centered care under the medical home concept. It remains to be seen how much, if any, of these reforms will be directed to subspecialty teams. This clearly presents a challenge when the pulmonologist plays such a critical role in maintaining what may essentially be life support for a child who is living at home.

There are always roles for the pulmonologist that are critical to the health of the ventilator-dependent child and will not change: initiation of the ventilation support, ventilator management, oversight of equipment, and management of the lung disease. **It is important to understand, however, that meeting the needs of the family of a ventilator-dependent child is generally greater than what any one individual can provide, whether it be the pulmonologist, the family, or the primary care provider.** No one individual has the complete expertise to meet all of the medical and supportive service needs of the ventilator-dependent child. In addition, the designated Medical Home provider should act as the main contact for the family, facilitating and coordinating access to all necessary services, including those services that the provider is not an expert in. At the minimum, implementing effective care through the medical home concept for the ventilator-dependent child presents a daunting challenge for the family, pulmonologist, PCP, and all related services. Provider and family roles need to be defined to ensure comprehensive needs are met and overlap minimized; staff need to be appropriately supported (often with a dedicated point person who acts as a care coordinator) and trained; families need to be supported as partners; and systems need to be operated efficiently.

In the following section, we present examples of potential models of care, along with the operationalization and the steps necessary to implement such care that meet the needs of the child and family and support effective healthcare delivery. It is important to recognize that while successful programs, by many measures, do exist, the research on what components are necessary and the financial models to bring them up to scale for a larger population remains subpar. This situation, however, does present the opportunity for the pulmonologist, the family, and supporting partners to innovate and be creative about how care is delivered effectively for the ventilator-dependent child. Readers of this chapter are encouraged to be knowledgeable about the state and local medical home initiatives and partner with other providers to improve care delivery for ventilator-dependent children who live at home.

Operationalizing Care Models for Ventilator-Dependent Children: The Current State

Ethan is a 3-year-old child with metatrophic dystrophy and a cervical spine injury requiring continuous ventilation. You get a call from the primary care physician, who has just assumed care of Ethan because his mother was not happy with the previous primary care physician. This physician notes that Ethan has lost weight since his last visit and sometimes appears short of breath. Ethan lives 200 miles away from you and his parents have transportation difficulties. His physician would like to speak with your nutritionist and he wants to know where to fax the results of his blood work today, and find out when you would like to see him next. The primary care physician does not know what to recommend about evaluating the shortness of breath or altering the vent settings but offers to work with you on co-managing the ventilator.

The successful care model of the ventilator-dependent child should be able to translate best care practices into effective care delivery and better health. Such care should have technical and medical expertise, embrace the Medical Home concept, and address the care partnership needs of the family. However, local contexts vary; family-centered care, too, can be messy because care plans should be negotiated and tailored to specific situations. This means that ultimately, the treating physician may be willing to agree to a care plan that may not be his or her first choice of options, but is acceptable to all to move forward.

It is crucial to understand that the pulmonologist plays a very specific and important role in the care of the ventilator-dependent child. Many aspects of the medical care can ONLY be done by the pulmonologist, such as the assessment of ventilation, ventilator management, acute respiratory illness assessment, and management of airway disease. By default, the pulmonary orders are written by the pulmonologist, and when the child is sick, the pulmonologist may be called first. The pulmonologist, as the expert in a field of subspecialty medical knowledge that applies to a small number of children, may be responsible for medical decisions for where there may be little precedent because of the ongoing advances in technology.

The intensity of the pulmonary team involvement can also lead, often by default, to the pulmonary team managing nutrition, social services, and case management, particularly with speech, swallowing, and behavior management. This may occur because either the primary care physician may not have the expertise or familiarity, or these services were initiated in the hospital while the child was under the care of the pulmonologist. In any event, the family may come to see the pulmonologist as the primary contact and, in fact, the de facto "Medical Home" provider as the contact for all care. Some pulmonary services have accordingly developed multidisciplinary programs dedicated to the care of the child with ventilator dependency, including dedicated staff roles and time. Reimbursement frequently does not adequately cover the operating expenses of such programs. Nonetheless, such programs offer an identity for a central location for pulmonary services dedicated to ventilator-dependent children.

The risk of centering so much care within the pulmonary team can lead to the ventilator-dependent child not establishing a close relationship with the primary care physician in the community. The absence of a close relationship with the primary care physician can lead to missed immunizations, missed preventive care visits, and missed opportunities to assess behavior, nutrition, and many other care aspects that are best performed in the primary care setting. A further complication may occur given the regionalization of subspecialty care. The pulmonary team may be far from the child's place of residence, sometimes hundreds of miles away. In that situation the pulmonologist is not readily accessible for a clinic visit when the child is acutely ill. In the absence of a close relationship with the primary care team, the local physician may not be comfortable assessing an acute pulmonary problem in a ventilator-dependent child. Alternatively, the local physician may feel comfortable assessing but may not have the training to render the optimal management decision. Thus, in the absence of a local physician willing to evaluate the child during acute respiratory illnesses and partner with the pulmonary team, the family must rely on limited, telephone-only evaluation by the pulmonary team or travel long distances to the tertiary care center every time the child is acutely ill. Neither scenario will substitute for a qualified physician providing hands-on assessment and up-to-date timely management. The lack of having a qualified physician with access to optimal decision-making is not ideal for the ventilator-dependent child.

One alternative is to co-locate services in individual care settings. Some pulmonologists may be more comfortable providing primary care-type preventive services such as immunizations and anticipatory guidance in behavior and development, just as some primary care physicians may be comfortable even managing ventilator support or weaning oxygen; there is the occasional primary care physician that has subspecialty training, for example. However, reimbursement models do not support the time needed for primary care delivery in the pulmonary setting. In addition, the stakes are too high with the ventilator-dependent child to routinely have pulmonary care outside of the subspecialty clinical setting for the following reasons:

- The tracheostomy /ventilator is complex technology
- The tracheostomy /ventilator is intimidating to families and providers alike
- Improper management of tracheostomy /ventilator may be life-threatening
- Most providers who are not pulmonologists have no experience with home ventilator support
- The pulmonary team is multidisciplinary, including the physician, respiratory therapist, social worker, specialty nurse, and other managing subspecialists; with so many moving parts, there is a larger margin for error with miscommunication

In summary, the ideal model of care for the ventilator-dependent child should thus:

- Acknowledge the unique and critical role of the pulmonary team
- Acknowledge the unique and critical role of the primary care team
- Clearly delineate the responsibilities of each member of the care team
- Support a partnering approach for the families, who will also bring the integrated view of all other needed care and support services
- Support timely and ongoing communication between all parties
- Acknowledge that the roles that all parties have will change over time as the child grows and develops.

Encouraging the best care from all services usually entails supporting families and providers to provide the best care in their own settings. The realities of reimbursement make building multidisciplinary care programs difficult. The challenge for pulmonologists is to work with families and primary care physicians to have the best care possible in their own settings while coordinating care so that the family sees efficient and effective care throughout. Remember that the family sees the entire care system and all moving parts — including parts that the pulmonary team or primary care team may not be familiar with!

Co-Management between Primary and Specialty Care: Building the Family-Centered Gold Standard

Co-management reflects a care model in which multiple providers, usually the primary care provider and specialty provider, work together in a planned, coordinated manner to deliver seamless care [30]. Co-management, however, does not happen by accident. Co-management is planned between providers and families, delineates roles, and utilizes a number of tools such as comprehensive written care plans. When well implemented, co-management can address the gaps that occur if care is centered completely on the primary care OR the pulmonary settings.

Antonelli [31] outlined three models of care for children for CYSHCN that reflect the interplay between primary care physician (PCP) and specialty care that is usually found [31]. Each model has its benefits and drawbacks that should be considered in assessing the care plan for the ventilator-dependent child, as illustrated below.

PCP as the Primary Manager. This care model emphasizes that the primary care physician is the first point of contact and the main decision maker for the medical issues of the child. In the case of the ventilator-dependent child, this is not a model that will typically be used, because it is extremely rare for the primary care physician to be comfortable with management. Some primary care settings may have an external care coordinator that provides additional care coordination support for families, but it would be extremely unusual for such external care coordination support to have sufficient expertise in managing home ventilation.

Specialist as Primary Manager. The specialist is the primary manager of the child's medical needs. In the case of the ventilator-dependent child, this may happen by default to the pulmonary service because of the frequency and intensity of the care management, at least initially. This model, however, acknowledges that the specialist must be able to coordinate *all* aspects of the child's medical care *and* non-medical service needs. For example, assessments for school, education, other organ systems, and psychosocial needs should be regularly assessed, as well as immunizations, behaviors, and even toileting. It also asks for 24/7 access as in the Medical Home concept for all of these situations.

PCP and Specialist as Co-Managers. Recent studies favor co-management, as when it is executed successfully, it enhances access for families since the primary care physician can be an effective first contact. That does not mean the primary care physician is the medical decision maker when it comes to pulmonary issues. Rather, the primary care physician acts as the eyes and ears of the pulmonologist, for example, during evaluation of an acute pulmonary illness. This setup works best if the pulmonologist is familiar with the comfort level and experience of the primary care physician. Co-management works well IF the following are achieved: [30]

- Good relationship with the primary care physician
- Clear delineation of roles
- Clear protocols of care
- Data sharing

Families, if co-management works well, prefer this arrangement because it is able to merge the best of both worlds. PCPs can also become increasingly comfortable with certain aspects of care with co-management [32].

Factors that will drive decisions about which model of care to implement include the family's preference, resources in the community, distance to the tertiary care center, and the PCP's level of training and comfort. All of this needs to be individually assessed. With any co-management agreement, a phone call with mutual care planning should be considered at the minimum. The challenge of co-management is being able to develop the necessary relationships with the primary care providers, as these typically develop over time and entail building confidence among all providers in their care.

One additional emerging model is the comprehensive complex care service at the tertiary care center [33]. Such services offer multidisciplinary, team-based care and care coordination to children who are deemed as "complex" because of multi-organ disease and frequent hospitalization. In contrast to a ventilator-dependent program, such complex care services often admit children based on medical care need and not by diagnosis. In certain situations, the whole-child orientation of the complex care clinic may be a helpful adjunct to the care of the ventilator-dependent child. Emerging evidence suggests that such clinical services may be helpful in making care more efficient, effective, and family-centered [19], and thus the number of such services are gaining popularity. Complex care services have the same challenges as any other multidisciplinary service: inadequate reimbursement, staff training, and need to coordinate with the primary care service, although some do provide primary care services. Payment models to support this care model vary considerably, although efforts on the federal level are being considered that could potentially standardize this care delivery model in the future. The pulmonary team may consider the complex care service as an additional resource for patients and families.

Implementation of Collaborative, Co-Management Care between Primary and Subspecialty Care

When implementing co-management, it is important to recognize that the pulmonologist is likely going to initiate a substantial portion of the medical care plan. The pulmonologist will have initiated the ventilator support in-house, and will design the transition plan from hospital to home. The pulmonologist will also be viewed as the expert on the critical portions of the life-sustaining ventilator support. Even the most capable and involved primary care physician and family will defer to the leadership of the pulmonary team with these key aspects of care.

The experience and desire of primary care physicians to care for the ventilator-dependent child will vary considerably. Some primary care physicians are experienced in caring for critically ill children and will readily be able to co-manage by providing preventive care, anticipatory guidance, immunizations, and acting as the local "eyes and ears" for the pulmonologist. These practices may also be staffed with dedicated care coordinators. Other practices may be less capable with staffing and experience. **The pulmonologist will need to be able to assess not only the family's ability to assume home care, but also the capability and comfort of the primary care physician, and initiate co-management accordingly.**

This section of the chapter is thus geared towards the pulmonologist, but in some cases, the primary care physician may initiate the conversation towards better co-management of medical issues. What follows is a general guide for implementing co-management, including the tools that the pulmonologist, primary care physician, and family may wish to utilize.

1. Pulmonologist reaches out to PCP upon discharge. At a minimum, the pulmonologist should identify a primary care physician and ensure that there is a primary care physician or a team at the PCP office that self-identifies as "taking charge" of the medical care plan in the PCP setting. The pulmonologist should be able to speak with the PCP by phone to discuss the hospital course, care plan, and expectations for co-management.

2. Pulmonologist and PCP should clarify roles. At the initial phone call, the pulmonologist and PCP should identify their respective roles so that there is no confusion or duplication. The pulmonologist will clearly maintain oversight and management of the ventilator. The primary care physician should follow the routine well-child visit schedule as outlined by Bright Futures [34]. Roles to clarify include: who will adjust the medications? The nutrition plan? Swallowing evaluation and therapy?

Developmental assessment and referral? Who should be the primary contact in case of specific illnesses? The PCP may also be expected to learn aspects of care of the ventilator-dependent child over time. Finally, the role of the family and the roles of office staff should be clarified as well. The PCP and the pulmonologist may both have dedicated staff members, such as a nurse or a social worker that acts as the primary contact for care coordination and information sharing.

3. Develop written care plan and red flags for PCP. The PCP should have a documented written care plan, including the summary of the initial hospital stay. Also documented should be specific contact information for the pulmonologist and all related hospital care team members, including nutrition, social work, respiratory therapy, and others. The list of red flags should include baseline vital signs and ventilator settings, with specific reasons for both family and PCP to contact pulmonologist immediately. Emergency contact information and plans, including emergency room, should be clarified.

4. Pulmonologist and PCP agree on routine visit schedule. The pulmonologist and the PCP should agree on a routine follow-up schedule that is tailored to the needs of the patient and family. This schedule may be tailored for distance, family ability to transport equipment, and comfort of the PCP. For example, a pulmonologist and PCP may opt to see the child every 2 weeks, alternating between the two, with a phone contact between the two physicians after the visit.

5. Pulmonologist, family, and PCP should clarify how information will be shared, the frequency of sharing and by whom. Co-management is optimized if there is immediate communication of clinical assessments, changes in care plans, medication changes, or setting of new goals. The optimal method, which is not always available, would be a shared electronic medical record or patient portal. Alternatives may include phone calls, secure email, fax-back forms, and letters that are dictated and mailed in a timely fashion.

6. Pulmonologist, family, and PCP should clarify care plan goals. A written care plan that is formulated by the "medical home provider"—which may be the PCP or the pulmonologist—is an essential tool that helps set care plan goals. The family should participate in developing care plan as it offers the opportunity for all parties to clarify short- and long-term goals of the care of the child.

A number of tools are available to support the implementation of co-management and the medical home. Examples of written care plans and care summaries can be easily found on medical home resource web pages such as the National Center for Medical Home Implementation: www.medicahomeinfo.org. Examples of tools that practices may wish to avail themselves of include:

- Medical home assessment tools
- Family partnership tools
- Cultural competency assessments and tools
- Billing and coding help for care coordination
- Staffing plans
- Family support groups

Finally, this section highlights the specific relationship between the pulmonologist and PCP. It is important to recognize that many ventilator-dependent children receive care from multiple other specialists, such as ENT for dysphagia and/or tracheostomy care, cardiology for pulmonary hypertension, and nephrology for hypertension. It is unlikely that anyone other than the pulmonologist or PCP will be considered the "Medical Home" provider for ventilator-dependent children. However, the logistics of coordinating multiple plans become more complicated and time-consuming. It is imperative that one provider acts as the primary "Medical Home" provider [35] and that is agreed upon between the pulmonologist and PCP. The "Medical Home" provider ideally has the dedicated time and resources, such as a designated care coordinator, to coordinate a care plan that accounts for multiple specialists. This means that the "Medical Home" provider works with the family to continually update the care plan, accounting for the input of multiple specialists, and reaches out to the specialists individually through email or phone if necessary. Tools, secure messaging and communication methods, and dedicated staff become even more important in this regard. Another option available to some pulmonologists and PCPs may be to utilize a tertiary care center-based comprehensive care clinic for the child with medical complexity.

Summary

Effective care for ventilator-dependent children entails being able to implement recommended care in the community setting. Research supports a comprehensive care approach, embracing the role of the primary care provider and providing family-centered care within the medical home concept. Multiple providers and care components need to be successfully coordinated. The pulmonologist, however, is crucial to keeping the child healthy, due to the direct management of life-sustaining treatment. Multidisciplinary programs are frequently valuable in coordinating multiple services that work with the child and family, and care can be coordinated in a co-management protocol by the PCP, family, and pulmonologist. Reimbursement remains a challenge, particularly for sustaining the multidisciplinary programs that may need to be supported by the individual service or the hospital, but healthcare reform may encourage new opportunities for reimbursing supportive services and effective health delivery.

Optimal care models should incorporate the strengths of all providers that are needed to provide comprehensive, medical home-based care for the ventilator-dependent child. A variety of tools exist to help the pulmonologist, primary care physician, and family jointly plan care that provides timely, effective medical care and the needs of the child and family. If successful, the Medical Homecare concept is likely to result in the effective care delivery sought by all: improved quality of life, better health, and family need that are met. However, the critical role of the pulmonologist will mean that the pulmonary team needs to take a lead role in setting the tone for co-management, including patient and family assessments, working relationships with primary care providers, care protocols, and care access.

Much future research continues to be needed. Specific research questions include: what are the important care components associated with improved healthcare outcomes? What services and care arrangements should be supported by innovative payment mechanisms? What is the return of investment on multidisciplinary care services? What are the metrics that accurately assess family-needs and outcomes?

References

1. Com G, Kuo DZ, Bauer ML, et al. Outcomes of children treated with tracheostomy and positive-pressure ventilation at home. Clin Pediatr (Phila). 2013;52(1):54–61.
2. Quint RD, Chesterman E, Crain LS, Winkleby M, Boyce WT. Home care for ventilator-dependent children. Psychosocial impact on the family. Am J Dis Child. 1990;144(11): 1238–41.
3. Carnevale FA, Alexander E, Davis M, Rennick J, Troini R. Daily living with distress and enrichment: the moral experience of families with ventilator-assisted children at home. Pediatrics. 2006;117(1):e48–60.
4. McPherson M, Arango P, Fox H, et al. A new definition of children with special health care needs. Pediatrics. 1998;102(1 Pt 1):137–40.
5. U.S. Department of Health and Human Services. Children with Special Health Care Needs. Campaign '87. Surgeon General's Report. Commitment to: Family-Centered, Community-Based, Coordinated Care. Rockville, MD: U.S. Department of Health and Human Services; 1987.
6. Kratz L, Uding N, Trahms CM, Villareale N, Kieckhefer GM. Managing childhood chronic illness: parent perspectives and implications for parent-provider relationships. Fam Syst Health. 2009;27(4):303–13.
7. MacKean GL, Thurston WE, Scott CM. Bridging the divide between families and health professionals' perspectives on family-centred care. Health Expect. 2005;8(1):74–85.
8. Sia C, Tonniges TF, Osterhus E, Taba S. History of the medical home concept. Pediatrics. 2004;113(5 Suppl):1473–8.
9. American Academy of Pediatrics. The medical home. Pediatrics. 2002;110(1 Pt 1):184–6.
10. Cooley WC, McAllister JW, Sherrieb K, Kuhlthau K. Improved outcomes associated with medical home implementation in pediatric primary care. Pediatrics. 2009;124(1):358–64.
11. McAllister JW, Sherrieb K, Cooley WC. Improvement in the family-centered medical home enhances outcomes for children and youth with special healthcare needs. J Ambul Care Manage. 2009;32(3):188–96.
12. Cooley WC, McAllister JW, Sherrieb K, Clark RE. The medical home index: development and validation of a new practice-level measure of implementation of the medical home model. Ambul Pediatr. 2003;3(4):173–80.
13. Homer CJ, Klatka K, Romm D, et al. A review of the evidence for the medical home for children with special health care needs. Pediatrics. 2008;122(4):e922–37.
14. US Department of Health and Human Services. Healthy People 2020. http://healthypeople. gov/2020/topicsobjectives2020/objectiveslist.aspx?topicId=26. Accessed 5 Aug 2013.
15. American Academy of Family Physicians, American Academy of Pediatrics, American College of Physicians, American Osteopathic Association. Joint principles of the patient centered medical home. Washington, DC: American Academy of Family Physicians/American Academy of Pediatrics/American College of Physicians/American Osteopathic Association; 2007.

16. Stille C, Turchi RM, Antonelli R, et al. The family-centered medical home: specific considerations for child health research and policy. Acad Pediatr. 2010;10(4):211–7.
17. Perrin JM, Romm D, Bloom SR, et al. A family-centered, community-based system of services for children and youth with special health care needs. Arch Pediatr Adolesc Med. 2007; 161(10):933–6.
18. Cohen E, Kuo DZ, Agrawal R, et al. Children with medical complexity: an emerging population for clinical and research initiatives. Pediatrics. 2011;127(3):529–38.
19. Cohen E, Jovcevska V, Kuo DZ, Mahant S. Hospital-based comprehensive care programs for Children with Special Health Care Needs (CSHCN): a systematic review. Arch Pediatr Adolesc Med. 2011;165(6):554–61.
20. Leiter V. Dilemmas in sharing care: maternal provision of professionally driven therapy for children with disabilities. Soc Sci Med. 2004;58(4):837–49.
21. Ray LD. Parenting and childhood chronicity: making visible the invisible work. J Pediatr Nurs. 2002;17(6):424–38.
22. Gordon J. An evidence-based approach for supporting parents experiencing chronic sorrow. Pediatr Nurs. 2009;35(2):115–9.
23. Kuo DZ, Houtrow AJ, Arango P, Kuhlthau KA, Simmons JM, Neff JM. Family-centered care: current applications and future directions in pediatric health care. Matern Child Health J. 2012;16(2):297–305.
24. Kuhlthau K, Bloom S, Van Cleave J, et al. Evidence for family-centered care for children with special health care needs: a systematic review. Acad Pediatr 2011;11(2):136–43.
25. Dunst CJ, Dempsy I. Family-professional partnerships and parenting competence, confidence, and enjoyment. Int J Disabi Dev Educ. 2007;54(3):305–18.
26. Bodenheimer T, Wagner EH, Grumbach K. Improving primary care for patients with chronic illness: the chronic care model, Part 2. JAMA. 2002;288(15):1909–14.
27. Liptak GS, Revell GM. Community physician's role in case management of children with chronic illnesses. Pediatrics. 1989;84(3):465–71.
28. McPherson M, Weissman G, Strickland BB, van Dyck PC, Blumberg SJ, Newacheck PW. Implementing community-based systems of services for children and youths with special health care needs: how well are we doing? Pediatrics. 2004;113(5 Suppl):1538–44.
29. Kuo DZ, Cohen E, Agrawal R, Berry JG, Casey PH. A national profile of caregiver challenges among more medically complex children with special health care needs. Arch Pediatr Adolesc Med. 2011;165(6):1020–6.
30. Stille CJ. Communication, comanagement, and collaborative care for children and youth with special healthcare needs. Pediatr Ann. 2009;38(9):498–504.
31. Antonelli R, Stille C, Freeman L. Enhancing collaboration between primary and subspecialty care providers for children and youth with special health care needs. Washington, DC: Georgetown University Center for Children and Human Development; 2005.
32. Kuo DZ, Cheng TL, Rowe PC. Successful use of a primary care practice-specialty collaboration in the care of an adolescent with chronic fatigue syndrome. Pediatrics. 2007;120(6):e1536–9.
33. Berry JG, Agrawal R, Kuo DZ, et al. Characteristics of hospitalizations for patients who utilize a structured clinical-care program for children with medical complexity. J Pediatr. 2011; 159(2):284–90.
34. Hagan JF, Shaw JS, Duncan P, editors. Bright futures: guidelines for health supervision of infants, children, and adolescents. 3rd ed. Elk Grove Village, IL: American Academy of Pediatrics; 2008.
35. Berry JG, Agrawal RK, Cohen E, Kuo DZ. The landscape of medical care for children with medical complexity. Overland Park, KS: Children's Hospital Association; 2013.

Chapter 8
Outpatient Care of the Ventilator Dependent Child

Nanci Yuan and Laura M. Sterni

Introduction

Invasive mechanical ventilation via tracheostomy and noninvasive ventilator support have become increasingly utilized treatment options for pediatric patients with a wide variety of diagnoses. This is due to multiple factors including advancements in available technology, improved access to technology and medical care, increased clinical expertise, and a paradigm shift in patients, caregivers, and physicians' attitudes towards quality of life and long-term care. Children who depend on chronic ventilator support are a medically complex and diverse group with high morbidity and mortality. The increased risk for severe illness and death in this group of patients is related both to progression of underlying conditions and to complications related to comorbid conditions or the presence of a tracheostomy (e.g., tracheal plugging or bleeding) [1–3]. Despite the complex healthcare needs of children who rely on chronic ventilator support, there are few guidelines and little published evidence available to guide the clinicians who care for these patients in the outpatient setting.

The goals of home care for patients with chronic respiratory disorders were outlined in an American Thoracic Society (ATS) statement approved in 2005 [4]. In this statement, home care was defined as including home healthcare, hospice, chronic homecare services such as nursing and home medical equipment. The general goals of home care for patients with respiratory disorders included increasing survival, decreasing morbidity, improving function and quality of life, supporting

N. Yuan, M.D. (✉)
Stanford Children's Health Sleep Center,
770 Welch Road, Suite 350, Palo Alto, CA 94304, USA
e-mail: nyuan@stanford.edu

L.M. Sterni, M.D.
Eudowood Division of Pediatric Respiratory Sciences, The Johns Hopkins University School of Medicine, 200 North Wolfe Street, Baltimore, MD 21287, USA
e-mail: lsterni1@jhmi.edu

© Springer Science+Business Media New York 2016
L.M. Sterni, J.L. Carroll (eds.), *Caring for the Ventilator Dependent Child*,
Respiratory Medicine, DOI 10.1007/978-1-4939-3749-3_8

self-management and independence, encouraging positive health behaviors, and promoting optimal growth and development in pediatric patients [4]. Minimizing recurrent hospitalizations is another very important goal in complex patients with technology dependencies [5]. To meet these goals, outpatient providers must help patients and their families navigate a complex array of providers and services. Professionals caring for children requiring chronic ventilator support require specialized clinical knowledge and an understanding of how to access the services and equipment that will be required for care in the home. Often care of these complex patients is accomplished through multidisciplinary care teams. The objective of this chapter is to review aspects of outpatient management that should be considered in all patients requiring ventilator support. While the indications for and methods used to provide respiratory support vary widely, there are many common themes in the outpatient care of these children.

The Importance of the Care Team

Multiple studies in the last several years show an increase in the prevalence of home mechanical ventilation worldwide. These retrospective studies and reviews from countries as diverse as Canada, Korea, Poland, and the United States demonstrate similar findings, as follows: (1) there have been significant increases in the number of patients treated with noninvasive mechanical ventilation; (2) there are an increasing variety of underlying diagnoses accepted as indications for chronic ventilator support; (3) there are an increasing number of pediatric patients utilizing chronic ventilator support leading to issues during the period of transition from pediatric to adult care; and (4) these patients are resource intense and have a significant impact on both hospital and community services [6–10]. Patients requiring home ventilator support have significant medical and technology requirements and care often involves a large number of medical professionals. The complexity of their care places them at risk of unmet medical needs and poor coordination of needed services [5, 11].

There is also evidence showing that providing care to a patient requiring chronic ventilator support in the home places a significant burden on the family. Several studies show the complex emotional impact of home care of a patient with either noninvasive or invasive mechanical ventilation on the caregiver and the individual members of the family [12–17]. These studies share common themes. The caregiver's obligations negatively impact their mental, physical, and sleep health as well as their family relationships. These issues worsen as the primary caregiver ages. Caregivers report a lack of support from the medical system and the community as well as from other members of the family, who may feel resentment towards the patient. There is a large gap between caregiver expectations and what the community healthcare services are able to provide, even when almost unlimited resources are available. Caregivers and extended family members usually see a negative impact on their ability to participate in school, employment, and in social activities due to the considerable time demands of caring for the patient. Families often have little or no access to suitably trained professional caregivers who can provide the technical care required by the patient, leaving family caregivers and the entire family without a respite from the continuous stresses associated with their home medical care responsibilities.

A number of support measures are needed to facilitate appropriate care of patients requiring chronic ventilator support and to reduce the burden on their family members. A healthcare team skilled in all aspects of care for these patients is important if the goals of home care are to be reached. Given the complexity of care required, the care teams for these patients often span multiple disciplines and, based on patient and family requirements, may include nurses, respiratory therapists, nutritionists, physical therapists, speech therapists, social workers, and psychologists.

The use of family-centered care and the Medical Home comprehensive care model are reviewed in Chap. 7. A dedicated pediatric palliative care team can play an important role for many of these patients (Chap. 5). While care team composition may vary from patient to patient and clinic to clinic, a team leader or case manager, responsible for ensuring multidisciplinary follow-up and working to address the changing needs of the patient and family, is recommended for children requiring chronic ventilator support [18].

Respiratory Care in the Outpatient Clinic

Respiratory care may be provided in a variety of outpatient settings but all children requiring chronic ventilation should have an involved respiratory specialist, usually a pediatric pulmonologist, but in some centers this may be a neonatologist or pediatric-intensive care physician. The goals of an outpatient visit to the clinic managing the child's respiratory care should be to evaluate the patient's stability and/or progress, manage the patient's respiratory illnesses, assess the adequacy of the prescribed ventilator support, and review the use and tolerance of the ventilator and other respiratory support equipment. Children who rely on chronic ventilator support utilize a wide variety of ventilators and interfaces. Troubleshooting the home equipment required for the patient's care has been addressed in Chap. 10. Clinic visits often provide the forum for patients and their caregivers to report equipment concerns or ask questions about the use of equipment they have been provided. When possible, asking caregivers to demonstrate the use of the equipment is valuable, providing an opportunity for medical professionals to reinforce the caregiver's skills. Requesting that patients bring their home ventilators to clinic when feasible allows clinic staff to check equipment settings and compliance monitors. During a quality control survey of 290 patients receiving home mechanical ventilation (primarily noninvasive ventilation) in Spain, significant differences were found between the ventilator settings prescribed and both the actual settings on the ventilator panel and the support (pressures or volume) provided by the ventilator [19]. Clinics caring for these complex children should be staffed not only by physicians but by respiratory therapists or alternative specially trained staff who can evaluate the home equipment and provide ongoing support and teaching to the home caregivers.

When using noninvasive positive airway pressure (PAP) ventilation in growing children, both continuous positive airway pressure (CPAP) and noninvasive positive pressure ventilation (NIPPV), the appropriateness of the interface should be reevaluated frequently. As children grow, mask sizes change. Review of the patient's mask is essential in the clinic as common complications of PAP therapy, such as skin and eye irritation, are often related to poor mask fit or placement. Nasal and facial masks frequently lead to skin irritation or ulceration [20, 21]. Skin complications in these patients can be significant leading to the need for wound care and resistance to using the mask. Overtightening of the mask to prevent leak often leads to pressure-related skin problems. Caregivers should be encouraged to clean the mask daily as accumulation of oils from the skin on the mask contributes to skin irritation. A change in the mask to avoid contact with injured areas of skin should be considered when possible. Nasal symptoms, including congestion, dryness, or rhinorrhea, are common complications of PAP therapy and can be managed with heated humidity and, if needed, intranasal steroids or other medical therapies [20, 22].

There have been published reports of children using nasal noninvasive ventilator support for long periods developing mid-face hypoplasia, likely secondary to the prolonged application of force exerted by the mask and headgear on growing facial features [21, 23, 24]. Fauroux et al. evaluated 40 children using nasal masks for noninvasive pressure support and found 68 % had facial flattening when assessed by physical examination [21]. Children using PAP therapy for long periods of time should have regular assessment of their facial development during their physical examination. In our clinics, when the development of facial deformities is noted, patients are provided with an alternate interface to change where pressure is applied on the face. We also stress the importance of avoiding mask and headgear overtightening, and review the appropriate mask fit and placement at each visit. In the Fauroux study, spontaneous regression of a facial deformity that had developed in a 3.5-year-old patient who had been using NIPPV since infancy was seen after the support was discontinued.

Patients prescribed noninvasive PAP support must be monitored closely to assess and encourage adherence with therapy. Best studied in children with obstructive sleep apnea syndrome (OSAS), adherence with PAP is known to be poor and is a limitation to effective treatment for many patients [25, 26]. Multiple factors influence adherence, including patient and family characteristics, disease characteristics, equipment features, and side effects [27]. A recent study in children and adolescents with OSAS treated with PAP found that PAP adherence was primarily related to demographic and family factors. The strongest predictor of poor PAP use in this study was low maternal education [28]. Time in outpatient clinic can be spent discussing PAP use and when available reviewing compliance data obtained from the patient's equipment. Programs to encourage adherence with PAP therapy have focused on behavioral therapy, intensive family education, and counseling and equipment modification with treatment of complications [27, 29–31]. Many clinics caring for children requiring noninvasive ventilator support are staffed with behavioral psychologists or respiratory therapists who work with families and patients. The addition of a specially trained respiratory therapist to provide education and evaluate the patient's PAP equipment during visits to a multidisciplinary sleep clinic improved adherence in pediatric patients with OSAS and poor adherence at baseline [32]. Adherence in children requiring NIPPV for treatment of hypoventilation related to neuromuscular or lung disease has not been extensively studied. A recent study examining CPAP and noninvasive ventilator use in patients with a variety of diagnoses who had been using the therapy at least 1 month did not find a difference in adherence when comparing OSAS patients to those with lung or neuromuscular disease [33]. In this study, however, very good compliance was noted in all groups and the number of non-OSAS patients was small. PAP compliance and strategies to improve adherence are addressed in Chap. 12.

Children receiving ventilation via tracheostomy should have regular evaluations of their airway to assess tracheostomy tube fit and to help detect and avoid any airway complications that may result from the indwelling tube, such as tracheal granulomas. Examination of the airway and tracheostomy tube size and curvature is often best accomplished with flexible bronchoscopy. An ATS consensus statement addressing care of the child with a tracheotomy recommended rigid or flexible bronchoscopy every 6–12 months although noted that there is little data to support the use of surveillance bronchoscopies in this setting [34]. Choosing the appropriate tracheostomy tube size for a patient involves evaluating the patient's airway size and shape and demonstrating that the tube provides an adequate airway for ventilation [35]. When possible, after considering the patient's medical stability, airway patency and cognitive status, a tracheostomy tube size that would allow for speech (not to exceed 2/3 of the tracheal lumen) can be chosen [34]. The ATS consensus statement referenced above recommends that all patients with a tracheostomy be referred to a speech pathologist for services, regardless of diagnosis, age, or expected length of time tracheostomy will be in place. Cuffed tracheostomy tubes are associated with complications caused by the localized pressure the inflatable cuff places on the airway wall. Cuff pressures higher than the capillary perfusion pressure of the tracheal mucosa can result in ulceration and ischemic necrosis of the airway which may lead to tracheal stenosis or tracheal dilatation [34, 36]. The indications for the use of cuffed tubes in pediatrics are limited, and careful monitoring and family education is needed if a cuffed tube is required [34].

An important component of the outpatient respiratory clinic visit is the evaluation of the patient's pulmonary status. A consensus statement on the respiratory care of patients with Duchenne muscular dystrophy recommended that clinics caring for these young men have the ability to perform and interpret specific tests that are important for monitoring the patient's respiratory status [37]. These recommendations seem generalizable to any clinic caring for children on chronic invasive and noninvasive ventilation, many of whom have neuromuscular disease. "Necessary" tests that should be available in clinic include pulse oximetry, capnography, peak cough flow, maximum inspiratory and expiratory pressure measurement and arterial blood gas analysis. Tests that the panel of experts felt should be available by referral outside of the clinic include polysomnography, overnight pulse oximetry or overnight pulse oximetry combined with capnography measured in the patient's home.

There are no published protocols outlining the routine pulmonary assessment of patients requiring chronic ventilator support and monitoring will be dependent on the patient's underlying diagnosis, comorbidities, and medical status. Consensus statements have outlined respiratory monitoring protocols for patients with Duchenne muscular dystrophy and spinal muscular atrophy [37, 38].

Polysomnography and home measurements of gas exchange are important in the ongoing care of pediatric patients requiring ventilator support as respiratory requirements may change with growth, with disease progression or as their underlying condition improves. A consensus statement from Australia recommended sleep studies, ideally full polysomnography, at regular intervals for all children on respiratory support [18]. Widger et al. found that titration studies performed to adjust both CPAP and bi-level ventilation in children using these therapies chronically frequently led to recommendations to optimize therapy [39]. Further, scores on a quality of life questionnaire were more likely to improve if the changes recommended had been implemented by the time of the patient's next sleep study (recommended yearly in their center). Useful guidelines for PAP titration in patients with OSAS and adjustment of noninvasive positive pressure ventilation in adults and children with stable hypoventilation syndromes have been published by the American Academy of Sleep Medicine [40, 41]. It should be noted that the availability of polysomnography to monitor gas exchange during sleep in ventilator-dependent patients is limited in some centers, while other centers prefer home measurement of oxyhemoglobin saturations and carbon dioxide levels to eliminate the risk of underestimating abnormalities in the laboratory setting due to poor sleep. The optimal method for monitoring and titrating ventilator support in children is an area requiring further investigation.

Regular assessment of a patient's respiratory status leads to informed discussions regarding the current plan of care, transition to the next stage of care and avoidance of "crisis" situations. The timing of clinical evaluations is dependent on many factors. Based on the consensus of the authors, a minimum of every 3 months for children on invasive ventilation and 3–6 months for patients on noninvasive ventilator support have been proposed in one guideline from Australia [18]. As noted above, the optimal schedule for routine respiratory clinic evaluation with the goal of improving outcomes for patients requiring chronic ventilator support has not been studied.

Liberating a patient from mechanical ventilator support, both invasive and noninvasive, is a realistic goal for many children, depending on the original indication for long-term ventilation. Often this is accomplished through a gradual decrease in ventilator settings, during which the patient is followed closely to be sure they are tolerating the reduction in provided support. This process, often called "weaning," may occur over weeks, months, or even years. There is little published evidence detailing how and when weaning should be attempted and the approach must take into account the underlying cause of the patient's respiratory failure. Weaning from mechanical ventilation may occur stepwise at home, in subacute facilities or in acute-care hospitals. Some patients are liberated from ventilators in favor of diaphragmatic pacing. Validated protocols for safely weaning appropriate patients from ventilator support have not been published. Further, it is not known if weaning algorithms will lead to improved patient outcomes. A consensus report from a workgroup of experts in the United States details a protocol for weaning patients from mechanical ventilation in a post-acute hospital setting; the authors note that further study to validate this approach is needed [42].

Smoking and Secondhand Smoke

Tobacco use harms children, and is even more dangerous for children with respiratory disorders. Tobacco use and secondhand smoke exposure increases the frequency of respiratory illnesses and infections and decreases lung function [43]. Smoking in the home is the leading cause of residential fire deaths in the United States and fatal home fires have been reported secondary to smoking in the presence of home oxygen therapy [44, 45]. The risk of fire related to oxygen use must be stressed with families and patients. Those caring for children with respiratory issues should work with families and patients to attain smoking-free environments, both in the home and out of the home, and help active tobacco users develop a plan and find resources for tobacco use cessation [46]. Information to help patients and families eliminate tobacco use can be found at Smokefree.gov [47].

Infection

In a study by Kun et al., pneumonia and tracheitis were found to be the most common reasons for hospital readmission during the year following the initiation of chronic ventilator support via tracheostomy [48]. Poor care of the tracheostomy and respiratory equipment may be responsible for some of these infections. Children dependent on invasive ventilator support and many children using noninvasive support may have complex chronic conditions which predispose them to serious infections even in the setting of excellent care. Prior to discharge home, caregivers must be trained in appropriate infection prevention practices. Routine handwashing and the use of alcohol-based hand cleansers should be encouraged. Use of the appropriate infection control techniques for procedures, such as tracheostomy suctioning, and appropriate care and cleaning of respiratory equipment should be stressed. Review of the importance of infection control practices in clinic may be useful. Demonstration and support of these practices by clinical staff while caring for the patients during outpatient visits is of utmost importance.

Children requiring ventilator support in the home may have difficulty with respiratory infections secondary to their underlying disorders. Patients that have undergone tracheostomy tube placement and require invasive mechanical ventilation have an increased risk for respiratory infections. Bypassing the nasopharynx and the protection provided by the nose, mouth, and upper airway contributes to recurrent tracheal infections. The tracheostomy tube also provides a direct entryway for infectious agents into the lower airway. Lastly, the presence of the tracheostomy tube in the airway and the need for suctioning of the tube to clear the airway may lead to tracheal ulceration, denudation, and inflammation predisposing to the development of infection. These factors lead to both serious acute respiratory infections and result in colonization of the trachea with multiple and potentially pathogenic bacteria. Colonization of the airway has been reported in 100 % of children with long-term tracheostomy with Staphylococcus aureus and Pseudomonas aeruginosa being among the most common organisms identified [49, 50].

Differentiating acute bacterial tracheobronchitis or pneumonia from colonization of the respiratory tract or a viral upper or lower airway infection can be difficult. A careful history and physical are important with acute infection often leading to deterioration in the patient's respiratory status which may manifest as an increased need for ventilator support, supplemental oxygen, or suctioning of the tracheostomy. Fever, leukocytosis or leukopenia, and an elevated CRP are consistent with an acute respiratory infection. Upper airway secretions can be tested for common viral pathogens. In patients with an appropriate clinical picture, tracheal aspirates demonstrating elevated leukocytes and high colony counts of pathogenic bacteria leads to a diagnosis of tracheobronchitis. If the patient has a new or progressive infiltrate on chest radiograph a diagnosis of pneumonia can be made.

A recent study examined the usefulness of surveillance tracheal aspirate cultures in children with tracheostomies for determining treatment during acute lower respiratory infections [51]. The study demonstrated significant changes in bacteria and antibiotic sensitivities when comparing cultures obtained during an acute exacerbation to the most recent previous culture (which may have been obtained when the child was healthy for surveillance or during a prior hospitalization). The authors found there was limited value in using previous tracheal aspirate cultures to guide antibiotic therapy for acute respiratory infections in children with tracheostomy tubes.

Ventilator-associated pneumonia (VAP) is a serious complication in intensive care units leading to significant morbidity and mortality. Chenoweth et al. performed a retrospective cohort study on adult and pediatric patients receiving mechanical ventilation at home to characterize VAP in this setting [52]. They found that the incidence of VAP is significantly lower in the home setting and that VAP was most common during the first 500 days of ventilation. The authors postulate that patients may be more acutely ill when initially discharged home or that the reduction in VAP over time may be due to improved care at home as providers learn needed skills. Patients that required ventilator support for longer periods per day had a higher risk of VAP, perhaps reflecting increased severity of underlying illness or increased opportunity for bacterial contamination. VAP did not lead to death in this small cohort but did result in hospitalization in 87 % of patients affected. Studies designed to identify interventions that may reduce tracheobronchitis and VAP in the home are needed.

Once a diagnosis of bacterial tracheobronchitis or pneumonia is made the antibiotics chosen should initially cover the organisms suspected based on the child's clinical picture and history and then be modified based on the most recent cultures and sensitivities.

Antibiotics are generally given enterally or intravenously in serious infections. Little data exists to support the use of aerosolized antibiotics in the treatment or prevention of airway infections in this home-based patient population [53, 54].

Children requiring chronic ventilator support should be carefully monitored to be sure that immunizations are up to date. The American Academy of Pediatrics currently recommends annual seasonal influenza vaccination for all children and adolescents over the age of 6 months with an emphasis on immunization of children at increased risk of complications from influenza including those with lung disease and chronic medical conditions [55]. Yearly influenza vaccination should also be provided to all household contacts and out-of-home caregivers of at-risk children. Antiviral medications, such as oseltamivir, can be considered for chemoprophylaxis in chronically ill patients with contraindications to vaccination or for treatment of influenza.

Respiratory syncytial virus (RSV) can lead to severe lower respiratory tract illness in many patients that require ventilator support. Infants with severe bronchopulmonary dysplasia, complex congenital heart disease, or immunodeficiency are at particular risk. Monthly intramuscular administration of Palivizumab, a humanized mouse monoclonal antibody, during the RSV season is recommended in infants and children under the age of 24 months with CLD requiring medical therapy and congenital heart disease to reduce the risk of severe lower respiratory tract infection [56]. Families caring for infants at high risk for severe respiratory viral infections, including RSV, should be counseled to reduce exposure to these viruses through handwashing and limiting time in high-risk settings (e.g., daycare), particularly during the respiratory viral season.

Many patients requiring chronic ventilator support will also be candidates for appropriate pneumococcal vaccinations. The type of pneumococcal vaccine that should be given depends on the age and prior immunization history of the child [57]. Recommendations for and types of vaccinations required may change with research and development, up to date information can be obtained from both the Centers for Disease Control (CDC) (http://cdc.gov) and the American Academy of Pediatrics (https://www.aap.org).

Cardiology

Chronic respiratory failure that is inadequately treated can result in pulmonary hypertension which may progress to right heart failure. Hypoxia and chronic inflammation appear to be the main factors that lead to vasoconstriction, vascular remodeling, and subsequent pulmonary hypertension in patients with chronic lung disease. Hypoxic pulmonary vasoconstriction, muscularization of previously nonmuscular arteries, and capillary endothelial and smooth muscle proliferation lead to increased tone in the small pulmonary arteries [58]. In patients with obstructive sleep apnea, repetitive falls in oxygen saturation, wide swings in intrathoracic pressures and increased sympathetic tone may lead to the development of pulmonary hypertension [58]. Close monitoring is needed by the pulmonologist to guarantee that ventilator settings, whether the patient is using invasive or noninvasive ventilation, are adequate to address the patient's respiratory issues and avoid cardiac complications. Cardiology evaluation should be considered in patients with signs or symptoms that may be consistent with pulmonary hypertension or right heart failure (e.g., reduced exercise tolerance, tachycardia, cardiac enlargement on chest radiograph) or for those at risk of significant hypoxemia (e.g., poor adherence with ventilator usage, very severe respiratory disease).

Orthopedic Problems/Scoliosis

Many patients who require chronic ventilator support have neuromuscular disorders (NMD) which place them at risk of developing musculoskeletal complications. The most frequently encountered problems are scoliosis, joint contractures, bony rotational deformities, and hip dysplasia [59–61]. Because of the added negative impact on respiratory function, surveillance for scoliosis is recommended for all patients and in particular, patients with NMD. In many cases the first indications for orthopedic evaluation and treatment are musculoskeletal complaints due to pelvic obliquity, dislocation of the hip, limited balance or ability to sit, and/or back pain [59–61].

Treatment options for scoliosis include bracing and surgery. The goals of surgical correction of scoliosis include correcting the deformity to obtain a balanced spine and level pelvis and stabilize the spine to prevent progression and delay secondary respiratory complications [61]. In the immediate postoperative period, thoracic surgery, including scoliosis surgery, results in decreased lung volumes, expiratory flow rates, and oxygenation as a result of the site of surgery itself, anesthesia, pain, and decreased mobility [62]. In one study examining children undergoing surgery to correct scoliosis, pulmonary function testing declined by 60 % after surgery, remained significantly decreased at 1 week and did not return to near baseline until 1–2 months after surgery [62]. A thorough preoperative pulmonary evaluation can obviate postoperative morbidity. Preoperative pulmonary function measurements and nutritional status have been validated in multiple studies as reliable predictors of postoperative respiratory morbidity in all patients but especially in those with NMD disorders [63, 64]. Polysomnography is the gold standard for documentation of sleep-disordered breathing (nocturnal hypoventilation, hypoxemia, and obstructive sleep apnea). While polysomnography has not yet been shown to be a reliable preoperative marker for postoperative complications, the detection of sleep-disordered breathing demonstrates existing pulmonary compromise and the necessity of initiating therapy such as noninvasive positive airway pressure ventilation pre- and/or postoperatively [65, 66].

A variety of surgical approaches have been used to correct scoliosis in patients with NMD, the type and timing of which require careful thought due to the increased risk of anesthetic and surgical complications (postoperative wound infections, bleeding, respiratory compromise) [59–61, 63, 67–73]. Preoperative assessment of surgical and anesthesia risk includes an understanding of the primary disease and its prognosis, the preoperative risk factors (i.e., poor baseline pulmonary function measurements, non-ambulatory status, preoperative curve magnitude, the presence of a ventriculoperitoneal shunt), and the goal for surgical correction (preservation of lung function versus performance and function in activities of daily living). The long-term effects of scoliosis surgery on lung function are debated. One study from Velasco et al. showed a significant decrease in the rate of decline in forced vital capacity (FVC) in Duchenne muscular dystrophy patients following surgical correction of scoliosis when compared to pre-surgery rates [74]. In contrast, an observational study from Alexander et al. did not show any reduction in the rate of FVC decline in Duchenne patients who had posterior spinal fusion compared to patients who had not undergone surgical correction [75]. Correction of scoliosis surgically can improve quality of life via improvement in pelvic obliquity and sitting balance [68, 73].

Bone health is an important consideration in the care of many of the patients requiring long-term ventilator support. Poor mobility, poor nutrition, and glucocorticoid therapy are factors which may place a patient on chronic ventilator support at risk of secondary osteoporosis resulting in bone pain or fractures [76]. Vitamin D deficiency has been shown to be common in adult patients with neuromuscular disease and chronic respiratory failure, likely due to inadequate intake of vitamin D and insufficient sun exposure [77]. Maintaining adequate Vitamin D and serum calcium levels is one component of bone care. Patients with clinical predictors of osteoporosis, including low-impact fractures or backache, or incidental osteopenia in radiographs should be referred to endocrinology for evaluation [76].

Nutrition in Patients Requiring Chronic Ventilator Support

Patients with chronic respiratory failure are at risk for a variety of nutritional complications. Malnutrition is commonly seen in children requiring long-term ventilator support. Along with poor somatic growth, patients who are undernourished may also have decreased respiratory muscle strength and be more prone to infection, increasing their dependence on mechanical ventilation. There are a number of factors that can lead to malnutrition in this group of patients. In patients with lung disease, upper airway obstruction or neuromuscular disease increased respiratory muscle work results in increased energy demands which enhance the risk of malnutrition [78]. Systemic inflammation is another important factor contributing to hypermetabolism and loss of body cell mass through catabolic activity [78, 79]. Many children requiring ventilator support are at risk of swallowing dysfunction which may lead to poor nutrition. Swallowing dysfunction is a common difficulty in many of the conditions that lead to chronic respiratory failure, for example neuromuscular disorders. Children requiring chronic invasive ventilator support may have swallowing dysfunction related to the tracheostomy. In patients with a tracheostomy swallowing dysfunction may be related to multiple factors including the anchoring of the trachea to the skin and neck muscles limiting the motion of the larynx, disruption of normal airway pressures which play a role in movement of a bolus through the pharynx and a decrease in the glottic closure response [80, 81]. The ATS consensus statement addressing the care of children with tracheostomy recommended swallowing evaluations after tracheostomy in all patients [34]. Gastrointestinal issues such as gastroesophageal reflux, diarrhea (e.g., related to medications such as antibiotics or infection with Clostridium difficile) or constipation (e.g., due to immobility, low fiber diets, dehydration) may also contribute to poor feeding and nutritional compromise.

The goal of treatment for nutritional failure in children on home chronic ventilation should be to provide adequate nutrition safely. Children with dysfunctional swallow may benefit from changes in food consistency such as thickened liquids or pureed diets. Videofluoroscopic swallow studies or clinical evaluation by an expert in feeding and swallowing can help objectively assess possible interventions. Some children with normal swallowing function may be unable to take in the calories they require secondary to fatigue related to chronic illness. When appropriate nutrition cannot be safely delivered by oral feeding, gastrostomy tube placement should be considered. Management of feeding plans by an expert in nutritional assessment and interventions is an important component of the outpatient care of patients in chronic respiratory failure.

Obesity is another common problem among patients with chronic respiratory disease and a requirement for ventilator support. Decreased mobility and treatment with glucocorticoids are some of the risk factors for excessive weight gain. Excessive weight gain can have negative effects on respiratory function and increase the risk of upper airway obstruction [82–84]. Nutritional counseling with the goal of maintaining ideal weight and body mass index should be part of the ongoing care of these patients.

CPAP or bi-level-positive airway pressure therapy is often provided to OSAS patients who are obese and either were not candidates for adenotonsillectomy or did not have resolution of their OSAS with adenotonsillectomy (Chap. 13). In these patients weight loss should be encouraged and can improve OSAS, possibly reducing their reliance on PAP therapy [85–87]. The amount of weight loss required to result in improvement in OSAS has not been determined but attaining and maintaining a healthy weight, both to improve OSAS and avoid the other many consequences of obesity, is a goal for all children.

Dentistry

There is growing medical literature supporting the need for instituting good oral health practices as a disease prevention strategy for both healthy adults and children. Good oral health includes care of the gums, teeth, and oral mucosa. Disease and decay may impair the ability to properly chew and swallow resulting in malnutrition and dehydration; impair the ability to socialize and communicate due to poor speech and smile; and cause pain resulting in poor sleep and behavior. Poor oral health can also lead to localized and then disseminated infection as well as increase the risk for chronic inflammatory-based systemic diseases [88, 89]. In the critical care setting, guidelines are being established for oral care protocols to reduce the incidence of ventilator-associated pneumonia (VAP) in critically ill patients with an endotracheal tube [90, 91]. However there is a paucity of peer-reviewed published medical literature showing the effectiveness of oral care in preventing VAP in patients mechanically ventilated with a tracheostomy. A recent article demonstrated the simple oral care in the form of tooth brushing with toothpaste and applying chlorhexidine gluconate 0.12 % oral rinse solution may be effective in reducing the VAP rate in patients with tracheostomies who were being mechanically ventilated in a step-down unit [92].

As modern healthcare has increased the lifespan of patients with special health-care needs, oral health has grown as an unmet healthcare need. Patients with special healthcare needs have a multifold risk for developing oral disease and decay. They are also more likely to have oral infections, periodontal disease, enamel irregularities, broken teeth, and moderate-to-severe malocclusion [93, 94]. Underlying medical conditions may place ventilator-dependent children at increased risk for developing oral disease. Other important factors which lead to poor oral health in this group of patients include the need to rely on a caregiver to provide routine oral care, impaired ability to effectively clear oral contents due to issues with chewing and/or swallowing, impaired salivary production, the type of diet with liquid nutrition having a higher sugar content, overindulgence of caretakers, gastroesophageal reflux disease, and facial deformities [95].

Patients with chronic, complex healthcare needs often have difficulty accessing appropriate dental care. Factors such as lack of or inadequate dental insurance, household income, parent-reported dental health, transportation issues, difficulty finding an appropriate and willing dental provider, and parents' perception regarding the need for oral healthcare can lead to poor oral health in complex children [96, 97].

Social Work and Community Resources

Guidelines providing criteria for home discharge of patients requiring chronic ventilator support list adequate financial resources to access care outside of the hospital and provide needed equipment as a criteria for discharge home [18, 98, 99]. For many families, changes in insurance coverage due to changes in employment, economic status or once the patient reaches adulthood brings challenges. Families often need help in the community, working with local school systems to develop appropriate educational plans for school-aged children, accessing transportation services for wheelchair or bed-bound patients or locating respite care services. A clinic social worker or team members skilled in addressing funding/insurance issues and in accessing community resources can be an invaluable member of the care team.

Transition to Adult Care

When children dependent on home mechanical ventilation reach adolescence, a successful transition of care from pediatric to adult healthcare providers must be provided. Providing services to transition children with complex medical needs to adult healthcare has been mandated by the Department of Health and Human Services, Maternal and Child Health Bureau as a core measure required to create a comprehensive system of services for youth with special healthcare needs and supported by the National Committee on Quality Assurance, the American Academy of Pediatrics, the American Academy of Family Physicians and the American College of Physicians [100–102]. This process can be difficult and patients are at risk of emotional and financial stress, interrupted healthcare and negative health outcomes during the transition period. Adult providers may be unfamiliar with chronic conditions that may have been limited to pediatrics in the past complicating the transition process. Poor healthcare funding for young adults (or a sudden change in insurance coverage) can limit access to physicians and needed services and equipment. A recent survey found that among academic pediatric pulmonary programs caring for respiratory technology-dependent patients, few had standardized transition programs for their patients [103]. Core elements for successful transition may include (1) a written transition policy for the clinic (2) a registry for identification and tracking of patients, (3) tools to facilitate transition planning, such as a transition readiness assessment and portable medical summary and (4) organized and timely transfer to adult providers [104]. Resources for clinics developing transition programs can be found at www.gottransition.org [105].

Children requiring chronic ventilator support in the home are a diverse and complex group of patients with many healthcare needs. Given the multiple medical issues that may be faced by these patients, families are often asked to navigate a medical system characterized by poor access to physicians or other needed medical professionals, significant variations in practice and fragmented care. For many patients, limited family and community resources also affect care. Outpatient clinic physicians and staff can play an important role in providing and coordinating the patient's care needs with the goal of improving outcomes. Funding, research, and clinical guidelines to assist practitioners caring for these patients are urgently needed.

References

1. Edwards JD, Kun SS, Keens TG. Outcomes and causes of death in children on home mechanical ventilation via tracheostomy: an institutional and literature review. J Pediatr. 2010;157(6):955–9. e2. Epub 2010/08/18. eng.
2. Reiter K, Pernath N, Pagel P, Hiedi S, Hoffmann F, Schoen C, et al. Risk factors for morbidity and mortality in pediatric home mechanical ventilation. Clin Pediatr. 2011;50(3):237–43. Epub 2010/12/04. eng.
3. Cristea AI, Carroll AE, Davis SD, Swigonski NL, Ackerman VL. Outcomes of children with severe bronchopulmonary dysplasia who were ventilator dependent at home. Pediatrics. 2013;132(3):e727–34. Pubmed Central PMCID: PMC3876749, Epub 2013/08/07. eng.

4. Statement on home care for patients with respiratory disorders. Am J Respir Crit Care Med. 2005;171(12):1443–64. Epub 2005/06/09. eng.
5. Elias ER, Murphy NA. Home care of children and youth with complex health care needs and technology dependencies. Pediatrics. 2012;129(5):996–1005. Epub 2012/05/02. eng.
6. King AC. Long-term home mechanical ventilation in the United States. Respir Care. 2012;57(6):921–30. discussion 30-2. Epub 2012/06/06. eng.
7. McDougall CM, Adderley RJ, Wensley DF, Seear MD. Long-term ventilation in children: longitudinal trends and outcomes. Arch Dis Child. 2013;98(9):660–5. Epub 2013/07/11. eng.
8. Amin R, Sayal P, Syed F, Chaves A, Moraes TJ, MacLusky I. Pediatric long-term home mechanical ventilation: twenty years of follow-up from one Canadian center. Pediatr Pulmonol. 2014;49(8):816–24. Epub 2013/09/04. eng.
9. Nasilowski J, Wachulski M, Trznadel W, Andrzejewski W, Migdal M, Drozd W, et al. The evolution of home mechanical ventilation in poland between 2000 and 2010. Respir Care. 2015;60(4):577–85. Epub 2014/12/11. eng.
10. Han YJ, Park JD, Lee B, Choi YH, Suh DI, Lim BC, et al. Home mechanical ventilation in childhood-onset hereditary neuromuscular diseases: 13 years' experience at a single center in Korea. PLoS One. 2015;10(3), e0122346. Pubmed Central PMCID: PMC4379105, Epub 2015/03/31. eng.
11. Kuo DZ, Goudie A, Cohen E, Houtrow A, Agrawal R, Carle AC, et al. Inequities in health care needs for children with medical complexity. Health Aff. 2014;33(12):2190–8. Pubmed Central PMCID: PMC4334319, Epub 2014/12/10. eng.
12. Heaton J, Noyes J, Sloper P, Shah R. Families' experiences of caring for technology-dependent children: a temporal perspective. Health Soc Care Community. 2005;13(5):441–50. Epub 2005/07/29. eng.
13. Tsara V, Serasli E, Voutsas V, Lazarides V, Christaki P. Burden and coping strategies in families of patients under noninvasive home mechanical ventilation. Respiration. 2006;73(1):61–7. Epub 2005/08/18. eng.
14. Mah JK, Thannhauser JE, McNeil DA, Dewey D. Being the lifeline: the parent experience of caring for a child with neuromuscular disease on home mechanical ventilation. Neuromuscul Disord. 2008;18(12):983–8. Epub 2008/11/01. eng.
15. Carnevale FA, Alexander E, Davis M, Rennick J, Troini R. Daily living with distress and enrichment: the moral experience of families with ventilator-assisted children at home. Pediatrics. 2006;117(1):e48–60. Epub 2006/01/07. eng.
16. Toly VB, Musil CM, Carl JC. Families with children who are technology dependent: normalization and family functioning. West J Nurs Res. 2012;34(1):52–71. Pubmed Central PMCID: PMC3271785, Epub 2010/12/15. eng.
17. van Huijzen S, van Staa A. Chronic ventilation and social participation: experiences of men with neuromuscular disorders. Scand J Occup Ther. 2013;20(3):209–16. Epub 2013/01/24. eng.
18. Nixon GM, Edwards EA, Cooper DM, Fitzgerald DA, Harris M, Martin J, et al. Ventilatory support at home for children: a consensus statement from the Australasian Paediatric Respiratory Group; 2008. http://www.thoracic.org.au/professional-information/position-papers-guidelines/oxygen-therapy-home-ventilation/.
19. Farre R, Navajas D, Prats E, Marti S, Guell R, Montserrat JM, et al. Performance of mechanical ventilators at the patient's home: a multicentre quality control study. Thorax. 2006;61(5):400–4. Pubmed Central PMCID: PMC2111198, Epub 2006/02/10. eng.
20. Marcus CL, Ward SL, Mallory GB, Rosen CL, Beckerman RC, Weese-Mayer DE, et al. Use of nasal continuous positive airway pressure as treatment of childhood obstructive sleep apnea. J Pediatr. 1995;127(1):88–94. Epub 1995/07/01. eng.
21. Fauroux B, Lavis JF, Nicot F, Picard A, Boelle PY, Clement A, et al. Facial side effects during noninvasive positive pressure ventilation in children. Intensive Care Med. 2005;31(7):965–9. Epub 2005/06/01. eng.
22. Massie CA, Hart RW, Peralez K, Richards GN. Effects of humidification on nasal symptoms and compliance in sleep apnea patients using continuous positive airway pressure. Chest. 1999;116(2):403–8. Epub 1999/08/24. eng.

23. Li KK, Riley RW, Guilleminault C. An unreported risk in the use of home nasal continuous positive airway pressure and home nasal ventilation in children: mid-face hypoplasia. Chest. 2000;117(3):916–8. Epub 2000/03/14. eng.
24. Villa MP, Pagani J, Ambrosio R, Ronchetti R, Bernkopf E. Mid-face hypoplasia after long-term nasal ventilation. Am J Respir Crit Care Med. 2002;166(8):1142–3. Epub 2002/10/16. eng.
25. Marcus CL, Rosen G, Ward SL, Halbower AC, Sterni L, Lutz J, et al. Adherence to and effectiveness of positive airway pressure therapy in children with obstructive sleep apnea. Pediatrics. 2006;117(3):e442–51. Epub 2006/03/03. eng.
26. Nixon GM, Mihai R, Verginis N, Davey MJ. Patterns of continuous positive airway pressure adherence during the first 3 months of treatment in children. J Pediatr. 2011;159(5):802–7. Epub 2011/05/24. eng.
27. Sawyer AM, Gooneratne NS, Marcus CL, Ofer D, Richards KC, Weaver TE. A systematic review of CPAP adherence across age groups: clinical and empiric insights for developing CPAP adherence interventions. Sleep Med Rev. 2011;15(6):343–56. Pubmed Central PMCID: PMC3202028, Epub 2011/06/10. eng.
28. DiFeo N, Meltzer LJ, Beck SE, Karamessinis LR, Cornaglia MA, Traylor J, et al. Predictors of positive airway pressure therapy adherence in children: a prospective study. J Clin Sleep Med. 2012;8(3):279–86. Pubmed Central PMCID: PMC3365086, Epub 2012/06/16. eng.
29. Uong EC, Epperson M, Bathon SA, Jeffe DB. Adherence to nasal positive airway pressure therapy among school-aged children and adolescents with obstructive sleep apnea syndrome. Pediatrics. 2007;120(5):e1203–11. Epub 2007/10/10. eng.
30. O'Donnell AR, Bjornson CL, Bohn SG, Kirk VG. Compliance rates in children using noninvasive continuous positive airway pressure. Sleep. 2006;29(5):651–8. Epub 2006/06/16. eng.
31. Koontz KL, Slifer KJ, Cataldo MD, Marcus CL. Improving pediatric compliance with positive airway pressure therapy: the impact of behavioral intervention. Sleep. 2003;26(8):1010–5. Epub 2004/01/30. eng.
32. Jambhekar SK, Com G, Tang X, Pruss KK, Jackson R, Bower C, et al. Role of a respiratory therapist in improving adherence to positive airway pressure treatment in a pediatric sleep apnea clinic. Respir Care. 2013;58(12):2038–44. Epub 2013/06/15. eng.
33. Ramirez A, Khirani S, Aloui S, Delord V, Borel JC, Pepin JL, et al. Continuous positive airway pressure and noninvasive ventilation adherence in children. Sleep Med. 2013;14(12):1290–4. Epub 2013/10/26. eng.
34. Sherman JM, Davis S, Albamonte-Petrick S, Chatburn RL, Fitton C, Green C, et al. Care of the child with a chronic tracheostomy. This official statement of the American Thoracic Society was adopted by the ATS Board of Directors, July 1999. Am J Respir Crit Care Med. 2000;161(1):297–308. Epub 2000/01/05. eng.
35. Mitchell RB, Hussey HM, Setzen G, Jacobs IN, Nussenbaum B, Dawson C, et al. Clinical consensus statement: tracheostomy care. Otolaryngol Head Neck Surg. 2013;148(1):6–20. Epub 2012/09/20. eng.
36. Papakostas K, Morar P, Fenton JE. Ballooned trachea caused by cuffed tracheostomy tube. J Laryngol Otol. 2000;114(9):724–6. Epub 2000/11/25. eng.
37. Birnkrant DJ, Bushby KM, Amin RS, Bach JR, Benditt JO, Eagle M, et al. The respiratory management of patients with duchenne muscular dystrophy: a DMD care considerations working group specialty article. Pediatr Pulmonol. 2010;45(8):739–48. Epub 2010/07/03. eng.
38. Wang CH, Finkel RS, Bertini ES, Schroth M, Simonds A, Wong B, et al. Consensus statement for standard of care in spinal muscular atrophy. J Child Neurol. 2007;22(8):1027–49. Epub 2007/09/01. eng.
39. Widger JA, Davey MJ, Nixon GM. Sleep studies in children on long-term non-invasive respiratory support. Sleep Breath. 2014;18(4):885–9. Epub 2014/02/25. eng.
40. Kushida CA, Chediak A, Berry RB, Brown LK, Gozal D, Iber C, et al. Clinical guidelines for the manual titration of positive airway pressure in patients with obstructive sleep apnea. J Clin Sleep Med. 2008;4(2):157–71. Pubmed Central PMCID: PMC2335396, Epub 2008/05/13. eng.

41. Berry RB, Chediak A, Brown LK, Finder J, Gozal D, Iber C, et al. Best clinical practices for the sleep center adjustment of noninvasive positive pressure ventilation (NPPV) in stable chronic alveolar hypoventilation syndromes. J Clin Sleep Med. 2010;6(5):491–509. Pubmed Central PMCID: PMC2952756, Epub 2010/10/21. eng.
42. O'Brien JE, Birnkrant DJ, Dumas HM, Haley SM, Burke SA, Graham RJ, et al. Weaning children from mechanical ventilation in a post-acute care setting. Pediatr Rehabil. 2006;9(4):365–72. Epub 2006/11/23. eng.
43. The health consequences of smoking: a report of the surgeon general. Atlanta GA2004.
44. Fatal fires associated with smoking during long-term oxygen therapy—Maine, MA, New Hampshire, and Oklahoma, 2000–2007. MMWR Morb Mortal Wkly Rep. 2008;57(31):852–4. Epub 2008/08/08. eng.
45. Hall JR, Ahrens M, Rohr K, Gamache S, Comoletti J. Behavioral mitigation of smoking fires through strategies based on statistical analysis. Emmitsburg: National Fire Protection Association for US Fire Administraton, Department of Homeland Security; 2006. http://www.usfa.dhs.gov/downloads/pdf/publications/fa-302-508.pdf.
46. From the American Academy of Pediatrics. Policy statement—Tobacco use: a pediatric disease. Pediatrics. 2009;124(5):1474–87. Epub 2009/10/21. eng.
47. Services UDoHaH, Health NIo, Institute NC, USA.gov. http://smokefree.gov. Accessed 14 July 2015.
48. Kun SS, Edwards JD, Ward SL, Keens TG. Hospital readmissions for newly discharged pediatric home mechanical ventilation patients. Pediatr Pulmonol. 2012;47(4):409–14. Pubmed Central PMCID: PMC3694986, Epub 2011/09/09. eng.
49. Morar P, Singh V, Jones AS, Hughes J, van Saene R. Impact of tracheotomy on colonization and infection of lower airways in children requiring long-term ventilation: a prospective observational cohort study. Chest. 1998;113(1):77–85. Epub 1998/01/24. eng.
50. Brook I. Bacterial colonization, tracheobronchitis, and pneumonia following tracheostomy and long-term intubation in pediatric patients. Chest. 1979;76(4):420–4. Epub 1979/10/01. eng.
51. Cline JM, Woods CR, Ervin SE, Rubin BK, Kirse DJ. Surveillance tracheal aspirate cultures do not reliably predict bacteria cultured at the time of an acute respiratory infection in children with tracheostomy tubes. Chest. 2012;141(3):625–31. Epub 2011/03/26. eng.
52. Chenoweth CE, Washer LL, Obeyesekera K, Friedman C, Brewer K, Fugitt GE, et al. Ventilator-associated pneumonia in the home care setting. Infect Control Hosp Epidemiol. 2007;28(8):910–5. Epub 2007/07/11. eng.
53. Hagerman JK, Hancock KE, Klepser ME. Aerosolised antibiotics: a critical appraisal of their use. Expert Opin Drug Deliv. 2006;3(1):71–86. Epub 2005/12/24. eng.
54. Abu-Salah T, Dhand R. Inhaled antibiotic therapy for ventilator-associated tracheobronchitis and ventilator-associated pneumonia: an update. Adv Ther. 2011;28(9):728–47. Epub 2011/08/13. eng.
55. Committee On Infectious Diseases, American Academy Pediatrics. Recommendations for prevention and control of influenza in children, 2014–2015. Pediatrics. 2014;134(5):e1503–19. Epub 2014/09/24. eng.
56. Kimberlin MD, Brady MT, Jackson M, Long SS. Respiratory Syncytial Virus. Red Book 2015: Report of the Committee on Infectious Diseases. 30th ed. Elk Grove Village: American Academy of Pediatrics; 2015. p. 667–76.
57. Kimberlin MD, Brady MT, Jackson M, Long SS. Pneumococcal infections. Red Book 2015: a report from the committee on infectious diseases. 30th ed. Elk Grove Village: American Academy of Pediatrics; 2015. p. 626–38.
58. Zangiabadi A, De Pasquale CG, Sajkov D. Pulmonary hypertension and right heart dysfunction in chronic lung disease. BioMed Res Int. 2014;2014:739674. Pubmed Central PMCID: PMC4140123, Epub 2014/08/29. eng.
59. Driscoll SW, Skinner J. Musculoskeletal complications of neuromuscular disease in children. Phys Med Rehabil Clin N Am. 2008;19(1):163–94. viii. Epub 2008/01/16. eng.
60. Ferrari A, Ferrara C, Balugani M, Sassi S. Severe scoliosis in neurodevelopmental disabilities: clinical signs and therapeutic proposals. Eur J Phys Rehabil Med. 2010;46(4):563–80. Epub 2011/01/13. eng.

61. Piazzolla A, Solarino G, De Giorgi S, Mori CM, Moretti L, De Giorgi G. Cotrel-Dubousset instrumentation in neuromuscular scoliosis. Eur Spine J. 2011;20 Suppl 1:S75–84. Pubmed Central PMCID: PMC3087033, Epub 2011/03/16. eng.
62. Yuan N, Fraire JA, Margetis MM, Skaggs DL, Tolo VT, Keens TG. The effect of scoliosis surgery on lung function in the immediate postoperative period. Spine. 2005;30(19):2182–5. Epub 2005/10/06. eng.
63. Yuan N, Skaggs DL, Dorey F, Keens TG. Preoperative predictors of prolonged postoperative mechanical ventilation in children following scoliosis repair. Pediatr Pulmonol. 2005;40(5):414–9. Epub 2005/09/08. eng.
64. Johnston CE. Preoperative medical and surgical planning for early onset scoliosis. Spine. 2010;35(25):2239–44. Epub 2010/11/26. eng.
65. Yuan N, Skaggs DL, Davidson Ward SL, Platzker AC, Keens TG. Preoperative polysomno-grams and infant pulmonary function tests do not predict prolonged postoperative mechanical ventilation in children following scoliosis repair. Pediatr Pulmonol. 2004;38(3):256–60. Epub 2004/07/27. eng.
66. Katz SL, Gaboury I, Keilty K, Banwell B, Vajsar J, Anderson P, et al. Nocturnal hypoventilation: predictors and outcomes in childhood progressive neuromuscular disease. Arch Dis Child. 2010;95(12):998–1003. Epub 2010/09/03. eng.
67. Lonstein JE, Koop SE, Novachek TF, Perra JH. Results and complications after spinal fusion for neuromuscular scoliosis in cerebral palsy and static encephalopathy using luque galveston instrumentation: experience in 93 patients. Spine. 2012;37(7):583–91. Epub 2011/06/16. eng.
68. Van Opstal N, Verlinden C, Myncke J, Goemans N, Moens P. The effect of Luque-Galveston fusion on curve, respiratory function and quality of life in Duchenne muscular dystrophy. Acta Orthop Belg. 2011;77(5):659–65. Epub 2011/12/23. eng.
69. White KK, Song KM, Frost N, Daines BK. VEPTR growing rods for early-onset neuromuscular scoliosis: feasible and effective. Clin Orthop Relat Res. 2011;469(5):1335–41. Pubmed Central PMCID: PMC3069260, Epub 2011/01/08. eng.
70. Kang GR, Suh SW, Lee IO. Preoperative predictors of postoperative pulmonary complications in neuromuscular scoliosis. J Orthop Sci. 2011;16(2):139–47. Epub 2011/02/12. eng.
71. Master DL, Poe-Kochert C, Son-Hing J, Armstrong DG, Thompson GH. Wound infections after surgery for neuromuscular scoliosis: risk factors and treatment outcomes. Spine. 2011;36(3):E179–85. Epub 2011/01/21. eng.
72. Master DL, Son-Hing JP, Poe-Kochert C, Armstrong DG, Thompson GH. Risk factors for major complications after surgery for neuromuscular scoliosis. Spine. 2011;36(7):564–71. Epub 2010/08/05. eng.
73. Moon ES, Nanda A, Park JO, Moon SH, Lee HM, Kim JY, et al. Pelvic obliquity in neuromuscular scoliosis: radiologic comparative results of single-stage posterior versus two-stage anterior and posterior approach. Spine. 2011;36(2):146–52. Epub 2010/07/17. eng.
74. Velasco MV, Colin AA, Zurakowski D, Darras BT, Shapiro F. Posterior spinal fusion for scoliosis in duchenne muscular dystrophy diminishes the rate of respiratory decline. Spine. 2007;32(4):459–65. Epub 2007/02/17. eng.
75. Alexander WM, Smith M, Freeman BJ, Sutherland LM, Kennedy JD, Cundy PJ. The effect of posterior spinal fusion on respiratory function in Duchenne muscular dystrophy. Eur Spine J. 2013;22(2):411–6. Pubmed Central PMCID: PMC3555614, Epub 2012/11/28. eng.
76. Saraff V, Hoegler WENDOCRINOLOGYANDADOLESCENCE. Osteoporosis in children: diagnosis and management. Eur J Endocrinol. 2015;173(6):R186–93. Epub 2015/06/05. Eng.
77. Badireddi S, Bercher AJ, Holder JB, Mireles-Cabodevila E. Vitamin D deficiency in patients with neuromuscular diseases with chronic respiratory failure. J Parenter Enteral Nutr. 2014;38(5):602–7. Epub 2013/06/12. eng.
78. Schols AMWJ. Nutrition and respiratory disease. Clin Nutr. 2001;20(Supplement 1):173–9.
79. Soeters PB, Reijven PL, van Bokhorst-de van der Schueren MA, Schols JM, Halfens RJ, Meijers JM, et al. A rational approach to nutritional assessment. Clin Nutr. 2008;27(5):706–16. Epub 2008/09/12. eng.

80. Bonanno PC. Swallowing dysfunction after tracheostomy. Ann Surg. 1971;174(1):29–33. Pubmed Central PMCID: PMC1397436, Epub 1971/07/01. eng.
81. Dikeman KJ, Kazandjian MS. Pathophysiology of swallowing. Communication and swallowing management of tracheostomized and ventilator dependent adults. San Diego, CA: Singular Publishing Group; 1995. p. 229–49.
82. Deane S, Thomson A. Obesity and the pulmonologist. Arch Dis Child. 2006;91(2):188–91. Pubmed Central PMCID: PMC2082679, Epub 2006/01/24. eng.
83. Davidson WJ, Mackenzie-Rife KA, Witmans MB, Montgomery MD, Ball GD, Egbogah S, et al. Obesity negatively impacts lung function in children and adolescents. Pediatr Pulmonol. 2014;49(10):1003–10. Epub 2013/10/30. eng.
84. Mathew JL, Narang I. Sleeping too close together: obesity and obstructive sleep apnea in childhood and adolescence. Paediatr Respir Rev. 2014;15(3):211–8. Epub 2013/10/08. eng.
85. Marcus CL, Brooks LJ, Draper KA, Gozal D, Halbower AC, Jones J, et al. Diagnosis and management of childhood obstructive sleep apnea syndrome. Pediatrics. 2012;130(3):576–84. Epub 2012/08/29. eng.
86. Verhulst S. Toward a multidisciplinary approach to the treatment of obstructive sleep apnea in the obese child. Otolaryngol Head Neck Surg. 2009;141(4):549. Epub 2009/09/30. eng.
87. Kalra M, Inge T. Effect of bariatric surgery on obstructive sleep apnoea in adolescents. Paediatr Respir Rev. 2006;7(4):260–7. Epub 2006/11/14. eng.
88. Offenbacher S, Barros SP, Altarawneh S, Beck JD, Loewy ZG. Impact of tooth loss on oral and systemic health. Gen Dent. 2012;60(6):494–500; quiz p 1–2. Epub 2012/12/12. eng.
89. Babu NC, Gomes AJ. Systemic manifestations of oral diseases. J Oral Maxillofacial Pathol. 2011;15(2):144–7. Pubmed Central PMCID: PMC3329699, Epub 2012/04/25. eng.
90. Shi Z, Xie H, Wang P, Zhang Q, Wu Y, Chen E, et al. Oral hygiene care for critically ill patients to prevent ventilator-associated pneumonia. Cochrane Database Syst Rev. 2013;8, CD008367. Epub 2013/08/14. eng.
91. Muscedere J, Dodek P, Keenan S, Fowler R, Cook D, Heyland D. Comprehensive evidence-based clinical practice guidelines for ventilator-associated pneumonia: prevention. J Crit Care. 2008;23(1):126–37. Epub 2008/03/25. eng.
92. Conley P, McKinsey D, Graff J, Ramsey AR. Does an oral care protocol reduce VAP in patients with a tracheostomy? Nursing. 2013;43(7):18–23. Epub 2013/06/20. eng.
93. da Fonseca MA. Dental and oral care for chronically ill children and adolescents. Gen Dent. 2010;58(3):204–9. quiz 10-1. Epub 2010/05/19. eng.
94. Norwood Jr KW, Slayton RL. Oral health care for children with developmental disabilities. Pediatrics. 2013;131(3):614–9. Epub 2013/02/27. eng.
95. Moursi AM, Fernandez JB, Daronch M, Zee L, Jones CL. Nutrition and oral health considerations in children with special health care needs: implications for oral health care providers. Pediatr Dent. 2010;32(4):333–42. Epub 2010/09/15. eng.
96. Kenney MK, Kogan MD, Crall JJ. Parental perceptions of dental/oral health among children with and without special health care needs. Ambul Pediatr. 2008;8(5):312–20. Epub 2008/10/17. eng.
97. Iida H, Lewis CW. Utility of a summative scale based on the Children with Special Health Care Needs (CSHCN) Screener to identify CSHCN with special dental care needs. Matern Child Health J. 2012;16(6):1164–72. Epub 2011/10/15. eng.
98. McKim DA, Road J, Avendano M, Abdool S, Cote F, Duguid N, et al. Home mechanical ventilation: a Canadian Thoracic Society clinical practice guideline. Can Respir J. 2011;18(4):197–215. Pubmed Central PMCID: PMC3205101, Epub 2011/11/08. eng.
99. Jardine E, Wallis C. Core guidelines for the discharge home of the child on long-term assisted ventilation in the United Kingdom. UK Working Party on Paediatric Long Term Ventilation. Thorax. 1998;53(9):762–7. Pubmed Central PMCID: PMC1745309, Epub 1999/05/13. eng.
100. Cooley WC, Sagerman PJ. Supporting the health care transition from adolescence to adulthood in the medical home. Pediatrics. 2011;128(1):182–200. Epub 2011/06/29. eng.
101. The National Survey of Children with Special Health Care Needs Chartbook 2005–2006: Core Outcomes 2012. www.mchb.hrsa.gov/cshcn05/MI/cokmp.pdf.

102. Assurance NCoQ. Standards for Patient-Centered Medical Home (PCMH). Washington DC: National Committee on Quality Assurance; 2011.
103. Agarwal A, Willis D, Tang X, Bauer M, Berlinski A, Com G, et al. Transition of respiratory technology dependent patients from pediatric to adult pulmonology care. Pediatr Pulmonol. 2015;50(12):1294–300. Epub 2015/02/06. Eng.
104. McManus MA, Pollack LR, Cooley WC, McAllister JW, Lotstein D, Strickland B, et al. Current status of transition preparation among youth with special needs in the United States. Pediatrics. 2013;131(6):1090–7. Epub 2013/05/15. eng.
105. Health TNAtAA. Got Transition Washington, DC: The National Alliance to Advance Adolescent Health; 2014. www.gottransition.org. Accessed 14 July 2015.

Chapter 9
In-Home Care of the Child on Chronic Mechanical Ventilation

Deborah S. Boroughs and Joan Dougherty

Introduction

In the United States, approximately one million persons per year receive mechanical ventilation during their stays in intensive care units. The number of patients requiring prolonged mechanical ventilation beyond the hospital stay is rapidly increasing [1]. There is no US national registry of ventilator-dependent patients at home; therefore, the exact number of home ventilator patients is unknown. A conservative estimate of approximately 21,000 persons receiving mechanical ventilation at home can be extrapolated from the existing US 2010 data. Of this total number, it was estimated that approximately 4800 were children under the age of 18 who were supported with invasive mechanical ventilation [2]. Drawing conclusions from the number of ventilator-dependent children reported in Pennsylvania in 2012 and US population data, it is estimated that there are as many as 8000 children, ages birth through 21 years who are dependent upon some type of mechanical ventilation at home [3].

Mechanical ventilation is a high-stakes, high-risk intervention, especially for pediatric patients in the home setting. Secondary to acute illnesses or the natural progression of disease, some of these patients will require rehospitalization. Some

D.S. Boroughs, R.N., M.S.N. (✉)
Bayada Home Health Care, Pediatric Specialty Practice, 360 Route 44,
Logan Township, NJ 08085, USA
e-mail: debbyboroughs@gmail.com

J. Dougherty, B.S.N., C.P.N., C.S.N.
Pennsylvania Ventilator Assisted Children's Home Program (VACHP),
Wanamaker Building, 9th Floor, One Hundred Penn Square East, Philadelphia,
PA 19107, USA
e-mail: doughertyj@email.chop.edu

© Springer Science+Business Media New York 2016
L.M. Sterni, J.L. Carroll (eds.), *Caring for the Ventilator Dependent Child*,
Respiratory Medicine, DOI 10.1007/978-1-4939-3749-3_9

readmissions, however, are avoidable and are directly related to the quality of care received in the home, including inappropriate caregiver interventions and responses. The consequences of recurrent illnesses and readmissions are significant and include morbidity, mortality, family stress, and financial implications for the family and the healthcare system. Providing quality homecare through caregiver training may reduce avoidable readmissions [4].

Despite technological advances in home monitoring of ventilated patients, the preventable death rate among children at home has not changed significantly during the last two decades. Analyses of the data indicate that the three primary causes of preventable death in ventilator-dependent children at home are inadequate caregiver preparation and training, improper emergency response by caregivers, and a lack of vigilance [3]. In order for families to be successful and to experience a sense of reward and fulfillment in caring for their ventilator-dependent child at home, many factors must be considered. Even when caregivers are willing and able to care for their child, they are often faced with a heroic task that can prove to be overwhelming if proper preparation and ongoing supports are inadequate. Since 1979, the Pennsylvania Ventilator-Assisted Children's Home Program (VACHP) has provided services to more than 1000 ventilator-dependent children. These children, ranging in age from birth to 22 years old, can be grouped into three diagnostic categories: chronic lung disease (CLD), congenital anomaly or syndrome (CA), and neuromuscular/nervous system disorders (NM/NS). Approximately 83 % of these ventilator-dependent patients receive invasive mechanical ventilation and 17 % receive noninvasive mechanical ventilation. All of the VACHP patients qualify for home nursing services. The death rate of the VACHP children while enrolled in the programme is 18–20 % and the preventable death rate has remained nearly the same at 27 % of all deaths [3]. This accidental death rate is similar to findings of a large study reviewing outcomes of children and young adults on invasive ventilation support over 22 years, which reported a cumulative 5- and 10-year survival rate of 80 %. In this study approximately one-third of the deaths of children on mechanical ventilation were due to progression of the underlying disorder [5].

Preparation for Mechanical Ventilation of a Child at Home

Many children's hospitals have developed criteria for discharge of a ventilator-dependent child to home. Discharge criteria may vary for children being discharged on invasive mechanical ventilation versus noninvasive mechanical ventilation, but for all children being discharged on mechanical ventilation, there are factors to consider in preparing for discharge including:

Medical stability—The patient's airway, whether natural or artificial (tracheostomy), must be stable. The patient should demonstrate respiratory stability, there should be no acute decompensation events for several weeks prior to discharge. The supplemental oxygen requirement should not exceed 40 % since it is difficult to maintain a home oxygen supply when children require >50 % [6]. Ideally, the patient would successfully use the home ventilator in the hospital for at least 2 weeks prior to discharge, but this varies according to availability of the home ventilator and insurance coverage.

Psychosocial considerations—The family caregivers must consistently visit in the hospital and agree to learn all of the child's medical care. The caregivers must be able to meet the basic needs of food, clothing, housing, safety, and stimulation at home.

Family caregiver training—At least two identified family caregivers must complete tracheostomy and ventilator management training in the hospital and achieve competency in all required skills, treatments, technologies, and cardiopulmonary resuscitation (CPR). Caregivers do not have to be the child's biological parents, and in homes with single caregivers, a relative, friend, or neighbor may be the identified backup caregiver. A successful independent 24-h stay with the child must be accomplished by the family caregivers. Although the length of training programmes vary, caregivers can expect the training to take 6–8 weeks [6].

Environmental safety—The home must have space for the child's equipment and caregivers. The home must be safe from fire, pest, and health hazards, have a working telephone, and have adequate electrical and heating systems. Homes should be geographically located within reasonable distance of emergency services, and backup generators should be considered for homes where power outages occur frequently [6].

Financial considerations—The family must have appropriate resources to provide all basic needs of the child. The child must have health insurance coverage and insurance authorizations for needed home equipment, and services must be obtained prior to discharge. Families should be prepared for increases in their electric and water bills once the child is at home, and the reality that they may lose income from missed work hours when the child is ill or no homecare nurse is available.

Home nursing care—Ideally, the family is able to select an accredited nursing agency that provides experienced, trained, and skilled nurses who will provide safe care according to the physician's plan of care, but unfortunately family choice may be limited or dictated by the insurer. The agency selected must be prepared to fill the number of authorized nursing shifts to the best of its ability. At a minimum, the agency nurse manager should meet the child and family prior to discharge. The family should have the opportunity to meet the homecare nurses assigned to the case prior to discharge from the hospital so that they may be able to ask questions about the nurses' experience and qualifications to care for their child.

Respiratory needs—A reliable respiratory company that specializes in ventilator equipment and that is available 24 h a day, 365 days a year must be selected. The clinicians employed by the company must be experienced, skilled, and prepared to provide ongoing training to caregivers in the home. A home visit by the respiratory therapist or other appropriately trained staff prior to discharge from the hospital must include an environmental assessment and complete set up of all equipment and supplies. The company must make a commitment to supply, monitor, and replace equipment as it is needed and on a routine schedule. If the respiratory company cannot provide all the child's non-respiratory equipment needs, a durable medical equipment company (DME) must also be identified.

Proper Preparation of Caregivers

In order to ensure the best outcomes for a child who is supported by mechanical ventilation at home, proper preparation of all caregivers is essential.

Preparation of Family Caregivers

For caregivers of children receiving invasive mechanical ventilation, Storgion suggests that the formalized tracheostomy and ventilator management training provided by hospital staff to family caregivers include:

- Routine and emergency tracheostomy care with return demonstration on the patient
- Routine and emergency ventilator management using the home ventilator with the patient
- Responding to hypothetical emergency scenarios
- Demonstration of equipment management—pulse oximetry, assistive coughing and suction devices, respiratory therapy equipment including oxygen and nebulizer equipment
- Independent, overnight care of child while in hospital with a feedback and evaluation session
- CPR certification and specialized emergency training using the tracheostomy as the primary airway
- Instruction for safe transport of child and care outside of the home [7]

For caregivers of children receiving noninvasive mechanical ventilation, the same training principles apply except in place of tracheostomy training, there must be discussion and return demonstration of routine and emergency airway care, including preventing and treating appliance-related complications of nasal mask, oronasal mask, nasal pillows, or other facial appliances [8].

Preparation of Homecare Nurses

Ideally, preparation of the nurses who will care for the child in the home includes:

- A refresher course in anatomy/physiology of the pediatric respiratory system and pediatric respiratory assessment
- A mechanical ventilation theory course
- Training in routine and emergency airway care with a stepwise response
- Training in routine and emergency ventilator care and response with a stepwise response
- Instruction in hands-on operation of ventilators and airway clearance devices

- Simulation practice using emergency scenarios
- Knowledge of respiratory medications and proper sequence of administration
- A course in psychosocial aspects of homecare
- Precepting of the nurses by a qualified supervisor in the home prior to working independently with the patient [9].

Preparation by Nursing Agencies

Physicians and hospital discharge staff should require accountability from the nursing agency for the nurses working in the home [10]. Unfortunately, due to restrictions imposed by insurers or lack of available nursing agencies, physicians and discharge planning staff may work with agencies that are unfamiliar to them; therefore, it is important for the hospital staff discharging the patients and their families to meet with the nursing agencies and discuss their expectations. In centers with home ventilator programmes, staff should familiarize themselves with nursing agency policies and records before recommending them to patients and families. Although there are no national standards or certifications for nurses caring for tracheostomy and ventilator patients, we recommend the nursing agency be accountable for the following provisions to promote quality home nursing care:

- Comprehensive training for all agency nurses
- Validation of nurse skills with simulated return demonstration
- Provision for ongoing evidenced-based practice (EPB) training for nurses
- Arrangement for equipment in-servicing by DME companies
- Provision of formalized preceptor programme for each nurse with each patient
- Monitoring and documenting nurse performance and providing remedial training as needed
- Annual skill recertification and specialized CPR for nurses
- Meticulous record keeping of education, licensure, CPR certification, and DME training for each staff nurse
- Nurse performance evaluations and satisfaction surveys from families

Monitoring Mechanically ventilated Children in the Home

Monitoring Devices

A well-trained, alert caregiver provides the best monitoring of a ventilator-dependent child. Electronic monitoring devices alert caregivers when continuous and direct visualization of the child is not possible. The goal of home monitoring is to provide an early, reliable warning sign that the child's airway is compromised. In their 1999 clinical consensus statement, the American Thoracic Society reported that although there was wide variation in the use of monitoring devices for patients with chronic tracheostomy, most physicians prescribed monitoring devices for at least some of their patients. The role of home monitoring devices was included in their areas for future research [11].

A Duke University study by Peterson-Carmichael & Cheifetz examined the monitoring needs of ventilator-dependent children at home. Recommendations included determining each individual child's need for cardiorespiratory monitoring, pulse oximetry (continuous or intermittent), and/or capnography (time-based or volume-based); as no standard guidelines exist [12]. At Children's Hospital of Philadelphia, each patient requiring home ventilator support is provided a pulse oximeter for continuous or intermittent use to identify hypoxemia, a sensitive and early indicator of potential respiratory distress.

A home monitor must be reliable and routinely tested for accuracy. It is essential that the monitor has a battery backup for portability and for use during power outages. Monitors with download capabilities may be useful in certain homes to review collected data to assess patient trends over time and to evaluate episodic periods of clinical instability such as bradycardia, apnea, or desaturation. Monitors that have the capability of remotely downloading data via telephone or Internet provide the opportunity for medical providers to readily assess the data, especially for those patients who live a substantial distance from their medical team.

The monitors chosen for use in a patient's home should be maintained and serviced by the respiratory or DME company routinely and replaced as needed. In-home training for new monitoring technology for the family caregivers and homecare nurses should be provided. When monitors with download capability are employed, data can be downloaded by respiratory therapists or other DME staff at specified intervals to ensure that the monitor is being used appropriately and as ordered on the plan of care [12].

One of the key concerns regarding the most appropriate method for monitoring the chronically ventilated pediatric patient at home involves alarms. Loose leads are a frequent cause of false cardiorespiratory alarms. Patient movement can cause false pulse oximeter alarms. These false alarms, as well as ventilator alarms, both real and false, can quickly lead to sensory overload for family caregivers that may lead to an inability to distinguish real alarms from false ones. Conversely, the alarms on the various devices may not be adequately sensitive and fail to trigger an alarm during the occurrence of a genuine problem. The lack of a triggered alarm can provide caregivers with a false sense of the child's well-being in the event of a real problem. Given the possibility that a monitor may fail to alarm for a serious event, physicians often choose to utilize at least two forms of monitoring such as ventilator alarms plus pulse oximetry, for the care of their patients.

For children with small uncuffed tracheostomy tubes, high-tube resistance may prevent the low-pressure alarm from detecting accidental decannulation [13]. For these infants and children with small tracheostomy tubes, a decannulation test can be performed to demonstrate the risk of a child being decannulated without detection. A spare tracheostomy tube is attached to the ventilator tubing while the ventilator is in operation with all prescribed parameters set. If the low-pressure alarm fails to indicate decannulation, the infant is at risk for accidental harm or death. In a 2001 study done by Kun et al., it was reported that the tracheostomy tube size and ventilator settings must be considered when prescribing the low-inspiratory pressure alarms [13]. When the low-pressure alarms were set at 4 cm H_2O below peak-inspiratory pressure (PIP) for tracheostomy tubes <4.5 mm on low and medium settings, and <4.0 mm on high settings, and when the low inspiratory pressure alarm was set at 10 cm H_2O below PIP for tracheostomy tubes <6.0 mm, they failed to alarm for decannulation. Therefore, appropriate setting of ventilator low-pressure alarms, use of low minute volume alarms that detect leaks in the system, and consideration of additional forms of monitoring, such as pulse oximetry, should be considered for children with smaller tracheostomy tubes.

As technology advances, the reliability and accuracy of alarms will improve. Currently, the debate over how best to monitor chronically ventilated pediatric patients at home, and to what degree, will continue.

The Human Factor

A vigilant, well-trained caregiver is the best prevention for pediatric tracheostomy and ventilator emergencies in the home. This is equally true for both professional home nurses and family caregivers [14].

Nurses

The nursing profession and the public are concerned with the capacity for nurses to be consistent, vigilant caregivers. Families report that a primary frustration of homecare is a lack of vigilance by the nurses who monitor their children, especially when nurses sleep on the job. It is difficult for families to develop trust, confidence, and rapport with a nurse who has been found asleep. In its extreme, a lack of vigilance due to sleeping by a nurse can lead to the preventable death of a patient [15]. Nursing agencies are responsible for ensuring that work schedules for nurses allow for proper rest between shifts. Agencies are accountable for taking corrective action after families report a nurse sleeping on the job. For the nurse who commits a serious nursing error or is found asleep on the job we recommend reassessment of skill levels, followed by remedial instruction and documentation of completed remedial training by the nursing agency supervisor or clinical educator prior to the nurse returning to the child's home.

Family caregivers assume most of the responsibility of caring for their medically complex child. Home nursing support, especially night nursing, is vital for the health and well-being of family caregivers of ventilator-dependent children. Studies since the late 1980s have regularly reported sleep disturbances in parental caregivers of technology-dependent children [16–18]. A more recent study found a distinct relationship between home nursing coverage, sleep, and daytime functioning in parents of ventilator-assisted children. In the study, parents with clinically significant symptoms of depression and sleepiness received significantly fewer hours of night nursing [19]. Families rely on nursing agencies to provide enough qualified nurses to fill the number of approved nursing shifts for the child, especially during the night.

Family Caregivers

Ideally, preparation for discharge to home includes an independent 24-h provision of care by the family caregivers that is monitored, evaluated, documented, and determined to be safe by the hospital training team. Before discharge from the hospital, family caregivers should be certified in CPR and demonstrate proficiency in emergency care procedures including CPR with the tracheostomy as the primary airway for those children with tracheostomies.

Once at home, family caregivers require ongoing training by nurses, respiratory therapists, or physicians to maintain their skills in preparation for an emergency. Future educational needs should be anticipated and planned for, especially for children with progressive neurodegenerative disorders. Formalized continuing education in the home for family caregivers, however, rarely exists. Portable electronic simulation education may offer a promising solution for training family caregivers in the community [20]. Some homecare nursing agencies are currently exploring the potential for utilizing portable electronic simulation technology to provide continuing education to family caregivers at home.

Alternate Caregivers

The use of non-professional caregivers in the home is a topic that requires further investigation. An Australian study of 168 ventilator-dependent children at home followed 69 children that were provided care by alternative caregivers in place of skilled nurses [21]. Most of the children in the study received noninvasive ventilation; only 30 % were mechanically ventilated via tracheostomy tube. The study revealed that care given by trained "carers" was "safe and efficient" for children using either invasive or noninvasive ventilation. Potential benefits of using non-professional caregivers include: increasing the pool of available caregivers for families, providing care at a lower cost, and allowing families to use relatives and friends that they trust to provide the care [21]. Possible drawbacks to consider for using non-professional caregivers include: the responsibility of parents to train the lay caregivers; a lack of clinical oversight and accountability by professional agencies; the risk of improper or inadequate response to highly complex medical issues associated with invasive mechanical ventilation and tracheostomy emergencies; proper understanding, operation and monitoring of sophisticated ventilator equipment; and conflict of interest issues related to hiring relatives to provide care.

Preventing Accidental Deaths of Ventilator-Dependent Children in the Home

Noninvasive mechanical ventilation has fewer complications compared to invasive mechanical ventilation; however, it is essential that caregivers be able to address clearance of airway secretions and understand how to properly apply and fit facial appliances to prevent emergencies. For children who are invasively ventilated, the tracheostomy tube adds significant risk. The four most common life-threatening emergencies for ventilator-dependent children with tracheostomies are accidental decannulation, mucus plugging of tracheostomy, difficult insertion of tracheostomy tube, and water entering the tracheostomy tube. The key to preventing accidental deaths of ventilator-dependent children in the home is comprehensive preparation of the nurses and family caregivers. Family caregivers often rely on the knowledge, skill, and vigilance of homecare nurses. In a recent study, pediatric home nurses caring for ventilator-dependent children scored poorly when presented with online case-based, emergency ventilator alarm scenarios, regardless of the years of nursing experience. The vast majority of nurses surveyed for the study favored having more training opportunities [10]. The preventable death rate of ventilator-dependent children at home will decrease only when nurses are committed to maintaining high, evidence-based standards of care [3].

Proper Emergency Response by Caregivers

An efficient, stepwise response to each of the four primary emergencies should be rehearsed routinely by all care providers in anticipation of a true emergency. Without practice, complacency may develop during daily routine care. All caregivers need to maintain alertness so that response to a genuine emergency will be automatic and effective. In addition to specific well-defined steps taken during each possible emergency, some precautions and practices can help avoid emergency situations:

- Ensure that the child is receiving adequate systemic hydration and airway humidification at all times to prevent dehydration and thick secretions.
- Confirm that the child is wearing a humidification and moisture exchange device (HME) when off the ventilator or using stationary humidification.
- Change tracheostomy tube as ordered by the physician.
- Keep all scheduled doctor's appointments for routine airway evaluations.
- Ensure that caregivers report to the child's physician any difficulty they experience during a suctioning procedure or routine tracheostomy tube change that may indicate airway abnormalities such as new granulation tissue at the stoma or granulomas in the trachea.
- Prevent water from entering the tracheostomy tube by securing ventilator tubing, regularly emptying water from the tubing, and avoiding situations where the child is at risk for excess water in the tracheostomy tube, particularly when bathing. Swimming presents an unnecessary risk that should be avoided in children with tracheostomy tubes.

- Have a working phone with preprogrammed emergency numbers nearby at all times.
- Always carry portable oxygen, suction machine, resuscitation bag, and a "Go-Bag" of emergency supplies and extra tracheostomy tubes when outside the home.
- Ensure that all caregivers have current CPR certification and have demonstrated emergency responses and CPR using the tracheostomy as the primary airway [22].

Psychosocial Aspects of Care in the Home

Families use multiple strategies to manage the stress of perpetual care giving. They draw on informal and formal social supports that include friends, nurses, and physicians. They utilize emotional expression, physical exercise, distraction, humor, and prayer to cope [23].

Homecare nurses can play a vital role in creating a healthy psychosocial environment for the child receiving mechanical ventilation. Insight into the child's perceptions of self and ability, prepares the nurse to foster resiliency and a sense of self-worth in the child. The essential components of a relationship that allow psychosocial support to the child and family by the nurse are:

- The nurse and family participate in consistent, frequent communication.
- Household and parenting rules are established at the first encounter between the family and the nursing agency before the child leaves the hospital.
- Once home, give-and-take feedback between family and the nurse is ongoing.
- Supports for the nurses and families from the nursing agency that are consistent and appropriate.
- Scheduled routine assessment of care delivered in the home by nurse agency supervisors to reveal concerns that may be developing.

The effective homecare nurse recognizes the distinct differences between homecare and hospital care. A nurse who applies a "person approach" rather than a "patient approach" is able to provide supportive, appropriate homecare. Maintaining a flexible "way of doing" to accommodate family culture is important in home healthcare. The homecare nurse should recognize that the trained family members are the health team leaders and respect their authority in the home.

Trust may not develop between the nurse and family unless the nurse possesses clinical proficiency in each skill required by the patient prior to assuming care. Families cannot be held accountable for nurse training at home. Family caregivers should demonstrate to the homecare nurses how they were trained by hospital staff, relating techniques, schedules, and equipment that were used for their preparation to go home. Nurses should adapt their delivery of care to the family's wishes as much as is safely possible. A partnership between family and nurse needs to be firmly established for cohesive care. Once a trusting relationship develops, parents will be more responsive to nursing's suggestions of new, more effective protocols that may have developed since the child's initial discharge from the hospital.

Table 9.1 Professional boundaries that may be crossed by nurses

- Undermining parental authority with the child
- Ingratiating themselves to the child or family by buying gifts, bringing food, or doing non-nursing tasks in the home
- Becoming involved in family psychosocial dynamics unrelated to the child
- Disciplining or providing care to siblings
- Discussing the family with other nurses on the case
- Creating a personal mess in the home

Homecare nurses need to maintain professional boundaries. Family members often perceive non-professional behavior and gestures by nurses as smokescreens to mask poor clinical skills. Table 9.1 lists the common professional boundaries nurses may cross in the home. Trust between the nurse and family that has developed over time can be quickly destroyed when any of the professional boundaries are crossed. Nurses need to consciously guard against unprofessional behavior in the home.

The primary psychosocial goal for the nurse is to maintain the child's health and well-being in the most professional, supportive way possible. Valuing diversity has multiple benefits for homecare nurses that affect families in positive ways. The world view of the nurse cannot be imposed on the family. The nurse should have high regard for and an appreciation of the differences in culture and in other "ways of doing" that are important to the family. Appreciating diversity allows nurses to understand the family's frame of reference and adds valuable psychosocial skills to their nursing practice.

Nurses may provide valuable contributions that foster resiliency in a child who faces significant challenges in life. Resiliency in children with complex health needs is nurtured by helping them develop social competence, by assisting them in honing problem-solving skills, by encouraging their autonomy as much as possible, and by helping them to understand that they have worth and purpose in the world. Nurses can accomplish this with constructive thinking, encouragement, creative activities and by inspiring them, if possible, to reach out into the world rather than becoming isolated. Pity does not enhance resiliency.

Children often report that one of their favorite qualities in a nurse is a good sense of humor. All children, at all levels of development or cognition, want to laugh and have fun. Humor brings relaxation, distraction, positive influence on the immune system, pain reduction, temporary escape, positive self-image, and overall relief to the child [24].

Achieving Normalcy

A 2011 study that examined the challenges families of ventilator-dependent children face in the home revealed both positive and negative experiences. Parents described their overall experiences in caring for their ventilator-dependent children as deep and enriching. All of the participating family caregivers expressed a strong desire for their children to live as normal a life as possible; however, many problems that created roadblocks to achieving a sense of normalcy for families and children were identified. Family caregivers encountered difficulties with health and social services, a lack of privacy, a sense of isolation, inconsistent and incompetent nursing care, and the emotional stress, anxiety and exhaustion that accompanies the responsibility they had accepted. Despite these challenges, the value of life was so important to these families that all stated they would choose home mechanical ventilation again if faced with the same decision [25].

Normalization is the process of emphasizing the similarities between the experiences of families with children who are technology-dependent and those with healthy children [26]. Achieving normalcy requires providing supports to the family that establish a routine and consistency from the start. During the first week or so at home, 24-h in-home nursing is recommended to help the family adjust, gain confidence, and establish routines. Nurses can use this time to evaluate the learning needs of the family, review, and practice procedures with family caregivers, troubleshoot equipment, and organize supplies and emergency equipment for efficient accessibility. During this time period, it is not unusual for home caregivers to identify a need for additional supports, equipment, or home modifications. Having nurses in the home will help in the identification of those needs and funding sources. This transitional period is essential for families as they assume full responsibility for the child's care and become empowered to make decisions, advocate for the child, and navigate the healthcare system. After the first week of 24-h per day of nursing, skilled nursing care can be decreased in frequency as the child stabilizes and the family becomes accustomed to the routine of care. Skilled nursing care should only be decreased in frequency by the physician managing the child's mechanical ventilation. Unfilled nursing shifts need to be taken into consideration when the physician decreases the hours after the first week or two [7]. Many children will have an ongoing need for skilled care, and periodic reassessment of home nursing care needs by the managing physician is necessary [11]. Insurance approval for home nursing varies widely; patients are typically approved for 8–24 h of skilled nursing care per day [27]. In Pennsylvania, children enrolled in the Ventilator-Assisted Children's Home Program receive 12–16 h of skilled nursing care per day based on the child and family needs. The minimum number of nursing hours in the home should cover nighttime care to allow family caregivers the opportunity to sleep with the assurance that their child is being cared for and carefully monitored [3].

The child's evaluation by the primary care doctor in the first few weeks at home is important to ensure a normalized approach to childhood health at home. Open communication between practitioners is essential; however, families need to know who is managing which aspects of the child's care and what the expectations are for them in terms of their child's follow-up needs. The use of Medical Home models for ventilator-dependent children is discussed in Chap. 7. As the family develops a routine in their home and their confidence level in their ability to manage their child's care at home increases, medical caregivers, families, and the third-party payers should collaborate to develop an appropriate plan of care [28].

After the first few weeks, the family's focus will begin to transition from the child's medical condition to the child's growth and developmental needs. Families should participate in the educational and therapy evaluations of the child, and in many cases, the development of an individualized education plan (IEP) or 504 Plan. Decisions will include home versus center-based education and therapy and should be tailored to the child's needs and availability of resources in the home and community.

The value of respite care for the family cannot be underestimated. Respite services allow families additional time to attend to family needs other than the care of their ventilator-dependent child and to receive adequate rest to maintain physical, psychosocial, and emotional health. VACHP annually polls all families of ventilator-dependent children in the state to determine the benefits of the respite funds VACHP provides. Over the past three years, the three primary benefits of respite care identified by families were fewer hospital readmissions related to non-emergent medical care or caregiver fatigue; decreased rates of unemployment for one or both primary caregivers; and family stability when caregivers are given the opportunity temporarily to relinquish the responsibility of daily care that occupies most of the families' time and energy [23].

Despite the proven benefits of respite care for families, it is often difficult for families to obtain the required funding. When insurers deny respite funds, home health agencies and community agencies can help families identify alternate respite funding resources. Families typically prefer in-home respite services so the child can be cared for in a familiar environment; however, at times facility respite care is a necessary alternative [7].

Above all, if normalcy is to be achieved, professional homecare providers must make a conscious effort to validate the families' crucial role in care of the child and accept that the heroic efforts of family caregivers are driven by an abiding wish that their child experiences a meaningful life.

Traveling Outside of the Home

With a desire for normalcy, the ventilator-dependent child should have the opportunity to explore the world outside of the home domain as much as possible. Many children are able to attend school accompanied by a nurse. All of the children have physician appointments outside of the home. With proper preparation, most of the children are able to go outside. Leaving the home increases vulnerability and risk for the patient. Safe transport in non-emergency and emergency circumstances must be carefully planned and all the details conveyed to caregivers in the home [29]. Two caregivers should accompany the child, if possible, during transport. The caregiver must carry a working cell phone with preprogrammed emergency numbers. At a minimum, the equipment and supplies found in Table 9.2 should accompany the child when outside of the home. The resuscitation bag is a vital piece of equipment when traveling with a ventilator-dependent child. If the ventilator malfunctions or an electrical power source is unavailable, the child will require manual ventilation until help arrives. A spare, fully charged ventilator battery is helpful to bring along when traveling. When traveling to a distant location, the home respiratory company

Table 9.2 Essential equipment to carry outside of the home

• Resuscitation bag
• Portable suction machine that is charged and tested for good working order
• Portable oxygen, tubing, and tank holder (for patients receiving supplemental oxygen)
• A "Go-Bag" that contains an extra tracheostomy tube and obturator, a size smaller tracheostomy tube, suction catheters, scissors, tracheostomy tube ties, and lubricant
• Appropriately charged ventilator battery with backup if possible

should locate and contact a respiratory company at the intended location so that they may provide essential respiratory requirements for the child in the new location. The family will need a local source to call should there be equipment or supply problems. The travel destination must be accessible and able to accommodate the ventilator and other medical equipment. The physician in charge of the child's care plan should be aware of travel plans and approve the child for long distance travel. It is useful for the family to carry a full medical summary of the child.

Legal Issues

Families may require legal assistance to ensure that their child is receiving the benefits and resources to which they are entitled from third-party payers, school districts, and social services. Once the child is discharged from the hospital and adapts to life at home, some insurers seek to reduce services such as nursing or supplies. Some school districts prefer that ventilator-assisted children receive instruction at home; however, children should be given the opportunity to become part of the community and develop relationships outside of the home whenever possible. Most children who are supported by mechanical ventilation are able to attend school if accompanied by a nurse. They have the right to receive appropriate education in the least restrictive environment. Legal assistance may also be necessary to ensure safe housing that can accommodate the use of a ventilator and adaptive equipment.

Before leaving the hospital, families are educated about the risks of caring for their child at home, and despite those risks, most parents are eager to take their children home. Preparation of family members by the hospital staff is aimed at minimizing risks. The notion of risk becomes reality for parents when they find themselves alone at home for the first time without the support system they had in the hospital. In addition to trusting themselves and the level of skill they achieved during the child's hospital stay, they must be able to trust the agency that is supplying the homecare nurses. Most family caregivers who are new to homecare assume that risk is minimized when agencies send qualified nurses to care for their child. They expect that the homecare nurses will be as clinically proficient as the hospital nurses who cared for the child.

Among healthcare providers, physicians remain the main targets of medical malpractice lawsuits. Nurses account for about 2 % of all medical malpractice payments, accord-

Table 9.3 Six essential skills for nursing agencies to validate for their nurses

1.	A nursing skill exam to validate basic pediatric nursing skills
2.	An Introduction to Pediatrics or a Precepted Education for Pediatrics course. During this course, nurses should perform each skill on a mannequin; for example, proper suctioning technique and return demonstration of a tracheostomy change
3.	A Pediatric and Infant Care nursing exam—passing with an 80 % or better
4.	Guided practice of pediatric nursing skills in the home office by the nurse supervisor and competent skill validation by the clinical manager or nurse educator
5.	Simulation lab practice using emergency scenarios to validate critical thinking skills
6.	Oversight by a supervisor in patient home for at least three shifts, ensuring that critical nursing skills for that pediatric patient, particularly tracheostomy changes, are correctly performed on the patient by the nurse prior to working autonomously

ing to the National Practitioner Data Bank, operated by the US Department of Health and Human Services. Medical malpractice payments on behalf of nurses nearly doubled from 307 in 1997 to 586 in 2005. More and more nurses are being sued individually. The majority of these lawsuits were against non-advanced practice registered nurses [30].

In homecare, the most substantial legal risks are for the nurses and nursing agencies of mechanically ventilated children. Lawsuits resulting from harm, neglect, and deaths of ventilator-dependent children against homecare nurses and agencies are on the rise. The three primary types of lawsuits against homecare nurses are for incompetency, improper response to tracheostomy emergencies, and neglecting to properly assess and monitor patients.

In order for risks for the child and the nurse to be minimized, home agencies should develop a path to competency for every nurse they assign to a pediatric ventilator-dependent patient at home. Ideally, competency is confirmed and documented by the nursing agency after the nurse achieves all of the necessary skills to care for the patient at home. Simonds summarizes, "A key part of any homecare programme should be education of patients, families, and carers to help them use the equipment confidently and safely and to have a sensible plan of action once a problem arises [31]." Competency guidelines are being developed by many nursing agencies, but there is currently no national standard. Table 9.3 lists comprehensive training guidelines we recommend for homecare agencies.

Nurses should make it clear to the agency and family that they will not practice in a way they feel is unsafe or beyond their scope of practice. This includes turning down extra shifts if a nurse is fatigued or stressed. Nurses should thoroughly and accurately document the care they provide in the home. No patient or equipment alarms should be disabled without a thorough assessment of the situation. The patient should not be left unattended or unmonitored at any time. Nurses should report significant concerns about the patient and family to the agency supervisor and document those concerns.

Even the most cautious nurses sometimes may make mistakes. Occasionally, even when nurses provide competent care, pediatric patients can suffer setbacks or die, and their parents may sue. Nursing carries a risk, and homecare nursing of ventilator-dependent children carries additional risk, but risks in homecare are manageable. Nurses who achieve competency in all skills prior to delivering care assume control of their practice, and, thus, reduce risk. Most homecare nurses are aware of the risks, and yet they are committed to the care of their patients at home [32].

Outcomes

Mortality Rates

Outcomes for all children at home receiving mechanical ventilation need to be followed and reported by providers in order to identify barriers to and interventions for improving outcomes. Of the 1000 patients followed by VACHP over a 30-year period, approximately 44% are alive and remain mechanically ventilated. Thirty three percent are alive and liberated from mechanical ventilation. Eighteen percent are deceased and the outcomes of approximately 5% of the children are unknown. Of the deceased, approximately 27% of all the deaths were accidental and preventable [3].

Barriers to Improving Outcomes

The primary barrier to improving outcomes for children who receive mechanical ventilation at home is the insufficient preparation of all caregivers, especially preparation for effective emergency response. Monitoring devices are sometimes not used or are used improperly when alarms are silenced or when parameters are improperly set. Skill levels that are self-reported by nurses and by agencies may be overestimated and may lead to patient assignments for which nurses are not qualified. Nurse agencies may not provide routine and emergency tracheostomy and ventilator training to staff nurses. Ongoing assessment and continuous evidence-based education by agency educators may be lacking. Formalized family education may be non-existent for family caregivers once they leave the hospital.

Misperceptions about the role of a homecare nurse and fewer students choosing nursing as a career path have contributed to an insufficient pool of skilled nurses in an ever-growing homecare arena [33]. Nurses may regard the role of a pediatric homecare nurse as a less-than-desirable nurse specialty compared to hospital-based nursing positions. Recruitment of qualified nurses is a primary focus of most homecare agencies who diligently and creatively seek to hire highly-skilled clinicians to meet the need. For example, some agencies have developed formalized postgraduate nurse residency programmes to train newly graduated nurses for pediatric homecare. In the past, most nursing agencies required 1 or 2 years of hospital experience before nurses could apply for homecare positions. As the demand for pediatric homecare nurses increases, agencies will need to keep pace with a supply of qualified practitioners or funding for alternatives, such as training and use of non-professional caregivers, must be considered.

Interventions for Improving Outcomes

It is possible to improve outcomes for ventilator-dependent children at home if all caregivers are committed to the task. All homecare providers must be properly prepared for routine and emergency care. Skills should be validated for all caregivers. Consistent monitoring at home is essential. Homecare practices and protocols taught to families in the hospital prior to going home should be updated with evidence-based changes as they develop and when the child's medical condition changes. Physicians and families should demand nurse agency accountability for the nurses they send into the home [10].

Summary

All professional and family caregivers desire safe and healthy outcomes for children who are supported by mechanical ventilation at home. Family caregivers must be well-trained and confident they can handle both day-to-day care and emergencies. Nurses caring for ventilator-dependent children in the home require a specialized skill set; therefore, specialized and ongoing training well beyond their basic nursing education is necessary. Investing in the training of all caregivers and providing the support needed for adequate and appropriate care in the home will lead to improved outcomes for pediatric patients and their families, including a decrease in the number of accidental deaths at home. Accurate statistics need to be collected and recorded in a national database and shared among providers who oversee the care of mechanically ventilated children at home. These outcomes will reveal barriers to care and negative trends that impede progress towards safer care in the home. When barriers and negative trends are identified, interventions that result in safer, more effective homecare may be implemented.

References

1. Rivera A, Dasta J, Varon J. Critical care economics. Crit Care Shock. 2009;12(4):124–29.
2. King AC. Long-term home mechanical ventilation in the United States. Respir Care. 2012;57(6):921–30. discussion 30-2. Epub 2012/06/06. eng.
3. Boroughs D, Dougherty JA. Decreasing accidental mortality of ventilator-dependent children at home: a call to action. Home Healthc Nurse. 2012;30(2):103–11. quiz 12-3. Epub 2012/02/07. eng.
4. Kun SS, Edwards JD, Ward SL, Keens TG. Hospital readmissions for newly discharged pediatric home mechanical ventilation patients. Pediatr Pulmonol. 2012;47(4):409–14. Pubmed Central PMCID: PMC3694986, Epub 2011/09/09. eng.
5. Edwards JD, Kun SS, Keens TG. Outcomes and causes of death in children on home mechanical ventilation via tracheostomy: an institutional and literature review. J Pediatr. 2010;157(6):955–9. e2. Epub 2010/08/18. eng.

6. Panitch HB. Home ventilation. In: Light MJ, Homnick DN, Schechter MS, Blaisdell CJ, Weinberger MM, editors. Pediatric pulmonology. Illinois: American Academy of Pediatrics; 2011. p. 1100–27.
7. Storgion S. Care of children requiring home mechanical ventilation. In: Libby R, Imaizumi S, editors. Guidelines for pediatric home health care. 2nd ed. Illinois: American Academy of Pediatrics; 2009. p. 299–316.
8. Stick SM, Wilson A, Panitch HB. Home ventilation and respiratory support. In: Taussig L, Landau L, editors. Pediatric respiratory medicine. Philadelphia: Mosby Elsevier; 2008. p. 295–303.
9. Boroughs D, Dougherty JA. Care of technology-dependent children in the home. Home Healthc Nurse. 2009;27(1):37–42. Epub 2008/12/31. eng.
10. Kun SS, Beas VN, Keens TG, Ward SS, Gold JI. Examining pediatric emergency home ventilation practices in home health nurses: opportunities for improved care. Pediatr Pulmonol. 2014;7. Epub 2014/04/08. Eng.
11. Sherman JM, Davis S, Albamonte-Petrick S, Chatburn RL, Fitton C, Green C, et al. Care of the child with a chronic tracheostomy. This official statement of the American Thoracic Society was adopted by the ATS Board of Directors, July 1999. Am J Respir Crit Care Med. 2000;161(1):297–308. Epub 2000/01/05. eng.
12. Peterson-Carmichael SL, Cheifetz IM. The chronically critically ill patient: pediatric considerations. Respir Care. 2012;57(6):993–1002; discussion -3. Epub 2012/06/06. eng.
13. Kun SS, Nakamura CT, Ripka JF, Davidson Ward SL, Keens TG. Home ventilator low-pressure alarms fail to detect accidental decannulation with pediatric tracheostomy tubes. Chest. 2001;119(2):562–4. Epub 2001/02/15. eng.
14. Downes JJ, Boroughs DS, Dougherty J, Parra M. A statewide program for home care of children with chronic respiratory failure. Caring. 2007;26(9):16–8, 20, 2-3 passim. Epub 2007/10/24. eng.
15. Gaba DM, Howard SK. Patient safety: fatigue among clinicians and the safety of patients. N Engl J Med. 2002;347(16):1249–55. Epub 2002/10/24. eng.
16. Andrews MN, Nielson DH. Technology dependent children in the home. J Pediatr Nurs. 1988;14:111–51.
17. Kuster PA, Badr LK, Chang BL, Wuerker AK, Benjamin AE. Factors influencing health promoting activities of mothers caring for ventilator-assisted children. J Pediatr Nurs. 2004;19(4):276–87. Epub 2004/08/17. eng.
18. Heaton J, Noyes J, Sloper P, Shah R. The experiences of sleep disruption in families of technology-dependent children living at home. Child Soc. 2006;20:196–208.
19. Meltzer LJ, Boroughs DS, Downes JJ. The relationship between home nursing coverage, sleep, and daytime functioning in parents of ventilator-assisted children. J Pediatr Nurs. 2010;25(4):250–7. Pubmed Central PMCID: PMC2932665, Epub 2010/07/14. eng.
20. Galloway S. Simulation techniques to bridge the gap between novice and competent healthcare professionals. Online J Iss Nurs. 2009;14(2):3.
21. Tibballs J, Henning R, Robertson CF, Massie J, Hochmann M, Carter B, et al. A home respiratory support programme for children by parents and layperson careers. J Paediatr Child Health. 2010;46(1–2):57–62. Epub 2009/12/01. eng.
22. Kleinman ME, Chameides L, Schexnayder SM, Samson RA, Hazinski MF, Atkins DL, et al. Pediatric advanced life support: 2010 American Heart Association Guidelines for Cardiopulmonary Resuscitation and Emergency Cardiovascular Care. Pediatrics. 2010;126(5):e1361–99. Epub 2010/10/20. eng.
23. Statement on home care for patients with respiratory disorders. Am J Respir Crit Care Med. 2005;171(12):1443–64. Epub 2005/06/09.eng.
24. Boroughs D. Nurses who foster resiliency in chronically ill children; 2000. http://newsnurse.com/apps/pbcs.dll/article?AID=20002070374. Accessed 26 Mar 2013.
25. Dybwik K, Tollali T, Nielsen EW, Brinchmann BS. "Fighting the system": families caring for ventilator-dependent children and adults with complex health care needs at home. BMC Health Serv Res. 2011;11:156. Pubmed Central PMCID: PMC3146406, Epub 2011/07/06. eng.

26. Cockett A. Technology dependence and children: a review of the evidence. Nurs Children Young People. 2012;24(1):32–5. Epub 2012/04/12. eng.
27. De A, Kun SS, Keens TG. Home care ventilation for children: lessons learned at the Children's Hospital Los Angeles 2013. http://respiratory-care-sleep-medicine.advanceweb.com/features/articles/home-care-ventilation-for-children. aspx?CP=2. Accessed 21 July 2014.
28. Kun SS, Davidson-Ward SL, Hulse LM, Keens TG. How much do primary care givers know about tracheostomy and home ventilator emergency care? Pediatr Pulmonol. 2010;45(3):270–4. Epub 2010/02/11. eng.
29. Macdonald M, Boyle-King S. Transport of the child who is medically fragile. In: Libby R, Imaizumi S, editors. Guidelines for pediatric home health care. 2nd ed. Illinois: American Academy of Pediatrics; 2009. p. 205–14.
30. Services UDoHaH. The Data Bank-National Practitioner Healthcare Integrity and Protection Washington, DC; 2005. Available from: http://www.npdb.hrsa.gov/resources/aboutStatData.jsp. Accessed 26 Mar 2013.
31. Simonds AK. Risk management of the home ventilator dependent patient. Thorax. 2006;61(5):369–71. Pubmed Central PMCID: PMC2111178, Epub 2006/05/02. eng.
32. DeBartolomeo-Mager D. Unique bonds that form when visiting patients in their homes. Home Healthc Nurse. 2011;29(2):128.
33. Carter A. Nursing shortage predicted to be hardest on home healthcare. Home Healthc Nurse. 2009;27(3):198. Epub 2009/03/13. eng.

Chapter 10
Troubleshooting Common Ventilator and Related Equipment Issues in the Home

Denise Willis and Sherry L. Barnhart

Introduction

Advancements in neonatal and pediatric medicine have resulted in a rapidly growing number of children who require mechanical ventilation that extends beyond the acute care period. Improved portable ventilator technology and the increasing availability of home health-care professionals have provided more opportunities for these technology-dependent children to be cared for at home. The growing shift toward care at home is further supported by evidence that medically stable children experience improved psychosocial development and a better quality of life outside the hospital environment [1–5]. Studies show that the number of children receiving ventilatory support at home continues to increase [6–8].

A major factor in enabling ventilator-dependent children to live at home is the availability of portable ventilators and associated equipment. Whether ventilation is invasive or noninvasive and whether support is required continuously or only while asleep, appropriate medical equipment that is functioning properly is essential. The majority of these children, especially those who are also tracheostomy dependent, have complex chronic conditions that place them at high risk for critical illness and death. The addition of complicated medical equipment in the home brings this population at even higher risk for life-threatening events [9]. Despite the highest quality parental and professional health care provided, no home ventilator program is exempt from equipment-related problems or complications. This chapter addresses

D. Willis, B.S., R.R.T-.N.P.S. (✉)
Respiratory Care Services, Pulmonary Medicine Section, Arkansas Children's Hospital,
1 Children's Way, Little Rock, AR 72202, USA
e-mail: WillisDeniseL@uams.edu

S.L. Barnhart, R.R.T-.N.P.S., F.A.A.R.C.
Respiratory Care Discharge Planner, Respiratory Care Services, Arkansas Children's
Hospital, Little Rock, AR, USA

© Springer Science+Business Media New York 2016
L.M. Sterni, J.L. Carroll (eds.), *Caring for the Ventilator Dependent Child*,
Respiratory Medicine, DOI 10.1007/978-1-4939-3749-3_10

issues and problems related to the mechanical ventilator and other home medical equipment associated with the respiratory care of ventilator-dependent children.

The Mechanical Ventilator

Lack of a centralized database or registry for children receiving home ventilation makes it somewhat difficult to assess the extent of mechanical ventilator malfunction in ventilator-dependent children at home [10]. Although studies are limited, those available suggest that mechanical failure is infrequent and mortality relates most often to progression of the underlying disease or to complications associated with a tracheostomy [11]. In a 1-year study of 150 adult and pediatric ventilator-dependent patients in the United States, there were 189 reports of problems with the ventilator. Of these reports 39 % were due to defective equipment or mechanical failure, 30 % were due to caregivers improperly using the ventilator, 13 % were due to damage to or misuse of the ventilator, and in 3 % of the reports, the ventilator was functioning correctly but a change in the patient's condition was misinterpreted as ventilator malfunction. In 44 % of the cases, the problem was solved by completely replacing the ventilator; however, in 14 % of these no mechanical fault was actually identified, and replacement was done primarily to reassure the patient and caregivers. Adjusting ventilator settings alone corrected the problem in 21 % of the cases and replacing a part was the solution in 6 %. Fortunately patients were hospitalized in only 1 % of the reports [12].

A more recent study analyzed calls made to a dedicated respiratory support emergency telephone hotline for pediatric and adult ventilator-dependent patients [13].

Of the more than 1200 patients that called during the 6-month study period, the majority were receiving noninvasive ventilation with only 1 % having a tracheostomy and only 12 % requiring ventilation continuously. Half of the calls made to the on-call line after office hours were to report problems with the ventilator. Of these, 75 % were related to malfunction of the ventilator and alarms, while 25 % were reports that the ventilator alarm had identified a problem. During this same period, 188 home visits were made following the report of problems with the ventilator or associated equipment. Technical problems were solved in 64 % of the patients' homes, equipment was replaced in 22 % of the visits, and no problem with the ventilator or circuit was identified in 13 % of the visits. Problems associated with the alarms were mainly due to accumulation of water in the ventilator's pressure line. An increased malfunction rate was seen in ventilators that had been in service longer than 8 years and in those patients who required ventilator support for longer than 16 h per day. This may suggest a direct relationship between failure rate and the total hours of ventilator use. Most of the problems directly related to the ventilator were due to malfunction of the motor blower/bellows and circuit board. Interestingly, there was an increased rate of reported problems in ventilator models new to the market suggesting that problems may arise that were not identified in pre-market testing.

Although reports of ventilator malfunction are infrequent, there remain times when equipment fails. If there is a malfunction or an activated alarm cannot be corrected, the patient must be disconnected from the ventilator and either manually ventilated with the resuscitation bag until the problem is corrected or connected to a backup ventilator, if one is available. If the problem cannot be corrected and a backup ventilator is not available, the durable medical equipment company (DME) is immediately contacted for equipment replacement. Emergency medical assistance is contacted if the patient experiences acute respiratory distress.

Ventilators

Current microprocessor-driven ventilators are remarkably reliable and automatically undergo a safety check when the power is turned on. However, there is still the possibility of an electrical power failure or mechanical malfunction that may result in the ventilator failing to cycle on or failing to provide a set tidal volume or pressure. To ensure proper ventilator function and to confirm that ventilator settings and alarms are correctly set, ventilators must be regularly checked by the caregivers or home health-care professionals. Routine monitoring can identify potential equipment problems as well as determine if settings have been inadvertently changed [14]. Mechanical problems and incorrect ventilator settings can result in overdistention of the lungs, hypoxia, hypoventilation, respiratory failure, or death. Table 10.1 lists the settings and alarms that should be monitored with each ventilator check. If ventilator or alarm settings are found to be incorrect, a properly trained caregiver or health-care professional should immediately return them to the ordered settings. Using lockout features or protective covers over the control knobs can assist in preventing settings from being accidentally changed.

Ventilators must be plugged directly into grounded electrical outlets that are not used to supply power to a major appliance, such as a television, refrigerator, or air conditioner. Power strips and extension cords should not be used and the ventilator must be kept dry. Open containers of liquid should never be placed on the ventilator. If the ventilator is wet or damp, the moisture increases the potential for electrical shock. Using ungrounded outlets can result in voltage spikes that severely damage or destroy the ventilator. These electrical surges can also cause fires or electrical shock and pose a danger to both the patient and the caregivers.

Per the manufacturer's recommendations, all ventilators should undergo preventive maintenance to ensure proper functioning. This entails returning it to the manufacturer on a regularly scheduled basis, either after it has been in actual use for a specified number of hours (e.g., after every 10,000 h of use) or after it has been in the patient's home or in storage for a specified amount of time (e.g., every 2 years). Because the ventilator is physically removed from the home for an extended period, arrangements should be made for obtaining another ventilator to use while preventive maintenance is being performed.

Table 10.1 Ventilator checks

Date and time check is completed
Ventilator mode
Oxygen setting
Set ventilator rate
Total patient respiratory rate
Set tidal volume
Peak inspiratory pressure
Pressure control setting
Pressure support setting
PEEP setting
Inspiratory time setting
Sensitivity setting
Low-pressure alarm setting
Low-pressure alarm audible
High-pressure alarm setting
High-pressure alarm audible
Humidifier heater setting
Temperature
Battery check—internal
Battery check—external

When ventilator malfunction is suspected, the patient is disconnected from the ventilator and manually ventilated with the resuscitation bag. After confirming that the patient is receiving adequate ventilation, the caregiver can search for and attempt to correct the problem. Keeping a test lung at the bedside is helpful in being able to quickly determine if the problem is due to ventilator malfunction or due to a change in the patient's condition. If the problem cannot be resolved, another ventilator must be obtained for the patient to use.

Ventilator Alarms

Available alarm options vary widely depending upon the specific ventilator brand and/or model. Because ventilator nomenclature is not yet completely standardized, the same alarm may be named differently on different machines. For example, low pressure, low peak pressure, and low inspiratory pressure will in most cases all represent the same concept.

Ventilators are equipped with safety alarms that are sensitive to pressures and volumes, circuit disconnections, respiratory rates, and available electrical power. It is crucial that the alarms are set appropriately and can be heard in the intended area of use. Improper settings, electrical power failure, weak batteries, excessive leak associated with the interface, or alarms intentionally or inadvertently disabled may cause erroneous alarms or failure to sound in the presence of a true alarm condition. The alarm volume level can be adjusted on some but not all home ventilators but it should never be disabled. Some models have a feature where the alarm volume may have a different alert depending on the priority of the alarm. For example, there may be a low-, medium-, or high-priority alarm.

More than 2500 adverse events associated with the use of ventilators were reported to the Food and Drug Administration in 2010 alone. Of these events, nearly one-third were related to ventilator alarms, with many due to human error or audible ventilator alarm malfunctions that could have been prevented [15]. Regardless of the alarm activated, caregivers must immediately respond by first giving full attention to the patient, assessing the clinical status, and acting accordingly. This is done before taking steps to determine the cause of the alarm.

It has been reported that as much as 85–95 % of alarms occurring in the hospital setting do not require intervention and are considered a nuisance [16, 17]. This high percentage of false alarms has resulted in the phenomenon known as alarm fatigue and has led to many health-care providers becoming desensitized to the sound of alarms. Unfortunately, alarm fatigue has caused unnecessary deaths and other adverse outcomes. Caregivers in the home settings are not immune to becoming desensitized to alarms and must be educated on the potential for undesirable consequences associated with not appropriately responding to all alarms.

Low-Pressure Alarms

All home ventilators have a low-pressure alarm that may be referred to as low peak pressure or low peak inspiratory pressure. The low peak inspiratory pressure alarm is a set pressure threshold. The alarm will sound when the peak inspiratory pressure does not exceed this pressure threshold during the inspiratory time period. Some models also have an alert for low PEEP. The purpose of the low PEEP alarm is to detect a drop in PEEP, indicating a disconnection, leak in the circuit or airway, or that the patient is actively inspiring below the set PEEP. Additionally, some home ventilators also have the option to set the low peak pressure alarm to not sound for pressure-supported breaths.

When a low-pressure alarm is activated, it typically indicates that the patient has become disconnected from the ventilator (i.e., ventilator tubing is not connected to the interface or machine) or there is a leak in the circuit. Leaks occur most often around loose connections at the temperature probe, at the humidifier, and at the tracheostomy tube or mask interface. Tears, cracks, or holes in the circuit adaptors and tubing can also result in a leak. It is important to respond immediately to low-pressure alarms by first checking the patient to assure that the circuit is connected and the interface is secure and without leaks.

If the patient has a tracheostomy tube, it is critical that it is determined if decannulation has occurred. If the circuit is adequately connected and the airway stable, then the pressure line, exhalation line, oxygen connection, and humidifier should be examined for loose connections. This is best done by following the circuit, beginning at the patient's connection with the circuit, and then working back toward the ventilator, listening and feeling for leaks, cracks, and disconnects. Failure to quickly determine the reason for the low pressure can lead to severe hypoventilation and hypoxia with fatal consequences.

Table 10.2 Causes of
low-pressure alarm activation

Patient disconnected from ventilator
Disconnect or leak in ventilator circuit
Disconnect or leak in pressure line
Loose connection in ventilator circuit
Water in pressure line
Condensation in external PEEP valve
Faulty exhalation valve
Cracked or loose bacteria filter
Leak at the humidifier
Leak at patient's mouth
Deflated tracheostomy tube cuff
Loose inner cannula of tracheostomy tube
Inadvertent decannulation
Inadvertent ventilator setting change
Incorrect low-pressure alarm setting

It is important to remember that a leak or disconnect may be present yet no alarm is activated. The low-pressure alarm may not sound if the ventilator circuit becomes disconnected and tubing is occluded by bedding or the patient's soft tissue. It has been speculated that decannulation may be more readily detected when the low inspiratory pressure alarm is set at 4 cm H_2O below the peak inspiratory pressure instead of the more common practice of setting it at 10 cm H_2O or greater [18]. While the study by Kun and colleagues examined only small pediatric tracheostomy tubes, the possibility exists that a low-pressure alarm may fail to activate with any size tube when there is an inadvertent circuit disconnection and the tubing is occluded. Table 10.2 lists the most common causes for a low-pressure alarm to be activated.

Low Exhaled Minute Volume Alarm

A low exhaled minute volume alarm will function essentially in the same manner as a low-pressure alarm. It is activated when the volume of air exhaled is less than expected, most often indicating a disconnection from the circuit or a leak.

High-Pressure Alarms

The high-pressure alarm tends to be the one most often heard and is activated when the ventilator reaches a preset upper pressure limit. When this alarm is activated, inspiration is immediately terminated. The high-pressure alarm may be referred to as high peak pressure or high inspiratory pressure alarm. The purpose of this alarm

Table 10.3 Causes of high-pressure alarm activation	Mucus or mucous plugs in airway or tracheostomy tube
	Blockage in airway or tracheostomy tube
	Obstruction or kink in ventilator circuit
	Excessive water condensation in ventilator circuit
	Patient coughing
	Patient holding breath
	Condensation in external PEEP valve
	Inadvertent ventilator setting change
	Incorrect high-pressure alarm setting

is to alert caregivers to a potentially dangerous situation in which the inspiratory pressure has reached an unacceptably high level. Some models may also have a high PEEP or high expiratory pressure alarm, indicating the exhaled pressure has exceeded the set alarm threshold.

Activation is most often due to increased resistance or obstruction in the ventilator circuit or the patient's airway. The most common problems include increased pulmonary secretions requiring suctioning, coughing, mucous plugging in the inner cannula or in the heat and moisture exchanger, kinked or bent ventilator tubing, excessive water in the circuit, ventilator dyssynchrony, and physical activity such as kicking, squirming, or crying. Table 10.3 lists the most common causes for a high-pressure alarm to be activated. As an additional feature, some home ventilators offer a high-pressure breath delay in which the breath is terminated but the audible alarm will not sound until up to three consecutive breaths with high pressure have occurred.

High Exhaled Volume Alarm

The high exhaled volume alarm is activated when the volume that the patient exhales reaches a preset upper volume limit. Hyperventilation resulting from anxiety, pain, or hypoxemia is the most common cause for this alarm to sound.

Apnea Alarm

This alarm sounds when the time since the start of the last breath is longer than a preset apnea interval. Commonly available options for apnea alarm delay are 10–60 s. The prescribed setting will be based on multiple factors including age, patient condition, and need for ventilator support. Activation of this alarm usually indicates that the patient's respiratory rate has decreased or apnea is occurring; however, it may also occur when the patient becomes disconnected from the ventilator and breathing is not detected.

Disconnect Alarm

Some home ventilators have a disconnect alarm that is activated when a sensing line becomes disconnected or occluded. The alarm will also activate when the breathing circuit has become detached from either the child or the machine. Select models offer an option to either enable or disable this alarm. When enabled, it can be set to delay the audible alarm from 5 to 60 s. This could be useful when briefly disconnecting to replace the circuit or suction the tracheostomy tube. However, caution should be taken to ensure the child can sustain adequate ventilation when removed from ventilator support, and a manual resuscitation bag should be ready for use when necessary.

As with the low-pressure alarm, when the disconnect alarm sounds, the caregiver should immediately assess the patient and determine the reason for the alarm trigger. Failure of an alarm to activate, especially the low-pressure, apnea, and disconnect alarms, can result in life-threatening events. This is even more critical with patients who have little to no breathing autonomy or those who need the ventilator during sleep [19]. The manual resuscitation bag should be used to ventilate the patient if the disconnection status cannot be quickly determined.

Low Battery Alarm

Ventilators used in the home have both an internal battery and an external battery source. The low battery alarm is activated when the voltage in either of these batteries becomes low. Often the alarm begins as a slow beep or chirp. As the voltage gets lower, the alarm sounds louder and longer. The alarm will sound continuously if the battery is fully drained and the ventilator is not connected to an electrical power source.

Low Power/Power Failure Alarm

A low power alarm will be activated if there is an inadequate source of power. This may occur with an electrical power failure or loss of battery power. Immediate steps must be taken to determine the malfunction of the power system. The most common causes for this alarm are the electrical cord is not completely plugged in to the back of the ventilator, the cord has become disconnected at the electrical outlet, or the internal battery has drained and needs recharging. An electrical power failure may also be corrected by simply replacing a fuse, resetting the circuit breaker, or connecting the ventilator to a battery.

Ventilator Circuits

The patient breathing circuit includes the ventilator tubing and humidification system, mask or tracheostomy tube connector, and the parts that make up the tracheostomy tube or mask interface. Problems associated with circuits are usually due to cracked or loose adaptors that result in leaks or inadvertent disconnections. Water from condensation can collect in the tubing and cause alarms to be activated. Most circuits used in the home today are disposable and discarded after use. Ideally two caregivers should be present when changing out the ventilator circuit; however, this may not be possible if a circuit must be changed during an emergency situation. Prior to changing a circuit, the new circuit should be completely assembled and ready to use. Problems associated with a circuit often arise following a circuit change; therefore, caregivers are advised to perform a complete ventilator check immediately after a circuit is changed. Keeping a completely assembled clean circuit readily available at all times is also recommended. Except in an emergency situation, tape should never be used to secure adaptors within a circuit or to correct leaks within the tubing.

Batteries

Ventilators are electrically powered and can be run using a grounded electrical outlet with 120 V of alternating current (A/C), an internal direct current (D/C) battery located inside the ventilator, or an external D/C battery (see Fig. 10.1). Voltage may vary according to the country and region in which the ventilator is operating. Depending upon the battery type, age of the battery, and ventilator settings, a fully charged internal battery only supplies power for approximately 30–60 min, while an external battery may provide power for 4 up to 24 h. The internal battery is built into the ventilator and used mainly for short-term events or when there is a sudden drop in electrical power to the ventilator, which may occur during an electrical power failure or when the ventilator is accidentally unplugged. Internal batteries are recharged, while the ventilator is plugged into an electrical outlet; however, they may not recharge when the ventilator is plugged into an external battery. For this reason caregivers are advised to keep the ventilator plugged into an electrical outlet while at home.

Most home ventilator brands offer a portable, lightweight, external battery option. Deep cycle marine batteries are often also utilized. Battery performance and duration can be affected by age, amount of use, and the temperature in which it is operated. It is important to follow manufacturer instructions to preserve maximum battery life.

If electrical power is lost, the ventilator will automatically switch to the internal battery, unless the external battery is connected. Most ventilators audibly alarm and provide a visual indication that the internal or external battery is providing power. A malfunction occurs if the ventilator does not change over to the internal battery or if the external battery is not charged. If neither battery is functioning, the patient should be disconnected from the ventilator and manually ventilated with the resuscitation bag until the ventilator can be replaced.

It is good practice to mark the circuit breaker or fuse that controls the electrical outlet(s) frequently used for the ventilator and keep extra fuses readily available. Battery cables may break as a result of poor or rough care and should be immedi-

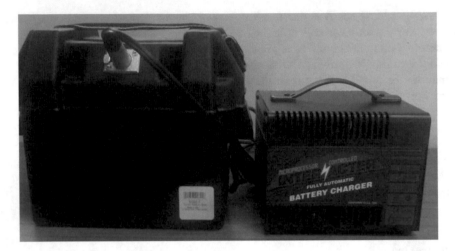

Fig. 10.1 External ventilator battery with charger

ately replaced. The use of extension cords cannot be recommended. Manufacturers recommend using only their product-specific cables and accessories.

Interface

Home mechanical ventilation can be accomplished either invasively with a tracheostomy tube or noninvasively with various interface options. The choice of invasive or noninvasive interface is dependent upon many factors including clinical condition, prognosis, underlying cause of need for ventilation, level of required support, and preference of the clinician, patient, and/or caregiver. Regardless of whether administered invasively or noninvasively, the need for ventilator support is not diminished by the choice of interface as some individuals are dependent upon noninvasive ventilation (NIV) on a continuous basis. In recent years there has been a trend toward NIV when it is a viable option due to the potential for fewer complications as compared to tracheostomy [20].

Tracheostomy Tubes

One of the most common problems encountered with the tracheostomy tube in respect to the ventilator is leak. Tracheostomy leak can cause a variety of issues including low-pressure and low minute volume alarms, low exhaled volumes, autocycling of the ventilator, and in some cases, inadequate ventilation leading to oxygen desaturation. Not only is leak around the stoma a contributing factor, but also mouth leak when attempting to speak or while sleeping. Tracheostomy leak tends to be more prominent during periods of sleep when the patient is more relaxed. The majority of the time a leak is more of a nuisance than a major concern. For minor leaks, simple repositioning of the head and/or neck or adding an extra layer of gauze padding around the stoma can help alleviate the problem. Ventilator settings can also be adjusted to help compensate for a leak but caution should be taken to not over ventilate if the leak is not consistent.

If the leak is causing inadequate ventilation and all other approaches to correct it have failed, a larger-sized tracheostomy tube may be needed. In pediatrics, uncuffed tracheostomy tubes are generally preferred [21]. However, a cuffed tube might be considered if upsizing the tube is not an option and ventilation is adversely affected, as evidenced by elevated carbon dioxide or decreased oxygen saturation. Oftentimes the cuff can be left deflated while the patient is awake to allow for vocalization. It is then inflated only during sleep using the least cuff volume necessary to correct the leak.

Noninvasive Ventilation Interfaces

The most crucial element to the success or failure of long-term NIV is the interface. The first factor that should be considered when NIV is poorly tolerated is the appropriateness and fit of the interface. There are many different styles, sizes, and varieties of NIV interface options including nasal and full face masks, nasal pillows, oral and oronasal interfaces, and mouthpieces (see Figs. 10.2, 10.3 and 10.4). Determining which one the patient will use and can tolerate is perhaps the biggest challenge. There are limited NIV interface options for children, and only over the past few years have masks been specifically designed for the pediatric patient. Previously, adult-sized masks were adapted for use in children. There is a helmet apparatus for NIV but it is not currently approved by the US Food and Drug Administration at the time of this writing.

Just as with a tracheostomy, leak is also a major issue with the mask interface. Leak with NIV is most often the result of an inappropriately fitting mask, the mouth falling open during sleep, or the need to adjust the headgear. A chin strap can be employed in cases where the leak is due to mouth opening (see Fig. 10.4). A full face mask can also be considered for this but caution must be taken as the mask must be removed quickly in the event of emesis so as to avoid aspiration. Many full face masks incorporate an air entrainment valve so the patient can breathe room air in the event of a power failure.

Mask adjustment can become a vicious cycle. The headgear is often over tightened to eliminate leaks, which in turn puts pressure on various points on the face including the forehead, bridge of the nose, and upper lip. Skin breakdown and pressure sores can also occur with long-term use, making it difficult for the patient to adhere to NIV. Alternating the mask with a nasal pillow style interface might be helpful to avoid this and allow time for the skin to heal. Additionally a skin barrier could be utilized. There are commercially available products specifically designed

Fig. 10.2 Nasal pillows

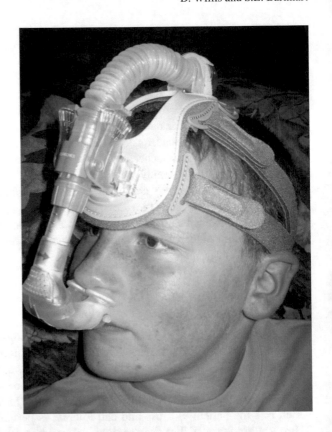

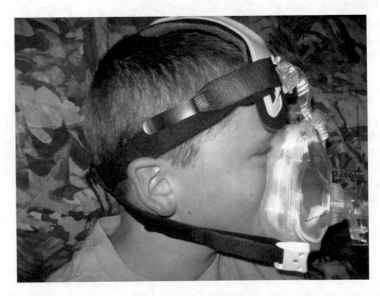

Fig. 10.3 Full face mask

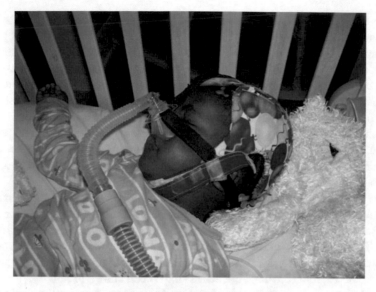

Fig. 10.4 Nasal mask with cap headgear and chin strap

Fig. 10.5 Skin barrier for use with nasal mask

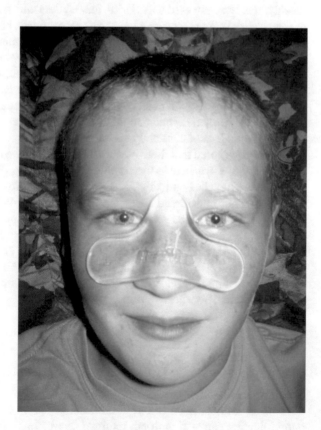

for this purpose (see Fig. 10.5). Despite the best precautions, facial hypoplasia and flattening can occur due to long-term use of a noninvasive interface [22–24].

When using a home mechanical ventilator for NIV, instead of a bi-level or CPAP device, consideration must be given as to whether the mask is vented or non-vented. A vented mask has an exhalation port, while a non-vented mask does not. If the ventilator circuit has an incorporated exhalation valve, a non-vented mask is the better option to avoid excessive leak. Otherwise the exhalation port on a vented mask should be occluded or the ventilator will never reach the prescribed pressure or volume setting. If the ventilator circuit does not employ an exhalation port, a vented mask would be the best choice; otherwise, an exhalation valve or port would have to be added if using a non-vented mask.

Many times patients have several masks they have used at home or sometimes even taken home after use during a hospitalization. The potential exists for a non-vented mask to be mistakenly used with a circuit that does not have an exhalation valve. Thorough education for caregivers is a must in order to avoid an adverse outcome in this scenario. If a non-vented mask is inadvertently used, a high-pressure alarm would most likely sound but alarms have been known to fail.

Mouthpiece or sip ventilation is becoming a more common practice for individuals with neuromuscular disease requiring some amount of ventilator support during the day. It is typically used only during the daytime with a mask worn during periods of sleep. These patients may not have use of their hands because of profound muscle weakness. This leads to problems in securing the mouthpiece in a manner in which it will be easily accessible to the patient. Previously there were no commercially available devices for this and parts had to be pieced together; however, new technology has made this more efficient (see Fig. 10.6). Another issue with sip ventilation is setting the machine appropriately, usually in a spontaneous mode, so the patient can trigger a breath when desired and thereby preventing the machine from blowing air in the patient's face or constantly alarming.

It should be noted that there are several limitations with using a bi-level device connected to a tracheostomy in the home setting. Bi-level devices are not approved by the US Food and Drug Administration for invasive use in the home as they are not considered life support equipment. While there is a particular brand of bi-level device specifically designed and approved for invasive use in the home, the manufacturer instructions state it is not intended for life support. Additionally, bi-level devices generally do not have an internal battery that will power the device in the event of electrical outage, and the alarm options vary considerably among brands. If bi-level-type settings are desired, there are home ventilators that offer these options.

Humidification

Humidification during mechanical ventilation is an absolute necessity in the presence of an artificial airway but is considered optional for NIV [25]. Inadequate humidification can lead to dried, retained secretions resulting in mucous plugging

Fig. 10.6 Sip ventilation circuit mounted on wheelchair (Used with permission of Philips Respironics, Murrysville, PA)

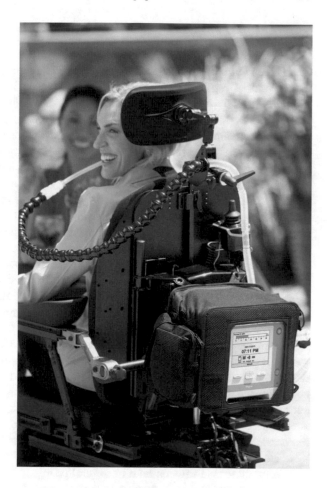

and atelectasis. Long-term consequences of inadequate humidification may result in mucosal dysfunction including slowed mucociliary transport and cell damage [26, 27]. However, excessive humidification can also be problematic. The goal is to deliver optimal humidification that mimics the normal physiological conditions present in the airway.

Humidification can be accomplished with either active or passive methods. Active humidification involves the use of a heated humidifier which works by increasing the heat and water vapor content of inspired gas. Passive humidification is the use of a heat and moisture exchanger (HME), often referred to as an "artificial nose."

Heated Humidifiers

The heated humidification system should provide a humidity level between 33 mg H_2O/L and 44 mg H_2O/L with a gas temperature of 34–41 °C at 100 % relative humidity (RH) for invasive ventilation. A maximum delivered temperature of 37 °C and 100 % RH at the circuit wye is recommended as condensation occurs with higher temperatures at 100 % saturation. Condensation can adversely affect muco-ciliary transport when mucus becomes thin and watery due to decreased mucus viscosity and increased pericellular fluid. Temperatures above 41 °C are considered a thermal hazard [25].

Inappropriate heater settings or heater malfunction may cause overheating of the inspired air to the patient and can result in thermal injury to the airways. The opposite may also occur in which the air delivered is too cool causing the pulmonary secretions to become thick and difficult to remove, which raises the risk of mucous plugging. It is important to ensure that the water chamber of a heated humidifier is not allowed to become dry, especially when used with a tracheostomy tube. Only sterile water should be utilized to minimize the chance of infection. If it is not available, tap water that has been boiled for 5 min can be used in its place. Distilled water should not be used as it can potentially be contaminated [28].

One of the more common problems in using heated humidification in the home setting is excessive condensation or "rain out" in the ventilator circuit. Circuit condensation actually represents under humidification and is a result of gas rapidly cooling in the tubing after leaving the chamber [27]. Causes include direct air drafts such as from fans or air-conditioning vents or a cool room temperature. Avoiding sources of drafts can help but this can be challenging for patients preferring cooler temperatures. Insulating the circuit with a wrap designed for tubing can also help alleviate much of the excess (see Fig. 10.7).

Circuit condensation can lead to several problems. It can cause the ventilator to auto-cycle and the high frequency/breath rate alarm to be activated. If condensation collects in the pressure lines of the circuit, it may also cause the ventilator to alarm. The potential also exists for accidental patient lavage. Circuit condensation should never be drained back into the humidifier as it is considered contaminated [25, 27, 29]. Although it may be difficult with heated wire circuits, a water trap can be used to remove condensation. Otherwise disconnect the tubing and drain the condensation on a towel or into a container to be discarded.

A heated tracheostomy collar, also referred to as a "mist collar," is frequently utilized during periods of sleep for those patients weaning from mechanical ventilation. It may also be used by patients during waking hours when more humidification is needed than an HME can provide. Bland aerosol, defined as delivery of sterile saline or water in aerosol form, is not a substitute for active humidification for patients receiving mechanical ventilation [30]. It should be avoided as a form of humidification because aerosol particles are capable of carrying particulate matter, whereas water vapor cannot, thereby increasing the

Fig. 10.7 Zippered insulation wrap for ventilator circuit

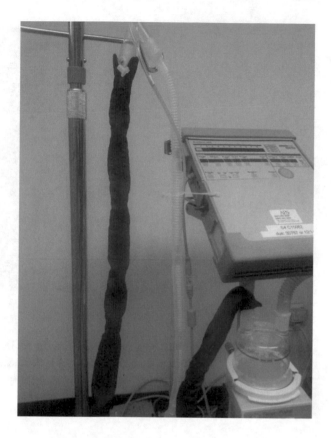

risk of infection [27]. Additionally, it has been shown in a tracheostomized, ventilated rabbit model that water administration via nebulizer (bland aerosol) may cause over-humidification, potentially leading to decreased alveolar air space, increased intra-alveolar and interstitial edema, and increased pulmonary arterial wall thickness [25–27, 31].

Heat Moisture Exchangers

While both active and passive humidification devices are acceptable for use with a tracheostomy tube, HMEs are more appropriate for short-term use (see Fig. 10.8). They may be inadequate for continuous use and are not recommended as a means of infection control in preventing ventilator-associated pneumonia [25]. The HME should deliver an absolute humidity of at least 30 mg H_2O/L for adequate humidification [25]. A fairly common practice is to utilize an HME during the day for portability and travel outside the home while using a heated humidifier at night. It also

Fig. 10.8 Heat moisture exchanger

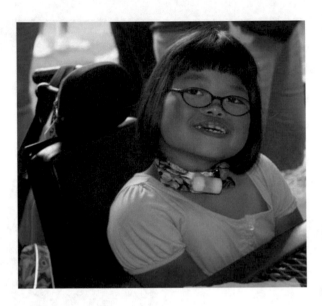

must be taken into account that the presence of an HME increases resistance and dead space which may lead to increased work of breathing in some patients [25, 29]. Additionally, an HME may cause the ventilator low-pressure alarm to be ineffective during disconnection [25].

Humidification with Noninvasive Ventilation

Although considered optional for NIV, humidification should not be disregarded. The high flows associated with NIV can disrupt the body's normal airway humidification process. Histopathological changes, increased vascularity of the nasal mucosa, and inspissated secretions have been reported in cases in which NIV was used without humidification [32–34].

Nasal congestion and oral dryness are common symptoms associated with use of NIV [35]. Leaks from both the mouth and around the mask can contribute to problems with humidification [33]. Use of heated humidification with NIV has been shown to increase comfort and adherence [25]. As standards have not yet been established, the temperature setting for the humidifier is generally based on patient preference [25, 33]. Heaters designed for use with NIV typically do not have a numerical temperature option but rather a dial to increase or decrease warmth. However, they are designed not to exceed 41 °C. Heated humidification is preferred over an HME for NIV because of decreased work of breathing due to less dead space [25, 32, 36].

Oxygen

With the exception of cystic fibrosis and other intrinsic lung diseases, the conditions seen in children who require supplemental oxygen often tend to improve with time such as with chronic lung disease of infancy. Those with neuromuscular diagnoses and congenital central hypoventilation syndrome (CCHS) generally do not utilize oxygen since the need for ventilator support is related to control of breathing for CCHS and respiratory muscle weakness in children with neuromuscular conditions rather than an underlying lung disease. Ventilator-dependent children are not always discharged home using continuous oxygen, but for those who are, many are weaned to needing it only at night and eventually not requiring it at all or just with acute illness.

Home oxygen is available in three forms: a liquid system, oxygen concentrators, and cylinders of oxygen. It is supplied by a DME provider who often makes the decision of which particular form to use. Required flow rate, patient mobility, and available space in the home are taken into consideration in choosing which option will be supplied. As children are rarely homebound, portable equipment should be provided as well as the stationary unit that remains in the home [37].

Liquid Oxygen System

A liquid oxygen system consists of a bulk storage reservoir unit and a small canister (see Figs. 10.9 and 10.10) that is refillable and portable for transport. While at home, the patient can use oxygen directly from the reservoir unit or can refill the canister and carry it from room to room in the home. Various style and sizes are manufactured but basically they all operate the same. There are several advantages to using a liquid system. They do not require electricity or generate heat, little noise is produced, and the canisters are lighter than oxygen cylinders and refillable at home using the reservoir unit. The main disadvantage to using the liquid oxygen system is that the DME provider must regularly refill the reservoir unit. How often this occurs depends upon the size of the reservoir unit and the required oxygen flow rate; however, it can be as frequent as once each week. Another disadvantage to the liquid system is that gas evaporates from the canisters whether the flow is on or off.

Most problems with a liquid oxygen system occur when refilling the canister. Ice crystals can form around the filling ports causing the connection to freeze and making it difficult to remove. It may take as long as 30 min for thawing to occur before the canister can be removed. This may be prevented by using a towel to dry the ports prior to connecting the canister. Caregivers are advised to allow for this possible delay when deciding when to refill the canister. White vapor spewing out of the fill port after removing the canister from the reservoir unit is another frequently encountered problem. This is usually an indication that the fill valve is stuck or frozen in the open position. This can be corrected by immediately reconnecting the canister

Fig. 10.9 Liquid oxygen reservoir unit

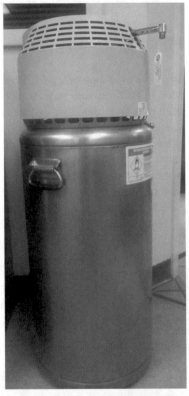

Fig. 10.10 Portable liquid oxygen canister

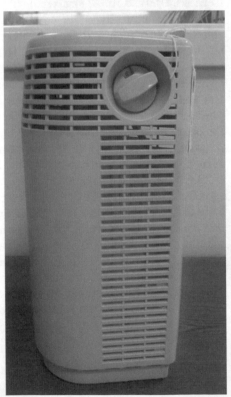

to the reservoir unit and waiting approximately 20 s before removing it. The greatest problem with liquid oxygen systems may simply be that the high cost of supply and delivery is causing many DME providers to no longer offer it as an option.

Oxygen Concentrators

Oxygen concentrators are electrically powered devices that separate oxygen from nitrogen in room air and then dispense the oxygen through a flow meter [38]. They include a colored visual alarm, which is triggered if the oxygen concentration falls below a certain level, and an audible alarm that is activated if there is a loss of electrical power. Concentrators are available as both stationary and portable units (see Fig. 10.11). Because they are cost prohibitive, most DME providers do not supply

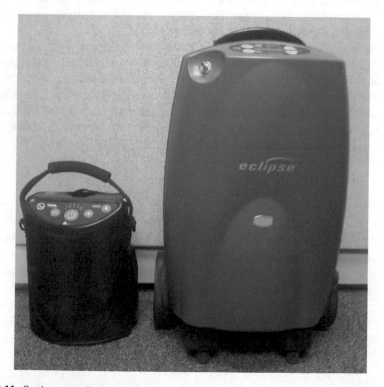

Fig. 10.11 Stationary and portable oxygen concentrators

the patient with portable concentrators except in special circumstances, such as airplane travel. Instead oxygen cylinders are usually provided to use for transport and as an alternative source in case of an electrical power outage or mechanical failure of the concentrator.

It should be appreciated that the oxygen purity delivered by a concentrator is lower than that from piped oxygen and is dependent upon the flow rate [39, 40]. The delivered concentration decreases as the liter flow requirement increases, making the concentrator unsuitable for some patients, especially those requiring higher flow rates. The concentration has also been found to decrease with increased working duration of the concentrator [41, 42]. The maximum concentration of oxygen obtained during studies was about 96 %, and a concentration greater than 90 % was usually attainable only when flow rates were less than 5 L/min. Oxygen concentration was found to decrease to less than 50 % when flow was maintained at 12 L/min or greater [43, 44].

Advantages to using oxygen concentrators are they can be easily moved from room to room, they cost less to use than bulk oxygen tanks, they do not require refilling, and they provide an unlimited supply of oxygen as long as there is available electrical power. Caregivers often complain that concentrators are noisy and that use results in an increase in their monthly electricity costs. Concentrators also generate heat which often causes the family to require additional cooling in the home, adding even more to their utility expense [45].

Stationary oxygen concentrators have minimal problems. Loss of electrical power that occurs during a storm or when the power cord becomes disconnected is the main reason the audible alarm is activated. The visual alarm may be activated if the intake filter is clogged with lint, in which case the filter should be replaced. It may also be activated if the concentrator's air intake area is blocked, for example, by furniture or curtains. It is important that caregivers provide the patient with another oxygen source before trying to determine the reason for the alarm.

Oxygen Cylinders

Oxygen cylinders are a very cost-effective option for providing oxygen in the home. They are less expensive than liquid oxygen and can be stored without gas evaporating. Unlike oxygen concentrators, cylinders do not require electricity or generate heat. Various sizes are available. The smaller cylinders have carrying cases which make for easy mobility, while E cylinders have a two-wheel cart that can be pulled. The major disadvantages of using oxygen cylinders are their frequent need for replacement, bulkiness which requires storage space, and the potential safety issues that arise when gas is contained under high pressure.

Monitoring

Standards of care are lacking regarding both the equipment utilized and the frequency of home monitoring for ventilator-dependent patients. Practices and recommendations differ among institutions and by region. Reimbursement, which varies from state to state, often determines what can be obtained for home. Options for monitoring the ventilator-dependent patient at home include the pulse oximeter, end-tidal carbon dioxide monitor, and apnea monitor. And although not considered monitors, ventilators today may be equipped with a smart card that can provide information about the patient and equipment. Data that is downloaded from the card may then assist with determining if problems exist. This can include identifying inappropriate ventilator settings, airway leaks, or patient dyssynchrony.

Pulse Oximeter

There are several potential problems that may be encountered with the pulse oximeter at home, most of which are related to the sensor. Table 10.4 lists factors that contribute to false results. A monitor that has a waveform display is helpful for distinguishing when signal strength is sufficient to produce a reliable reading. An accessory wrap can be utilized not only to reduce ambient light but also to help secure the probe in place. If the probe is placed on a toe, wearing a sock can help with keeping the probe securely in place. Nail polish should not be used on fingers or toes where the probe will be placed.

Most pulse oximeter probes are designed to be used on the fingers or toes. There are, however, probes designed for use on the forehead or nose. When placing the probe, the red light-emitting diode must directly align with the photodetector so one can communicate with the other. Inaccurate readings are likely to occur if they are not properly aligned.

A faulty sensor or cable should be suspected when the pulse oximeter will power on but a reading is either not displayed or shows only intermittently. This often occurs when the probe has become worn, is dirty, or the internal circuitry has been damaged. If replacing the probe does not resolve the problem, the next step would

Table 10.4 Factors contributing to false pulse oximetry readings	Low perfusion—weak pulse, hypotension, hypothermia
	Motion artifact—tremors, seizures, shivering, excessive movement
	Improper sensor placement
	Probe secured too tightly or too loose
	Bright ambient light
	Dirty probe
	Nail polish

be to change the cable which connects the probe to the pulse oximeter device. The probe should always be replaced if wires are exposed. Caregivers should be instructed on how to place the probe on themselves to test if it is working properly.

While usually a rare event, thermal burns and/or skin breakdown can occur if the sensor is not rotated at regular intervals [46, 47]. Infants and patients with fragile skin are more susceptible to this occurrence. The frequency of rotation may vary depending on manufacturer recommendations and the patient's individual needs. Establishing a schedule for changing the probe site at specific intervals can help avoid this problem.

Most pulse oximeter devices have an internal battery for portability. Caregivers should be aware of the battery capacity and plan accordingly when away from home. Ideally an oximeter with recording and downloading capabilities is preferred so usage and trends can be reviewed by the clinician.

End-tidal CO_2 Monitor

The use of routine monitoring of end-tidal carbon dioxide ($PETCO_2$) for home is not a common practice. However, there is evidence to support its use in monitoring patients with congenital central hypoventilation syndrome (CCHS) [48]. It is important to note that $PETCO_2$ may be underestimated in those with intrinsic lung disease. Breath-to-breath variation may also be observed depending on respiratory rate and effort. Typically the device will require calibration per the manufacturer specifications. Obtaining a reliable reading tends to be the most common problem with use of the end-tidal CO_2 monitor at home. Some models have a waveform display that may assist in determining if the reading is reliable. It is important to appreciate underestimation in the presence of lung disease and breath-to-breath variation.

Apnea Monitor

Since their introduction in the mid-1960s, apnea monitors, also known as cardiorespiratory monitors, have continued to be used at home by infants and children who have conditions that may result in episodes of prolonged apnea. A policy statement issued by the American Academy of Pediatrics in 2003 and reaffirmed in 2007 notes that apnea monitors may be warranted in patients who are at risk of sudden death. This includes infants with tracheostomies and those who require mechanical ventilation [49]. Current practice varies in the use of apnea monitors with ventilator-dependent infants and children. While monitors are believed by some to be an essential tool for detection of apnea, others feel that use is redundant with ventilators that have intrinsic apnea alarms.

Apnea monitors determine and display the patient's respiratory rate and heart rate. Alarms are activated when central apnea, bradycardia, or tachycardia occur.

Using impedance pneumography, the monitor detects respiratory movements by measuring the change in electrical impedance between two electrodes placed on the patient's chest. The electrode pads are maintained in place with a soft belt wrapped around the patient's chest and held together with a Velcro attachment. Failure to detect respiratory movement results in activation of an apnea alarm. It is critical to note that the apnea alarm will not be activated in the presence of obstructive apnea, such as occurs with an obstructed tracheostomy tube or occluded mask. However, obstruction that continues for an extended time eventually leads to bradycardia which will activate an alarm.

Although currently used mainly in the hospital setting, cardiorespiratory monitors are now available that monitor respiratory rate, heart rate, and SpO_2. With the additional ability to monitor oxygenation, these monitors may be capable of more quickly detecting obstructive events. Home apnea monitors include event-recording capabilities. This allows for interpretation of data that details the time and type of alarms, severity of apnea events, and hours of monitor use.

Problems encountered in the use of apnea monitors in the home are mostly related to activation of loose-lead or machine alarms. The loose-lead alarm may be activated when oil is present on the skin or the electrode pad, electrodes become detached from the pads, cable wires become detached from leads, or the belt is too loose causing the electrode pads to not be in close contact with the chest wall. Alarms may be activated if the electrode pads are not placed under the appropriate arm or if the monitor battery is low. Electronic or radio frequency from cordless phones or other devices may interfere with alarm function. If this is suspected, then the monitor should be placed at a sufficient distance from the devices.

Regardless of the type of monitor used in the home, caregivers should be reminded not to solely rely on the device but to also closely observe the patient for signs and symptoms of respiratory distress that may occur before an alarm is activated. Additionally, erroneous monitor readings could be mistaken for distress in the absence of other indicators of difficulty breathing. A vigilant and competent caregiver is often preferred over any monitoring device available. Without the knowledge to interpret the information from the monitor correctly, the best monitoring devices are useless.

Additional Equipment in the Home

Children dependent upon home mechanical ventilation are not a homogenous group. The etiology of the need for ventilator support can range from chronic lung diseases of infancy to neuromuscular disease to spinal cord injury and much more. Not all individuals requiring home ventilation have intrinsic lung disease or require additional respiratory modalities such as airway clearance. Therefore, additional equipment in the home, other than the ventilator, will vary in each case.

Suction Machine

If the patient has a tracheostomy, a portable suction machine is considered standard of care. In some cases the patient may have both a portable machine and a stationary machine that remains in the home. A leak or crack in the suction canister is the most common problem encountered and is cause for the canister to be immediately replaced. To prevent bacterial contamination, the canister should be cleaned at least once each week or whenever it requires emptying. Failure to empty the canister and allowing its contents to overflow can result in the filter becoming wet or even permanently damage the machine. The filter should be changed every 2 months or any time it becomes wet or soiled. If the machine does not provide a vacuum, it is most likely due to a kink in the connecting tubing. This tubing should be changed weekly or whenever it is heavily soiled. The portable machine relies on a battery for power and should be kept plugged into an AC power outlet when it is not in use. If the internal battery power is drained, the suction machine must be connected to AC power.

Resuscitation Bag

A self-inflating resuscitation bag is mandatory equipment for a ventilator-dependent child. Although flow-inflating bags are often used in the hospital setting, they require high flows and should be used with a pressure manometer. For these reasons they are not recommended for home use. There are several designs of resuscitation bags; however, the basic components include a valve head that connects to either a tracheostomy tube or a mask and the body that is squeezed. The most common problems experienced with a resuscitation bag include malfunction of the valve head and a leak in the body. The valve head can become cracked, disassembled, or disconnected from the body of the bag. A leak in the body will result in inadequate air filling the bag.

Caregivers should be instructed to test the bag daily for correct valve function and for leaks. Valve function can be tested by squeezing the bag completely and then releasing the bag while keeping the outlet occluded with the palm of the hand. If the bag does not refill, then the valve may be sticking. When this occurs the valve head should be taken apart, reassembled, and the test repeated. The bag should be replaced if it cannot refill freely.

To determine if the bag is free of leaks, the caregiver occludes the outlet of the bag with the palm of one hand while squeezing the bag with the other hand. Pressure will build in the bag if it is functioning correctly. Failure to do so indicates a leak. If a leak is present, then all connections should be checked and the test repeated. If the leak remains, then the bag should be replaced.

Resources When Equipment Fails

Educating parents and caregivers on the proper use of the home equipment and providing them with a plan of action should a problem occur is essential for successfully providing care at home. Identifying and troubleshooting problems with the ventilator and other respiratory equipment should be part of the competency training provided to parents and caregivers prior to discharging the patient from the hospital. Addressing when they should seek outside assistance and who to contact when advice is needed should be included. Although it varies as to whether or not a landline phone is mandatory, there must be twenty-four hour telephone access within the home.

Be it the DME company or the hospital, whoever provides the equipment in the home is the one who should be responsible for addressing mechanical issues or equipment failure. It is inappropriate to direct malfunction problems to the primary care physician or the home nursing company. Therefore, when selecting the DME provider, it is important to note if the company maintains therapists or nurses who are proficient in caring for and assessing a ventilator-dependent child and who can also solve equipment problems. Although delivery personnel and sales staff may provide home assistance, it is far better to have competent respiratory therapists or nurses available 24 h, 7 days per week to respond to issues concerning equipment malfunction.

Emergency and Disaster Preparedness

When preparing for the initial transition from hospital to home, emergency preparedness is not a subject to be taken lightly for this patient population. A survey of parents and caregivers of children dependent upon electrically powered medical devices at home found that most were not adequately prepared [50]. Unfortunately the importance is usually highlighted when a disaster has occurred but once a sense of normalcy returns, complacency often sets in until the next catastrophic event.

Depending on geographical location, natural disasters, such as tornadoes, hurricanes, earthquakes, and floods, are potential threats that may cause extended power outages. Another possible emergency event is a blackout. During the 2003 blackout in New York, emergency medical services and hospitals experienced an unexpected increase in calls and visits from patients dependent on electrically powered respiratory devices at home [51]. This was also the case during the 2011 Japan earthquake where 75 % of pediatric admissions were technology assisted patients [52].

Table 10.5 Contents of emergency travel bag

Ventilator circuit and adaptors
Heat moisture exchangers
List of ventilator settings
List of medications
Cleaning solution
Names and phone numbers of healthcare/community resources
• Hospital
• Clinic
• Physicians
• Durable medical equipment company
• Oxygen supply company
• Home care nursing company

Emergency Generators

During periods of prolonged power outage, a generator is one source of external power that can be utilized. While often recommended, it is not usually considered a necessity and many families are unable to obtain one. When a generator is available for use, one should be mindful that it is powered by gasoline. The cost of gasoline and the ability to obtain it during a disaster may become troublesome issues during a prolonged emergency or disaster.

Generators should be routinely maintained per manufacturer recommendations. They should also be periodically tested for proper function so that when the need arises to utilize it, caregivers are prepared and knowledgeable in its operation. Portable generators should be kept outside when in use to ensure adequate ventilation. Because the patient often requires equipment in addition to the ventilator, the generator's wattage rating should be noted, especially if the family plans to use it to power other devices. Consideration should be given to other equipment that requires an electrical power source. This includes oxygen concentrators, suction machines, air and aerosol compressors, airway clearance devices, and feeding pumps. Some of these devices have an internal battery backup but others do not. Other potential sources of external power supply include an inverter and car adapters.

Emergency Plans

Just as public schools and businesses have drills and emergency preparation plans in place to use in the event of a prolonged power failure or need for evacuation, a similar plan should exist for technology-dependent children living at home. Practicing drills in the home setting can help avoid additional problems that might be encountered should a disaster actually occur. A Japanese study of evacuation

Table 10.6 Future investigative issues concerning home equipment

Use and availability of generators in the home
Requirements concerning a "backup" ventilator
Cost-effectiveness and necessity of home monitoring
Home surveillance with videophone monitoring
Determination of which to use—apnea monitor, pulse oximeter, or both
Humidification practices with noninvasive ventilation
Safety and effectiveness of oxygen placement within the ventilator circuit
Frequency of home visit impact on hospital readmissions
Time frame post-discharge in which caregivers experience most technical problems
Time frame post-discharge in which DME company and nursing staff receive most calls concerning equipment problems
Effectiveness of training caregivers prior to discharge
• Various teaching methods—e.g., simulation, online instruction, bedside instruction, written manuals, videos
• Requirements concerning the mandatory number of caregivers to be instructed on equipment use and operation
• Rooming-in with patient prior to discharge—frequency, duration, location, responsibilities

disaster drills for those receiving home ventilation revealed three crucial elements for preparedness: the need for community awareness of the ventilator-dependent child, the family's practice of emergently leaving the home, and involvement of home nurses [53].

The family's emergency plan should include a list of places and addresses close to home where they can expect to obtain power. Hotels, hospitals, fire houses, and emergency halls are often able to maintain power during widespread outages. Out-of-town family and friends should also be listed. A travel bag should be packed and readily available to take along with the tracheostomy go bag. Table 10.5 lists the suggested contents of this bag.

The American Academy of Pediatrics policy statement regarding emergency preparedness for children with special needs recommends the use of an emergency information form (EIF) [54]. The EIF is a medical summary that includes information such as medical condition, medications, and health-care needs to facilitate emergency care. It should include disaster planning and be routinely maintained and updated every 6 months [54].

Summary and Future Research Needs

In summary, there are many potential problems that may occur in the home of the child dependent upon mechanical ventilation. The majority of issues tend to be equipment related; however, a properly trained and alert caregiver is critical for the ventilator-dependent child to safely remain at home. Despite the type of interface used and length of time dependent upon ventilator support, it is always important to respond to all alarms in a timely manner. Adequate humidification, appropriate oxygen use, and monitoring are also vital elements. History has shown that emergency and disaster preparedness should not be taken lightly.

Care of the ventilator-dependent child remains complex partially due to technological advances that have created more options and availability of equipment in the home. This includes not only the ability to provide additional types of equipment but to also provide more complex models of equipment currently used. And as technology changes, so do the questions concerning availability and appropriateness of the equipment and care provided at home. Although practice patterns are evolving in accordance with an expanding evidence base, there is still room for improvement and the need for further clinical studies. Table 10.6 lists areas in which future investigation may be warranted to determine guidelines concerning the type and amount of equipment placed in the home of the ventilator-dependent child.

Acknowledgments We thank Tammy Hall RRT and Michelle Mantuano RRT for sharing their expertise in caring for ventilator-dependent children at home.

References

1. Baldwin-Myers AS, Oppenheimer EA. Quality of life and quality of care data from a 7-year pilot project for home ventilator patients. J Ambul Care Manage. 1996;19:46–59.
2. Hammer J. Home mechanical ventilation in children: indications and practical aspects. Schweiz Med Wochenschr. 2000;130:1894–902.
3. Markström A, Sundell K, Lysdahl M, et al. Quality-of-life evaluation of patients with neuromuscular and skeletal diseases treated with noninvasive and invasive home mechanical ventilation. Chest. 2002;122:1695–700.
4. Murphy J. Medically Stable Children in PICU: better at home. Paediatr Nurs. 2008;20:14–6.
5. Warner J, Norwood S. Psychosocial concerns of the ventilator-dependent child in the pediatric intensive care unit. AACN Clin Issues Crit Care Nurs. 1991;2:432–45.
6. Gowans M, Keenan HT, Bratton SL. The population prevalence of children receiving invasive home ventilation in Utah. Pediatr Pulmonol. 2007;42:231–6.
7. Graham RJ, Fleegler EW, Robinson WM. Chronic ventilator need in the community: a 2005 pediatric census of Massachusetts. Pediatrics. 2007;119:e1280–7.
8. Racca F, Berta G, Sequi M, et al. Long-term home ventilation of children in Italy: a national survey. Pediatr Pulmonol. 2011;46:566–72.
9. Boroughs D, Dougherty JA. Decreasing accidental mortality of ventilator-dependent children at home: a call to action. Home Healthc Nurse. 2012;30:103–11.
10. Simonds AK. Risk management of the home ventilator dependent patient. Thorax. 2006;61:369–71.
11. Edwards JD, Kun SS, Keens TG. Outcomes and causes of death in children on home mechanical ventilation via tracheostomy: an institutional and literature review. J Pediatr. 2010;157(955-959), e2.
12. Srinivasan S, Doty SM, White TR, et al. Frequency, causes and outcome of home ventilator failure. Chest. 1998;114:1363–7.
13. Chatwin M, Heather S, Hanak A, et al. Analysis of home support and ventilator malfunction in 1,211 ventilator-dependent patients. Eur Respir J. 2010;35:310–6.
14. AARC Respiratory Home Focus Group. AARC clinical practice guideline: long-term invasive mechanical ventilation in the home – 2007 revision & update. Respir Care. 2007;52:1056–62.
15. Love LC, Millin CJ, Kerns CD. Take precautions with audible alarms on ventilators. Nursing. 2011;41:65.

16. Graham KC, Cvach M. Monitor alarm fatigue: standardizing use of physiological monitors and decreasing nuisance alarms. Am J Crit Care. 2010;19:28–34.
17. Management ED. Citing reports of alarm-related deaths, The Joint Commission issues a sentinel event alert for hospitals to improve medical device alarm safety. ED Manage. 2013;26(suppl):1–3.
18. Kun SS, Nakamura CT, Ripka JF, et al. Home ventilator low-pressure alarms fail to detect accidental decannulation with pediatric tracheostomy tubes. Chest. 2001;119:562–4.
19. Farre R, Navajas D, Prats E, et al. Performance of mechanical ventilators at the patient's home: a multicenter quality control study. Thorax. 2006;61:400–4.
20. Dohna-Schwake C, Podlewski P, Voit T, et al. Non-invasive ventilation reduces respiratory tract infections in children with neuromuscular disorders. Pediatr Pulmonol. 2008;43:67–71.
21. Sherman JM, Davis S, Albamonte-Petrick S, et al. Care of the child with a chronic tracheostomy. This official statement of the American Thoracic Society was adopted by the ATS Board of Directors, July 199. Am J Respir Crit Care Med. 2000;161:297–308.
22. Fauroux B, Lavis JF, Nicot F, et al. Facial side effects during noninvasive positive pressure ventilation in children. Intens Care Med. 2005;31:965–9.
23. Li KK, Riley RW, Guilleminault C. An unreported risk in the use of home nasal continuous positive airway pressure and home nasal ventilation in children: mid face hypoplasia. Chest. 2000;117:916–8.
24. Tsuda H, Almeida FR, Tsuda T, et al. Craniofacial changes after 2 years of nasal continuous positive pressure use in patients with obstructive sleep apnea. Chest. 2010;138:870–4.
25. Restrepo RD, Walsh BK. AARC clinical practice guideline: humidification during invasive and noninvasive mechanical ventilation 2012. Respir Care. 2012;57:782–8.
26. Ryan SN, Peterson BD. The ins and outs of humidification. J Respir Care Pract. 2003;27(1):37–40.
27. Schulze A. Respiratory gas conditioning in infants with an artificial airway. Semin Neonatol. 2002;7:369–77.
28. Saiman L, Siegel J. Infection control in cystic fibrosis. Clin Microbiol Rev. 2004;17:57–71.
29. Branson RD. Humidification for patients with artificial airways. Respir Care. 1999;44:630–41.
30. Kallstrom J. AARC clinical practice guideline. Bland aerosol administration—2003 revision & update. Respir Care. 2003;48:529–33.
31. John E, Ermocilla R, Goden J, et al. Effects of gas temperature and particulate water on rabbit lungs during ventilation. Pediatr Res. 1980;14:1186–91.
32. Nava S, Navalesi P, Gregoretti C. Interfaces and humidification for noninvasive mechanical ventilation. Respir Care. 2009;54:71–84.
33. Rodrigues AME, Scala R, Soroksky A, et al. Clinical review: humidifiers during non-invasive ventilation—key topics and practical implications. Crit Care. 2012;16:203.
34. Wood KE, Flaten AL, Backes WJ. Inspissated secretions: a life-threatening complication of prolonged noninvasive ventilation. Respir Care. 2000;45:491–3.
35. Oto J, Imanaka H, Nishimura M. Clinical factors affecting inspired gas humidification and oral dryness during noninvasive ventilation. J Crit Care. 2011;26:535.e9–535.e15.
36. Lellouche F, Pignataro C, Maggiore SM, et al. Short-term effects of humidification devices on respiratory pattern and arterial blood gases during noninvasive ventilation. Respir Care. 2012;57:1879–86.
37. Balfour-Lynn IM, Field DJ, Gringras P, on behalf of the Paediatric Section of the Home Oxygen Guideline Development Group of the BTS Standards of Care Committee, et al. BTS Guidelines for home oxygen in children. Thorax. 2009;64:ii1–26.
38. Harris ND, Stamp JM. Current developments in oxygen concentrator technology. J Med Eng Technol. 1987;11:103–7.
39. Bolton CE, Annandale JA, Ebden P. Comparison of an oxygen concentrator and wall oxygen in the assessment of patients undergoing long term oxygen therapy assessment. Chron Respir Dis. 2006;3:49–51.
40. Gould GA, Scott W, Hayhurst MD, et al. Technical and clinical assessment of oxygen concentrators. Thorax. 1985;40:811–6.
41. Bongard JP, Pahud C, De Haller R. Insufficient oxygen concentration obtained at domiciliary controls of 18 concentrators. Eur Respir J. 1989;2:280–2.

42. Sous-Commission Technique ANTADIR. Home controls of a sample of 2,414 oxygen concentrators. Eur Respir J. 1991;4:227–31.
43. Johns DP, Rochford PD, Streeton JA. Evaluation of six oxygen concentrators. Thorax. 1985;40:806–10.
44. Rathgeber J, Züchner K, Keitzmann D, et al. Efficiency of a mobile oxygen concentrator for mechanical ventilation in anesthesia. Studies with a metabolic lung model and early clinical results. Anaesthesist. 1995;44:643–50.
45. Munhoz AS, Adde FV, Nakaie CM, et al. Long-term home oxygen therapy in children and adolescents: analysis of clinical use and costs of a home care program. J Pediatr. 2011;87:13–8.
46. Bunker DLJ, Kumar R, Martin A, et al. Thermal injuries caused by medical instruments: a case report of burns caused by a pulse oximeter. 2013. J Burn Care Res, [Epub ahead of print].
47. Ceran C, Taner OF, Tekin F, et al. Management of pulse oximeter probe-induced finger injuries in children: report of two consecutive cases and review of the literature. J Pediatr Surg. 2012;47:e27–9.
48. Weese-Mayer DE, Berry-Kravis EM, Ceccherini I, et al. An official ATS clinical policy statement: congenital central hypoventilation syndrome: genetic basis, diagnosis and management. Am J Respir Crit Care Med. 2010;181:626–44.
49. American Academy of Pediatrics, Committee on Fetus and Newborn. Apnea, sudden infant death syndrome, and home monitoring. Pediatrics. 2003;111:914–7.
50. Sakashita K, Matthews WJ, Yamaoto LG. Disaster preparedness for technology and electricity-dependent children and youth with special health care needs. Clin Pediatr. 2013;52(6):549–56.
51. Prezant DJ, Stanislav Belyaev JC, Alleyene D, et al. Effects of the August 2003 blackout on the New York City healthcare delivery system: a lesson for disaster preparedness. Crit Care Med. 2005;33:S96–101.
52. Nakayama T, Tanaka S, Uematsu M, et al. Effect of a blackout in pediatric patients with home medical devices during the 2011 eastern Japan earthquake. 2013. Brain Dev, [Epub ahead of print].
53. Hatanaka H, Miki S, Yuasa N, et al. Conducting disaster assistance drills for patients who receive a home ventilator care. Gan To Kagaku Ryoho (Cancer and Chemotherapy). 2010;37:S201–3 [article in Japanese].
54. American Academy of Pediatrics, Committee on Pediatric Emergency Medicine and Council on Clinical Information Technology, American College of Emergency Physicians, Pediatric Emergency Medicine Committee. Policy statement—emergency information forms and emergency preparedness for children with special health care needs. Pediatrics. 2010;125:829–37.

Chapter 11
Inhaled Drug Delivery for Children on Long-term Mechanical Ventilation

Ariel Berlinski

Background

Improvements in neonatal and pediatric intensive care knowledge, skills, and technology have contributed to the development of a population that relies on technology for their health maintenance and survival. Many of these patients receive some type of respiratory support either as invasive or noninvasive ventilation. Most of these patients are prescribed inhaled therapeutic aerosols for chronic and acute management of their respiratory disease [1, 2]. To make matters more complex, this population is very heterogeneous making "one way fits all" not a viable approach. This population includes patients with different degrees of ventilator dependence (total vs. partial), patients with or without tracheostomy, patients with and without intrinsic lung disease, and patients with and without normal cognitive abilities.

The use of inhaled bronchodilators, corticosteroids, antibiotics, and mucolytics has been reported in this population [1–11]. Little evidence is available regarding optimization of aerosol delivery in this population. Several surveys have demonstrated variability in practice regarding administration of aerosol to patients receiving mechanical ventilation and with tracheostomies across different centers [1, 12].

Different types of ventilators, ventilation modality, circuits, aerosol generators, add-on devices, and connectors and their combination are responsible for the severalfold difference in drug delivery that has been found in several studies. For example, the same aerosol generator placed in a different position on a ventilator circuit can result in a severalfold difference in delivered drug. To make matters more complex, the optimization of drug delivery in invasive ventilation is not similar to that of using noninvasive ventilation. The same patient might start receiving noninvasive ventilation, then progress to tracheostomy and invasive ventilation or vice versa.

A. Berlinski, M.D. (✉)
College of Medicine, Arkansas Children's Hospital, University of Arkansas for Medical Sciences, 1 Children's Way, Slot 512-17, Little Rock, AR 72202, USA
e-mail: berlinskiariel@uams.edu

© Springer Science+Business Media New York 2016
L.M. Sterni, J.L. Carroll (eds.), *Caring for the Ventilator Dependent Child*,
Respiratory Medicine, DOI 10.1007/978-1-4939-3749-3_11

This might require changing the type and position of delivery device. Practitioners need to become proficient on how to optimize aerosol drug delivery under different clinical situations/device combinations.

In this chapter we will first discuss the basics of aerosol delivery. A description of the different available delivery devices will follow. Finally the use of aerosols will be discussed for different clinical scenarios that practitioners frequently encounter in the management of respiratory technology-dependent children (invasive vs. noninvasive ventilation and with either total or partial ventilation dependence).

The use of aerosols in the neonatal age group will not be discussed since the small size of the artificial airways and the low tidal volumes preclude any extrapolation of results to older children who are receiving chronic mechanical ventilation.

A Brief Primer on Principles of Respiratory Aerosol Delivery

Aerosol deposition is dependent on aerosol-related and patient-related factors [13]. The former include particle size, velocity, hygroscopic properties, type of aerosol generator, and availability of the drug. Patient-related factors include airway size, disease state, breathing pattern, and cognitive and physical ability. Additionally, patients receiving mechanical ventilation incorporate other factors such as type of ventilator support (noninvasive vs. invasive), endotracheal tube (ETT) size, tracheostomy size, bias flow, heated and humidified air, ventilation mode, gas properties, circuit size, and others (Table 11.1) [14, 15].

Aerosols are characterized by several parameters such as mass median aerodynamic diameter (MMAD), geometric standard deviation (GSD), and the fine-particle fraction [13, 16]. The latter is the ratio between the mass of particles <5 μm and the mass of the emitted dose. The MMAD is a measure of central tendency, while the GSD is a unitless measure of dispersion. Most medicinal aerosols are composed of particles of different sizes. When the GSD is greater than 1.22, they are considered polydispersed. Particles with an MMAD between 1 and 3 μm will be deposited in the peripheral airways, while particles with an MMAD smaller than 1 μm and especially those with an MMAD smaller than 0.5 μm tend to be exhaled. Aerosols with an MMAD between 1 and 5 μm are considered more likely to favor intrapulmonary deposition. However, it is not clear if these principles would apply to aerosols delivered during invasive mechanical ventilation via an endotracheal tube or a tracheostomy tube. Aerosols leave the generator at a certain size that increases by exposure to humidity present in the circuit and decreases through impaction with the circuit, connectors, and endotracheal tubes. In addition to particle size, inspiratory flow plays an important role in intrapulmonary drug deposition with lower flows resulting in larger deposition irrespective of the MMAD [17]. There are three main mechanisms of aerosol deposition in the lungs: impaction, sedimentation, and diffusion [13]. The latter is the mechanism mostly responsible for deposition of submicronic aerosols (MMAD < 1 μm). While impaction is responsible for deposition of aerosols traveling at high velocity and those larger than 3 μm,

Table 11.1 Factors influencing aerosol drug delivery during mechanical ventilation

| | | Device | | | |
Ventilator	Circuit	MDI	Nebulizer	Drug	Patient
Mode	Circuit size	Adapter/spacer	Type	Particle size	Disease state
Tidal volume	ETT size	Timing of actuation	Position		
Duty cycle	Humidity	Position	Mode of operation		
Flow pattern	Bias flow	Compatibility of actuator canister			
	Gas density				

Modified from [14]

sedimentation is responsible for slower aerosols and those with an MMAD between 0.5 and 3 μm. An increase in the time the aerosol stays in the airways favors its deposition via this mechanism and constitutes the basis for the breath-holding maneuver used when using pressurized metered-dose inhalers and dry powder inhalers. The presence of artificial airways (ETT and tracheostomies) increases airway resistance and airflow turbulence. Therefore, impaction plays a significant role in deposition in the circuit and artificial airways.

Delivery Devices

There are three main types of aerosol generators: nebulizers, metered-dose inhalers (pressurized and soft mist), and dry powder inhalers [13, 16].

Nebulizers can be classified into jet, ultrasonic, and vibrating mesh nebulizers. Jet nebulizers use an external air source to convert a solution or suspension into a mist [13, 16]. During that process aerosols decrease their temperature by 10 °C [18]. Jet nebulizers can be further classified as continuous-output (aerosol generated and released during inspiratory and expiratory cycle), breath-enhanced (drug output increases during inspiration due to incorporation of one-way valve in the nebulizer's design), and breath-actuated (drug delivery occurs only during inspiration) nebulizer [13, 16]. The latter requires a threshold flow to open the inspiratory valve and may not be suitable for use in children especially those with small tidal volumes and inspiratory flows.

The performance of disposable nebulizers can vary significantly even between units of the same brand [19]. Their filling volume is optimal between 3 and 4 mL [20]. The volume that remains in the nebulizer after the treatment is completed (residual volume) ranges between 0.8 and 1.5 mL [21]. Conversely, vibrating mesh nebulizers have minimal to no dead volume [22]. They require an external power source and they are nearly noiseless. Liquid is forced either actively or passively through a membrane with precision-drilled holes [23]. They produce a low-velocity and soft mist that keeps a constant temperature. Proper care of the mesh is crucial to avoid clogging of the holes. Lastly, ultrasonic nebulizers use an electrical source to vibrate a piezoelectric crystal at high frequency, which generates sound waves resulting in the production of an aerosol at the fluid surface [13, 16]. This technology heats the fluid up to 15 °C during nebulization and could potentially denature proteins [22]. The device has been also found to be inefficient to deliver budesonide due to the large size of the particles [24].

In addition to the complexity of aerosol delivery via nebulizers, its used attached ventilator circuits and tracheostomies introduce another set of problems that will be discussed later in the chapter. Nebulizers are connected to either T-pieces or spring-loaded T-pieces when used in tracheostomized patients and when placed in ventilator circuits. Additionally, some practitioners use a resuscitation bag to assist drug delivery when connected to either a tracheostomy or an ETT [1].

Pressurized metered-dose inhalers (pMDI) have a drug in suspension/solution mixed with a propellant. Currently, almost all pMDIs in the United States contain hydrofluoroalkanes (HFA) as propellant. These inhalers require specific care to properly function [13, 16]. Lack of proper care leads to the blockage of the actuator's nozzle. Unfortunately, each brand has specific instructions for initial and repeat priming as well as cleaning of the plastic booth. The canisters of medications containing HFA can't be submerged in water because it can cause obstruction of the metering valve. In addition, some brands changed the canister configuration to accommodate the presence of a dose counter [16]. Pressurized MDIs are used in combination with either holding chambers, spacers, or adapters when they are used in tracheostomized patients and when placed in ventilator circuits [1, 14, 15]. Additionally, some practitioners use a resuscitation bag to assist drug delivery when connected to either tracheostomy or an ETT [1]. This could be detrimental to aerosol delivery due to increased aerosol impaction caused by the generated high flows.

Recently, a soft metered-dose inhaler containing a combination of albuterol and ipratropium bromide was released in the United States. The device utilizes the mechanical energy provided by a spring to force a propellant-free solution through a very small nozzle generating a slow mist [25]. The development of an adapter for its use in an adult-type mechanical ventilation circuit has been reported [26].

Currently available dry powder inhalers (DPI) are breath-actuated devices that use the patient's inspiratory flow to disaggregate the drug [13, 16]. A clinical study in adults and an in vitro study using an adult model demonstrated the feasibility of delivering drug through tracheostomies and ETTs with this type of delivery device [27–29]. However, a recent survey reported its lack of use in pediatric population [1]. The need for large inhalation flows to disaggregate the powder does not make them a suitable alternative for drug delivery in children. In addition, the performance of these devices is adversely affected by humidity [30].

One of the major challenges in developing evidence-based recommendations for aerosol delivery in pediatric patients receiving invasive and noninvasive mechanical ventilation is the scarcity of clinical data due to the ethical considerations of use of radio-labeled aerosols and sequential blood draws in that age group [31]. In addition, age- and size-related changes in anatomy and physiology make matters more difficult. Few data are available with small- and medium-size animals [32–35]. Researchers have developed in vitro models to investigate the behavior of aerosols under different conditions. A good correlation between in vivo and in vitro data has been established [36–38].

Based on the type of ventilation and tolerance to being disconnected from it, the following clinical scenarios are possible: (1) patients receiving invasive mechanical ventilation who do not tolerate being disconnected from the ventilator, (2) patients receiving invasive mechanical ventilation who tolerate being disconnected from the ventilator, (3) patients who are tracheostomized and breath spontaneously, (4) patients receiving noninvasive mechanical ventilation who do not tolerate being disconnected from the ventilator, and (5) patients receiving noninvasive mechanical ventilation who tolerate being disconnected from the ventilator. Each of these scenarios presents unique challenges for effective aerosol delivery and will be discussed individually.

Patients Receiving Mechanical Ventilation Who Do Not Tolerate Being Disconnected from the Ventilator

Patients who are unable to be disconnected from the ventilator to receive inhaled therapy will have adaptor and connectors that will allow the aerosol to be generated and transported through the circuit (in-line therapy). Filters should be placed between the ventilator and the tubing that connects to the humidifier and between the expiratory limb of the circuit and the ventilator to prevent damage of the ventilator components by the aerosols (Figs. 11.1 and 11.5). The use of heated wired circuits further limits the potential placement of aerosol delivery devices.

Metered-Dose Inhalers

The pMDIs are generally placed between the Y-piece and the ETT or in the inspiratory limb just before the Y-piece (Fig. 11.1) [14]. Placing the pMDI after the Y-piece is less efficient and requires breaking the integrity of the circuit potentially causing lung de-recruitment and increasing the risk of ventilator-associated pneumonia [30]. This configuration also increases dead space. The pMDIs are connected to either adapters or spacers (Fig. 11.2) [14]. Spacers can be either rigid or collapsible and some offer the advantage that when not in use, they lead to minimal rain out (Fig. 11.2a–c). Adapters are small plastic connectors that serve as actuators of the pMDIs and are very inefficient and their use should be discouraged (Fig. 11.2d) [39–41]. In an ex vivo study using a porcine model of mechanical ventilation, a fourfold difference in drug delivery between the adapter and the spacer was recently reported [35]. A disadvantage of using in-line pMDIs is that the canister of aerosol is removed from its manufacturer designed actuator and placed in a generic actuator.

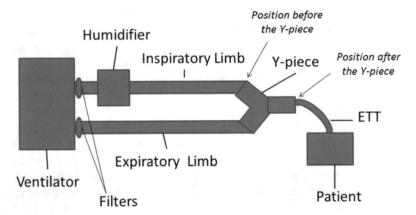

Fig. 11.1 Ventilator setup with different positions where adapters/spacer/holding chambers for pMDIs can be placed

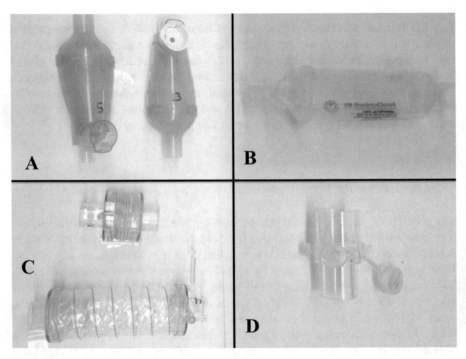

Fig. 11.2 Examples of adapters and rigid and collapsible spacers used for in-line administration on pMDIs. (**a**) Small-volume chamber made of antistatic material that accepts different canisters (with and without counters). (**b**) Rigid spacer. (**c**) Collapsible spacer (expanded and collapsed). (**d**) Adapter

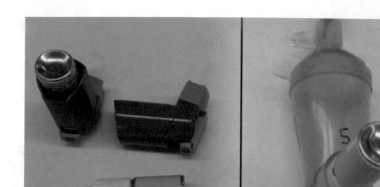

Fig. 11.3 Example of a pMDIs with incorporated counters requiring special adapters. (**a**) Canister with incorporated counter and plastic actuator of the pMDI together and disassembled. (**b**) Chamber with the pMDI's canister placed in it

Poor compatibility between the stem of the canister and the spacer/adapter actuator can reduce aerosol output [36–43]. The development of new pMDIs formulated with HFA and the incorporation of counters to the canister have aggravated this problem (Fig. 11.3). The material used to build the spacer is one more variable that needs to be considered. Similar to what is described for spontaneously breathing patients, spacers made of non-electrostatic material are more efficient than the others [13, 14].

The timing of actuation is critical and failure to actuate the pMDI during inspiration reduces albuterol delivery by at least 35 % (Fig. 11.4) [44]. The reduction is even more dramatic when an adaptor is used (86 %).

The presence of humidity in the ventilator circuit decreases albuterol delivery between 30 and 60 % due to hygroscopic growth of the aerosol particles and increased impaction (Fig. 11.4) [40, 45]. In addition, the use of helium-oxygen combination instead of nitrogen-oxygen combination in a pediatric ventilator in vitro model (tidal volume 200 mL, rr=25, and I:E 1:2.6) resulted in a 65 % increase in albuterol delivery from an pMDI/spacer placed between the ETT and the Y-piece (Fig. 11.4) [46, 47]. This increment was seen in models that had either humidified or non-humidified circuits, and it is due to a decrease in turbulence of the air in the circuit leading to a decrease in aerosol impaction.

The size of the ETT also plays a significant role in limiting aerosol delivery. A decrease from a 6 to a 4-mm internal diameter tube reduced albuterol delivery between 40 and 60 % (Fig. 11.4) [40, 45]. This effect is even more pronounced with smaller-size ETTs [49].

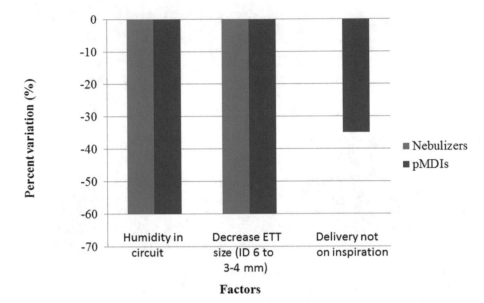

Fig. 11.4 Effect of several variables on drug delivery with pMDIs and nebulizers in pediatric ventilator circuits. From references [40, 42, 44–48]

The size of the aerosol is also an important factor determining aerosol delivery. In an in vitro study using a ventilator model, a beclomethasone aerosol with an MMAD of 1.2 µm resulted in significantly higher delivery than a formulation with an MMAD of 4.5 µm [50, 51]. This is consistent with Taylor et al. who reported that the MMAD of albuterol pMDI aerosol measured at the tip of an ETT with a 6-mm internal diameter was 1.1 µm [52]. The endotracheal tube acts as a filter letting the small particles go through, while the large particles impact against the walls. One could speculate that the use of a pMDI with small MMAD might be more appropriate for drug delivery through endotracheal tubes.

Although no pediatric data are available, adult studies suggest that neither flow patterns (decelerating vs. square wave), ventilator mode, nor end expiratory pause significantly affects drug delivery and clinical response [53–55].

Nebulizers

The position of nebulizers in the ventilator circuit also significantly affects albuterol delivery. Placement at the Y-piece or 30 cm before is significantly less efficient than placement on either the dry or wet side of the humidifier irrespective of the type of nebulizer used (Fig. 11.5) [56].

The choice of type of aerosol generator also significantly affects albuterol delivery (Fig. 11.6). Differences in albuterol delivery range from four- to tenfold

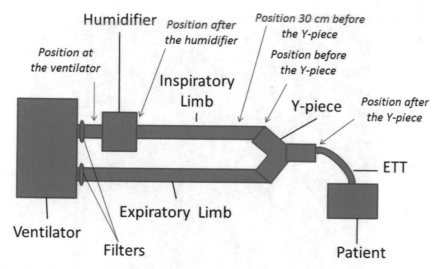

Fig. 11.5 Ventilator setup with different positions where nebulizer can be placed

depending on the location where different devices were placed [56–58]. Vibrating mesh and ultrasonic nebulizers are more efficient than jet nebulizers, but the latter are more efficient than the intrapulmonary percussive ventilator (IPV) [56–58]. This device is a modified ventilator that delivers a burst of air at high frequencies (100–300 Hz) and is used to aid with mobilization of airway secretions [57]. Goldstein et al. reported efficient delivery and bactericidal activity of inhaled amikacin delivered with an ultrasonic nebulizer placed in the inspiratory limb 40 cm before the Y-piece in a porcine model (21 kg) [33]. Ferrari et al. using the same model reported that the same nebulizer/placement yielded delivery of inhaled ceftazidime equivalent to a vibrating mesh nebulizer placed 15 cm from the Y-piece [34].

In contrast to findings reported in adult ventilator models, increasing the duty cycle (percentage of time spent delivering positive inspiratory pressure by the ventilator) does not enhance aerosol delivery with nebulizers during mechanical ventilation in pediatric models [40, 59].

Although once thought to be an effective modality to enhance aerosol delivery, increasing the tidal volume has been later shown not to be applicable to pediatrics. Both clinical studies in adults and pediatric in vitro studies agree on this subject [57, 58]. An in vitro study reported no increase in drug delivery after increasing tidal volume from 100 to 200 mL with a resulting increase in minute ventilation [57]. A follow-up study expanded these findings to the 100–300 mL range with similar results [unpublished data Berlinski et al.].

The mode of operation of the nebulizer (continuous vs. intermittent) could also influence drug delivery during mechanical ventilation in pediatric ventilator models. However, the currently available data are conflicting [39, 48, 60].

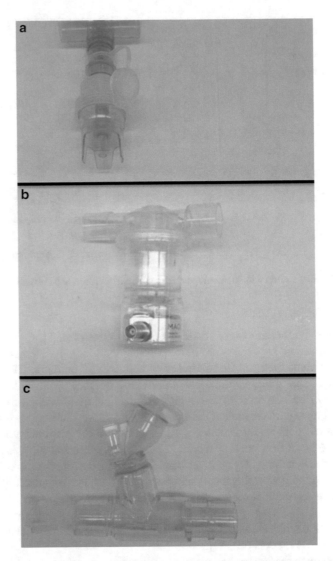

Fig. 11.6 Examples of nebulizers used for in-line administration of inhaled aerosols. (**a**) Continuous-output nebulizer attached to a spring-loaded T-piece. (**b**) Ultrasonic nebulizer. (**c**) Disposable single patient use vibrating mesh nebulizer placed on its adapter

The effect of bias flow (2–5 L/min) on aerosol delivery in pediatric circuits is not significant when low-flow jet nebulizers (2 L/min) and vibrating mesh nebulizers are used [58]. However, the use of higher nebulizer flows combined with high bias flow could be detrimental. The increase in flow used to power the nebulizer results in a decrease in albuterol delivery [39, 61]. Moreover, the flow interferes with the functioning of the ventilation and requires adjustment of the settings (i.e., decreasing tidal volume to avoid barotrauma) [62, 63]. Some nebulizers are powered by the ventilator and inadequate flow has been documented in several instances [64]. Therefore, either low-flow jet nebulizer or vibrating mesh nebulizers are preferred for patients unable to be disconnected from invasive ventilator support.

The size of the ETT also plays a significant role in limiting drug delivered by nebulizers. Reducing the ETT internal diameter size from 6 to 3 mm resulted in a reduction of 60 % in aerosol delivery (Fig. 11.4) [48].

Aerosols with larger MMAD suffer impaction against the tube walls that leads to a reduction of particle size. Ahrens et al. reported a decrease in aerosol MMAD from 3.4 μm at the exit of the jet nebulizer to 0.42–1.20 μm at the tip of the ETT [61]. These data are in agreement with similar decrease in MMAD for both jet and vibrating mesh nebulizers found by Berlinski and Kesser (unpublished data). However, when submicronic aerosols are used, no change in MMAD is noted [61].

The use of a heated/humidified circuit reduces aerosol delivery by 60 % (Fig. 11.4) [42].

Very few human studies comparing devices in pediatric population are available. Garner et al. found similar clinical effects and serum albuterol concentrations when pediatric ventilated patients received the drug via pMDI with spacer placed between the Y-piece and the ETT and a nebulizer placed in the inspiratory circuit 10 to 20 cm before the Y-piece [65].

In summary, aerosol delivery in children receiving mechanical ventilation who do not tolerate being disconnected from the ventilator can be optimized by placing the nebulizer between the ventilator and the humidifier and using low bias flows. Vibrating mesh nebulizers are more effective and expensive than jet nebulizers, but if chronic therapy is required, the cost per treatment might be similar [56]. If pMDIs are used, they should be actuated at the beginning of the inhalation and a holding chamber should be used instead of an adapter.

Patients Receiving Invasive Mechanical Ventilation Who Tolerate Being Disconnected From the Ventilator and Tracheostomized Patients Who Breathe Spontaneously

Limited guidance is available regarding optimization of aerosol delivery in this population. Most of the available information is derived from in vitro studies [32, 66–72]. A recent survey revealed a wide variation in practice patterns in aerosol delivery in that population [1]. Of note, some of the reported practices have been found to reduce delivery efficiency. One study compared aerosolization versus instillation of 40 mg of gentamicin solution through the tracheostomy in pediatric patients [6]. They found a 28-fold higher blood concentration and a 24-fold higher sputum concentration when the instillation modality was used.

Although no pediatric data are available, adult data comparing drug delivery between ETTs and tracheostomy tubes show that the latter delivers 50 % more drug than the former [66].

Metered-Dose Inhaler

Several factors have been reported to affect aerosol delivery with pMDIs to children with tracheostomies (Table 11.2). Similar to what has been reported in invasive mechanical ventilation, there is an inverse correlation between artificial airway size and drug delivery [52]. Breathing patterns with larger tidal volumes result in higher drug deposition as it is seen in models of spontaneously breathing children [70]. In agreement with adult-type ventilator studies, a relatively low percentage of drug (7.4 % of nominal dose) is deposited in the tracheostomy tube [59, 67].

Berlinski et al. reported that the use of a self-inflating resuscitation bag (assisted technique) negatively influenced drug delivery resulting in decrease of delivery ranging from 18 to 54 % (Fig. 11.7) [67]. These findings were confirmed in a follow-up study [68]. Others reported enhancement of delivery in infants with small ETTs and low tidal volumes (<60 mL) [51, 73]. However, these findings are in contrast of small animal data [32]. Piccuito et al. in an adult-type tracheostomy model found that the addition of either dry, heated, or heated-humid high gas flow (30 L/min) resulted in a 65 % reduction in aerosol delivery [69].

Adapters were found to be very inefficient delivery devices with a reported nine-fold difference when compared to best performers [67]. A small-volume holding chamber made of antistatic material was the most efficient delivery device for all tracheostomy sizes (3.5, 4.5, and 5.5 mm internal diameter) and breathing patterns (tidal volume 80 mL, 155 mL, and 310 mL) [67]. This small-volume holding chamber does not require removal of the canister from the plastic actuator (Fig. 11.7).

Nebulizers

Several factors have been reported to affect aerosol delivery with nebulizers to children with tracheostomies (Table 11.2). In general, they deliver a low amount of drug beyond the tip of the tracheostomy [71].

Table 11.2 Factors affecting aerosol delivery through tracheostomies[a]

Metered-dose inhalers	Nebulizers
Adapter/spacer [67]	Nebulizer type [71, 72]
Tracheostomy size [67]	Tracheostomy size [71, 72]
Breathing pattern [67]	Breathing pattern [71]
Assisted breathing (−) [67, 68]	Assisted breathing (+) [66, 71]
Bias flow [69]	Interface [66, 71, 72]
	Bias flow [69]

[a]From references [66–69, 71, 72]

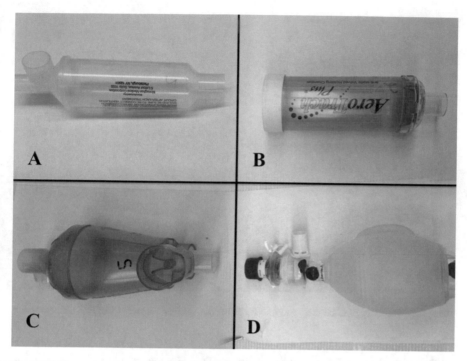

Fig. 11.7 Examples of adapters/spacers and holding chambers used with pMDIs and tracheostomies. (**a**) Plastic spacer. (**b**) Holding chamber made of non-electrostatic material that does not require removal of the canister from the plastic booth. (**c**) Small-volume chamber made of non-electrostatic material. (**d**) Self-inflating resuscitation bag used for assisted technique with (**a**) and (**c**). The bag is connected by adapter placed near the canister

Both pediatric and adult-type studies agree that a T-piece is a more efficient interface than a tracheostomy mask with reported differences ranging from 15 to 50 % (Fig. 11.8) [66, 69, 71].

The addition of either dry, heated, or heated-humid high gas flow (30 L/min) resulted in a three- to fivefold and three- to ninefold reduction in aerosol delivery when a T-piece and a tracheostomy mask were used, respectively [69]. This provides the basis for discouraging the use of in-line administration of aerosols in patients receiving humidification for their tracheostomy with a tracheal collar.

Similar to reports of aerosol delivery in invasive ventilation, the choice of device significantly affects the amount of aerosol that is delivered to the airways [71, 72]. In a pediatric in vitro model, a breath-enhanced nebulizer had higher delivery than a continuously operated and a breath-actuated nebulizer [71]. The latter had minimal delivery with breathing patterns with low tidal volume. Conversely, Pitance et al. in an in vitro model of an adult (internal diameter 6.5 mm) reported that a continuously operated nebulizer with an extension tube was slightly more efficient than a breath-assisted nebulizer [72]. The use of an extension tube coupled with the nebulizer resulted in an improvement in aerosol delivery between 12 and 22 % (Fig. 11.8) [72]. This phenomenon was more important in an adult model (53 %) possibly due to the larger tidal volume [72].

A. Berlinski

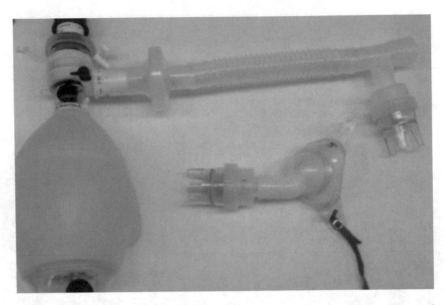

Fig. 11.8 Examples of nebulizers and interfaces used to deliver aerosols through tracheostomies

In contrast to findings reported with pMDIs, the use of assisted technique to deliver aerosols in tracheostomy models results in increased delivery (Fig. 11.8) [66–68, 71]. Moreover, the use of assisted technique with every other breath with the continuously operated nebulizer with an extension tube measured up to the breath-enhanced nebulizer's performance [71]. Every other breath-assisted delivery was found to be more efficient than assistance with every breath due to a possible reservoir effect generated with the former during the non-assisted breath [71]. The use of the assisted technique with every other breath resulted in a more proximal aerosol deposition [71]. This feature can be used to target the large airways during an episode of tracheitis. The differential behavior between MDIs and nebulizers regarding the effect of assistance on drug delivery could be explained in part by the continuous nature of the delivery that the latter provides.

Breathing pattern and tracheostomy size both influence drug delivery [71]. The former had a more important effect than the latter.

If assisted technique is used, it is recommended that a filter be placed after the resuscitation bag to avoid retrograde penetration of aerosols. This is critical with the administration of inhaled antibiotics.

Similar to what has been reported for aerosol delivery through ETTs, the passage of the aerosol through a tracheostomy tube significantly alters its size [48]. One study reported a 67 and 57 % reduction in MMAD after aerosols traveled through a tracheostomy tubes with internal diameter of 3.5 mm and 5.5 mm, respectively [71]. The final aerosols had an MMAD ranging from 1.22 to 1.77 µm with less than 1 % of the drug deposited in the tracheostomy tube [71].

The equivalence between pMDIs and nebulizers can be calculated from the data previously discussed. In an adult study (internal diameter 8 mm), Piccuito et al. reported that four puffs of albuterol led to 25 % of the drug deposited by a nebulizer (2.5 mg/3 mL loading dose) [71]. Berlinski et al. in a pediatric study (internal diameter 3.5 and 5.5 mm) found that two to three puffs delivered with a non-electrostatic holding chamber were equivalent to 2.5 mg/3 mL nebulized albuterol solution [67, 71].

In summary, aerosol delivery in children receiving mechanical ventilation who tolerate being disconnected from the ventilator can be optimized by either delivering drugs via pMDI using a holding chamber made of antistatic material and designed to be used with tracheostomies or using a jet nebulizer that connects through a T-piece to the tracheostomy and to an extension tube connected to a self-inflating resuscitation bag. The use of bias flow should be avoided. Practitioners need to be aware that tracheal instillation provides significantly higher doses than nebulized therapy.

Patient Receiving Noninvasive Mechanical Ventilation Who Do Not Tolerate Being Disconnected from the Ventilator

The current strategies used to optimize aerosol to patients receiving noninvasive mechanical ventilation who cannot tolerate being disconnected from the ventilator are mostly derived from in vitro data utilizing adult-type models [74–80].

A face mask with a good seal is important for optimization of aerosol delivery. Nasal masks are expected to be less efficient than oronasal masks due to loss of aerosol through the mouth and the fact that the aerosol goes through the nasal filter [81].

All data on aerosol delivery during noninvasive ventilation was obtained from in vivo and in vitro studies using a bi-level device with single limb circuit [74–80, 82–88]. These circuits incorporate either an exhalation port/leak or valve that can be located either in the circuit or at the mask. More recently, both home and hospital ventilators have noninvasive ventilation settings and use a double limb circuit with the Y-piece connected with a swivel valve to the mask. This is a setup similar to invasive mechanical ventilation except that a non-vented mask is placed where the ETT would have been placed. No data regarding aerosol delivery for that setup are currently available.

Metered-Dose Inhaler

The data on pMDI shows that timing of the actuation is as crucial as it is in invasive mechanical ventilation. A 50 % reduction in aerosol delivery results from actuation of the pMDI during expiration [74]. The same authors found similar albuterol delivery when the exhalation port/leak was at the mask or in the single limb circuit before the spacer and pMDI and the aerosol are actuated at the beginning of inhalation (Fig. 11.9).

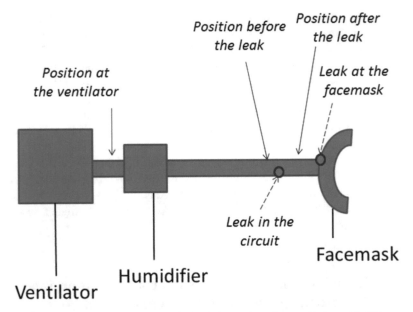

Fig. 11.9 Ventilator setup with single limb circuit for noninvasive ventilation with different positions where pMDIs and nebulizers can be placed and where leakage is found

Nebulizer

Calvert et al. reported that placing a jet nebulizer at the bi-level ventilator results in a 50–60 % reduction in aerosol delivery when compared to placement between the expiration port and the mask and between the expiration port and the ventilator (Fig. 11.9) [75]. These findings contradict those of Chatmongkolchart et al. who reported that placement at the ventilator was more efficient than placing it between the mask and the exhalation port [76]. In contrast to Calvert et al. who reported that aerosol output was larger if the jet nebulizer was right after the exhalation (away from the facemask), Abdelrahim et al. found the opposite (Fig. 11.9) [75, 77]. The difference in findings could be partially explained by the fact that Abdelrahim et al. placed the nebulizer closer to the leak port. In addition they tested both jet and vibrating mesh nebulizers and found that the vibrating mesh nebulizer delivered at least twice as much drug as the jet nebulizer [77]. In another study the amount of aerosol delivered by a jet nebulizer decreased by 56 % when the position of the leak was changed from the circuit (before the nebulizer) to the mask [74]. White et al. using a pediatric in vitro model reported that a single use disposable vibrating mesh nebulizer was more efficient when placed near the face mask than when placed between the bi-level ventilator and the humidifier [78]. The authors used a single limb circuit with a leak placed at the face mask. These authors also reported that a vibrating mesh nebulizer purposely designed to be placed in the mask was more efficient than the others [78].

The type of exhalation valve used also plays a role in determining the optimal position of the nebulizer [79]. In an adult in vitro model, Dai et al. compared drug delivery from a jet nebulizer during bi-level ventilation at different pressures, with different exhalation valves and two different positions [79]. The plateau valve provides a constant air leak, while the single arch and the whisper swivel increase their leak with higher pressures. The whisper swivel has a larger leak than the single arch. The authors reported that when a jet nebulizer was placed between the exhalation port and the patient, the single arch provided the largest and the swivel provided the lowest drug delivery. However, when the nebulizer was placed proximal to the ventilator, the single arch valve had the lowest drug delivery. The authors also reported that while higher inspiratory positive airway pressure increased aerosol delivery, the effect of expiratory positive airway pressure was not clear.

More recently, Michotte el al. compared the inhaled dose of three different vibrating mesh nebulizers, a jet nebulizer, and an ultrasonic nebulizer. The devices were placed between the ventilator and the leak on the circuit and between the leak and the mask [80]. They found that moving the ultrasonic and vibrating mesh nebulizers closer to ventilator decreased the inhaled mass 3.8-fold and the jet nebulizer 1.3-fold. However, the vibrating mesh nebulizers delivered an average of 3.5-fold more drug than the jet nebulizer. The delivery efficiency averaged 43, 12, and 12 % for the vibrating mesh, jet, and ultrasonic nebulizers, respectively, when the devices were placed between the leak and the mask.

The optimal position showed a delivery efficiency of ranging from 9.6 to 28.2 % for the jet nebulizer and 51 % for the vibrating mesh nebulizer [74–80].

Calvert el at. reported that operating a nebulizer into a bi-level ventilator circuit results in a 29% reduction of its particle size from an MMAD of 3.12–2.21 μm [75]. The high flows present in the circuit could generate aerosol impaction against the circuit walls [82].

The effect of the differential pressure (inspiratory–expiratory positive airway pressure) is quite complex and is affected by both placement of the nebulizer and respiratory rate [76]. The data that falls within pediatric range (tidal volume 300 mL) shows that a faster rate (20 vs. 10 bpm) and a larger differential pressure deliver more aerosol. This could be explained by the increase of the minute ventilation. At lower rates the proximal position is more efficient and at higher rates placement at the ventilator makes it more efficient.

Parkes et al. reported an 81 % decrease in aerosol delivery by a jet nebulizer when a CPAP system with a face mask was used compared to the nebulizer alone [82]. They also reported a similar bronchodilator response despite the decrease in intrapulmonary deposition. In an in vitro/in vivo study, Fauroux et al. demonstrated that in children with cystic fibrosis, a 30 % increase in aerosol deposition occurred when the delivery device was coupled to a pressure support system [83]. Conversely, Franca et al. in a study of healthy young adults found that delivering aerosol using a bi-level ventilation system (12/4) reduced aerosol deposition when compared to spontaneous breathing [84]. This was most likely due to the high flows that the bi-level ventilator generates. Reychler et al. had similar findings in a study comparing lung deposition (measured as urinary excretion) between nebulizer alone and a CPAP system (threefold difference) [85]. Brandao et al. reported a significantly higher improvement in asthmatic subjects inhaling aerosols into a bi-level ventilation system compared to nebulizer alone [86]. Abdelrahim et al. reported that systemic bioavailability of terbutaline was equivalent between a disposable vibrating mesh nebulizer (2 mg) and a breath-enhanced nebulizer (5 mg) when aerosols were delivered during bi-level ventilation [87]. More recently, Galindo-Filho et al. demonstrated that in asthmatic adult subjects experiencing an exacerbation, the delivery of aerosol in conjunction with noninvasive ventilation did not change intrapulmonary deposition despite achieving significant improvement in physiologic and spirometric outcomes compared to a control group receiving nebulization alone [88].

In summary, aerosol delivery in children receiving noninvasive mechanical ventilation who do not tolerate being disconnected from the ventilator can be optimized by coordinating pMDI actuation with the beginning of the inhalation, placing the nebulizer between the leak at the circuit and the face mask and by using vibrating mesh nebulizer. The in vivo data suggest a decrease in intrapulmonary deposition, although the net effect during acute bronchial obstruction might be beneficial.

Patients Receiving Noninvasive Mechanical Ventilation Who Tolerate Being Disconnected from the Ventilator

This subpopulation needs to be treated like other spontaneously breathing children [13]. In general, delivering aerosols with the patient disconnected from the ventilator is more efficient and less complicated. We prefer the used use of MDIs with holding chambers made of non-electrostatic material that do not require removal of the canister from the actuator. When a mask is needed, it should be soft and should provide minimum leak and dead space and should also provide feedback regarding inspiratory flow and proper seal [88]. Cognitive abilities and acceptance of the interface are more important factors in this subgroup.

Clinical Key Points

Like in real estate, in aerosol delivery during invasive and noninvasive ventilation, location of the device is paramount of value.

The choice of delivery device could represent a severalfold difference in drug delivery. Cost and availability should be considered when deciding which system to use.

Delivering aerosols with the patient disconnected from the ventilator is generally more efficient.

Assisted breathing is effective if nebulizers are used but not when MDIs are utilized.

The internal diameter of ETTs and tracheostomy tubes significantly affect the amount and the aerosol characteristics of the aerosol that exits their tips.

It is important to remember that proper instruction in the use of the chosen delivery devices is crucial. If the clinical scenario varies such as when a patient is decannulated, re-instruction of the delivery technique needs to be provided and should include cleaning and disinfection.

Summary

Aerosol delivery to children receiving chronic mechanical ventilation depends on multiple factors. Practitioner's knowledge of the variables that affect drug delivery are essential. The type of ventilator support and the tolerance of the child whom it should be removed from determine what delivery device/technique should be used. More clinical studies are necessary to improve our knowledge regarding optimization of aerosol delivery during mechanical ventilation in children.

References

1. Willis D, Berlinski A. Survey of aerosol delivery techniques to spontaneously breathing tracheostomized children. Respir Care. 2012;57(8):1234–41.
2. Sherman JM, Davis S, Albamonte-Petrick S, Chatburn RL, Fitton C, Green C, et al. Care of the child with a chronic tracheostomy. This official statement of the American Thoracic Society was adopted by the ATS Board of Directors, July 1999. Am J Respir Crit Care Med. 2000;161(1):297–308.
3. O'Callaghan C, Dryden S, Cert DN, Gibbin K. Asthma therapy and a tracheostomy. J Laryngol Otol. 1989;103(4):427–8.
4. Subhedar NV, Doyle C, Shaw NJ. Administration of inhaled medication via a tracheostomy in infants with chronic lung disease of prematurity. Pediatr Rehabil. 1999;3(2):41–2.
5. Monksfield P. Modification of a spacer device for paediatric tracheostomy. Clin Otolaryngol. 2008;33(2):193–4.
6. Baran D, Dachy A, Klastersky J. Concentration of gentamicin in bronchial secretions of children with cystic fibrosis or tracheostomy. Int J Clin Pharmacol Biopharm. 1975;12(3): 336–41.
7. Palmer LB, Smaldone GC, Simon SR, O'Riordan TG, Cuccia A. Aerosolized antibiotics in mechanically ventilated patients: delivery and response. Crit Care Med. 1998;26(1): 31–9.
8. Rusakow LS, Guarin M, Wegner CB, Rice TB, Mischler EH. Suspected respiratory tract infection in the tracheostomized child. Chest. 1998;113(6):1549–54.
9. Hamer DH. Treatment of nosocomial pneumonia and tracheobronchitis caused by multidrug-resistant pseudomonas aeruginosa with aerosolized colistin. Am J Respir Crit Care Med. 2000;162(1):328–30.
10. Falagas ME, Sideri G, Korbila IP, Vouloumanou EK, Papadatos JH, Kafetzis DA. Inhaled colistin for the treatment of tracheobronchitis and pneumonia in critically ill children without cystic fibrosis. Pediatr Pulmonol. 2010;45(11):1135–40.
11. Hendriks T, de Hoog M, Lequin MH, Devos AS, Merkus PJFM. DNase and atelectasis in non-cystic fibrosis pediatric patients. Crit Care. 2005;9(4):R351–6.
12. Salyer JW, Chatburn RL. Patterns of practice in neonatal and pediatric respiratory care. Respir Care. 1990;35(9):879–88.
13. Laube BL, Janssens HM, de Jongh FH, Devadason SG, Dhand R, Diot P, Everard ML, Horvath I, Navalesi P, Voshaar T, Chrystyn H, European Respiratory Society, International Society for

Aerosols in Medicine. What the pulmonary specialist should know about the new inhalation therapies. Eur Respir J. 2011;37(6):1308–31.

14. Dhand R. Aerosol delivery during mechanical ventilation: from basic techniques to new devices. J Aerosol Med Pulm Drug Deliv. 2008;21(1):45–60.

15. Dhand R. Aerosol therapy in patients receiving noninvasive positive pressure ventilation. J Aerosol Med Pulm Drug Deliv. 2012;25(2):63–78.

16. Dolovich MB, Dhand R. Aerosol drug delivery: developments in device design and clinical use. Lancet. 2011;377(9770):1032–45.

17. Laube BL, Jashnani R, Dalby RN, Zeitlin PL. Targeting aerosol deposition in patients with cystic fibrosis: effects of alterations in particle size and inspiratory flow rate. Chest. 2000;118(4):1069–76.

18. Clay MM, Pavia D, Newman SP, Lennard-Jones T, Clarke SW. Assessment of jet nebulisers for lung aerosol therapy. Lancet. 1983;2(8350):592–4.

19. Alvine GF, Rodgers P, Fitzsimmons KM, Ahrens RC. Disposable jet nebulizers. How reliable are they? Chest. 1992;101(2):316–9.

20. Hess D, Fisher D, Williams P, Pooler S, Kacmarek RM. Medication nebulizer performance. Effects of diluent volume, nebulizer flow, and nebulizer brand. Chest. 1996;110(2):498–505.

21. Kradjan WA, Lakshminarayan S. Efficiency of air compressor-driven nebulizers. CHEST. 1985;87:512–6.

22. Rau JL. Design principles of liquid nebulization devices currently in use. Respir Care. 2002;47(11):1275–8; discussion 1275–278.

23. Waldrep JC, Dhand R. Advanced nebulizer designs employing vibrating mesh/aperture plate technologies for aerosol generation. Curr Drug Deliv. 2008;5(2):114–9.

24. Berlinski A, Waldrep JC. Effect of aerosol delivery system and formulation on nebulized Budesonide output. J Aerosol Medicine. 1997;10(4):307–18.

25. Geller DE. New liquid aerosol generation devices: systems that force pressurized liquids through nozzles. Respir Care. 2002;47(12):1392–404; discussion 1404–5.

26. Dellweg D, Wachtel H, Höhn E, Pieper MP, Barchfeld T, Köhler D, Glaab T. In vitro validation of a Respimat® adapter for delivery of inhaled bronchodilators during mechanical ventilation. J Aerosol Med Pulm Drug Deliv. 2011;24(6):285–92.

27. García Pachón E, Casan P, Sanchís J. Bronchodilators through tracheostomy. Med Clin (Barc). 1992;99(10):396–7 [Article in Spanish].

28. Everard ML, Devadason SG, Le Souëf PN. In vitro assessment of drug delivery through an endotracheal tube using a dry powder inhaler delivery system. Thorax. 1996;51(1):75–7.

29. Johnson DC. Interfaces to connect the handihaler and aerolizer powder inhalers to a tracheostomy tube. Respir Care. 2007;52(2):166–70.

30. Young PM, Sung A, Traini D, Kwok P, Chiou H, Chan HK. Influence of humidity on the electrostatic charge and aerosol performance of dry powder inhaler carrier based systems. Pharm Res. 2007;24(5):963–70.

31. Everard ML. Ethical aspects of using radiolabelling in aerosol research. Arch Dis Child. 2003;88(8):659–61.

32. O'Callaghan C, Hardy J, Stammers J, Stephenson TJ, Hull D. Evaluation of techniques for delivery of steroids to lungs of neonates using a rabbit model. Arch Dis Child. 1992;67(1Spec No):20–4.

33. Goldstein I, Wallet F, Nicolas-Robin A, Ferrari F, Marquette CH, Rouby JJ. Lung deposition and efficiency of nebulized amikacin during Escherichia coli pneumonia in ventilated piglets. Am J Respir Crit Care Med. 2002;166(10):1375–81.

34. Ferrari F, Liu ZH, Lu Q, Becquemin MH, Louchahi K, Aymard G, Marquette CH, Rouby JJ. Comparison of lung tissue concentrations of nebulized ceftazidime in ventilated piglets: ultrasonic versus vibrating plate nebulizers. Intensive Care Med. 2008;34(9):1718–23.

35. Berlinski A, Holt S, Thurman T, Heulitt M. Albuterol delivery during mechanical ventilation in an ex-vivo porcine model. J Aerosol Med Pulm Drug Deliv. 2013;26(2):57.

36. Fink JB, Dhand R, Grychowski J, Fahey PJ, Tobin MJ. Reconciling in vitro and in vivo measurements of aerosol delivery from a metered-dose inhaler during mechanical ventilation and defining efficiency-enhancing factors. Am J Respir Crit Care Med. 1999;159(1):63–8.

37. Miller DD, Amin MM, Palmer LB, Shah AR, Smaldone GC. Aerosol delivery and modern mechanical ventilation: in vitro/in vivo evaluation. Am J Respir Crit Care Med. 2003;168(10):1205–9.
38. Watterberg KL, Clark AR, Kelly W, Murphy S. Delivery of aerosolized medication to intubated babies. Pediatr Pulmonol. 1991;10:136–41.
39. Coleman DM, Kelly HW, McWilliams BC. Determinants of aerosolized albuterol delivery to mechanically ventilated infants. Chest. 1996;109:1607–13.
40. Garner SS, Wiest DB, Bradley JW. Albuterol delivery by metered-dose inhaler with a pediatric mechanical ventilatory circuit model. Pharmacotherapy. 1994;14(2):210–4.
41. Wildhaber JH, Hayden MJ, Dore ND, Devadason SG, LeSouëf PN. Salbutamol delivery from a hydrofluoroalkane pressurized metered-dose inhaler in pediatric ventilator circuits: an in vitro study. Chest. 1998;113(1):186–91.
42. Ari A, Areabi H, Fink JB. Evaluation of aerosol generator devices at 3 locations in humidified and non-humidified circuits during adult mechanical ventilation. Respir Care. 2010;55(7): 837–44.
43. Berlinski A, Waldrep JC. Metering performance of several metered-dose inhalers with different spacers/holding chambers. J Aerosol Medicine. 2001;14(4):427–32.
44. Diot P, Morra L, Smaldone GC. Albuterol delivery in a model of mechanical ventilation. Comparison of metered-dose inhaler and nebulizer efficiency. Am J Respir Crit Care Med. 1995;152(4 Pt 1):1391–4.
45. Garner SS, Wiest DB, Bradley JW. Albuterol delivery by metered-dose inhaler in mechanically ventilated pediatric lung model. Crit Care Med. 1996;24(5):870–4.
46. Habib DM, Garner SS, Brandeburg S. Effect of helium-oxygen on delivery of albuterol in a pediatric, volume-cycled, ventilated lung model. Pharmacotherapy. 1999;19(2):143–9.
47. Garner SS, Wiest DB, Stevens CE, Habib DM. Effect of heliox on albuterol delivery by metered-dose inhaler in pediatric in vitro models of mechanical ventilation. Pharmacotherapy. 2006;26(10):1396–402.
48. Sidler-Moix AL, Dolci U, Berger-Gryllaki M, Pannatier A, Cotting J, Di Paolo ER. Albuterol delivery in an in vitro pediatric ventilator lung model: comparison of jet, ultrasonic, and mesh nebulizers. Pediatr Crit Care Med. 2013;14(2):e98–102.
49. Taylor RH, Lerman J. High-efficiency delivery of salbutamol with a metered-dose inhaler in narrow tracheal tubes and catheters. Anesthesiology. 1991;74(2):360–3.
50. Mitchell JP, Nagel MW, Wiersema KJ, Doyle CC, Migounov VA. The delivery of chlorofluorocarbon-propelled versus hydrofluoroalkane-propelled beclomethasone dipropionate aerosol to the mechanically ventilated patient: a laboratory study. Respir Care. 2003;48(11):1025–32.
51. Cole CH, Mitchell JP, Foley MP, Nagel MW. Hydrofluoroalkane-beclomethasone versus chlorofluorocarbon-beclomethasone delivery in neonatal models. Arch Dis Child Fetal Neonatal Ed. 2004;89(5):F417–8.
52. Taylor RH, Lerman J, Chambers C, Dolovich M. Dosing efficiency and particle-size characteristics of pressurized metered-dose inhaler aerosols in narrow catheters. Chest. 1993;103(3):920–4.
53. Fink JB, Dhand R, Duarte AG, Jenne JW, Tobin MJ. Aerosol delivery from a metered-dose inhaler during mechanical ventilation. An in vitro model. Am J Respir Crit Care Med. 1996;154(2 Pt 1):382–7.
54. Mouloudi E, Katsanoulas K, Anastasaki M, Askitopoulou E, Georgopoulos D. Bronchodilator delivery by metered-dose inhaler in mechanically ventilated COPD patients: influence of end-inspiratory pause. Eur Respir J. 1998;12(1):165–9.
55. Mouloudi E, Prinianakis G, Kondili E, Georgopoulos D. Bronchodilator delivery by metered-dose inhaler in mechanically ventilated COPD patients: influence of flow pattern. Eur Respir J. 2000;16(2):263–8.
56. Berlinski A, Willis RJ. Albuterol delivery by 4 different nebulizers placed in 4 different positions in a pediatric ventilator circuit. Respir Care. 2013;58(7):1124–33.

57. Berlinski A, Willis JR. Albuterol delivery by intrapulmonary percussive ventilator and jet nebulizer in a pediatric ventilator model. Respir Care. 2010;55(12):1699–704.
58. Ari A, Atalay OT, Harwood R, Sheard MM, Aljamhan EA, Fink JB. Influence of nebulizer type, position, and bias flow on aerosol drug delivery in simulated pediatric and adult lung models during mechanical ventilation. Respir Care. 2010;55(7):845–51.
59. O'Riordan TG, Greco MJ, Perry RJ, Smaldone GC. Nebulizer function during mechanical ventilation. Am Rev Respir Dis. 1992;145(5):1117–22.
60. Di Paolo ER, Pannatier A, Cotting J. In vitro evaluation of bronchodilator drug delivery by jet nebulization during pediatric mechanical ventilation. Pediatr Crit Care Med. 2005;6(4):462–9.
61. Ahrens RC, Ries RA, Popendorf W, Wiese JA. The delivery of therapeutic aerosols through endotracheal tubes. Pediatr Pulmonol. 1986;2(1):19–26.
62. Beaty CD, Ritz RH, Benson MS. Continuous in-line nebulizers complicate pressure support ventilation. Chest. 1989;96(6):1360–3.
63. Hanhan U, Kissoon N, Payne M, Taylor C, Murphy S, De Nicola LK. Effects of in-line nebulization on preset ventilator variables. Respir Care. 1993;38:474–8.
64. McPeck M, O'Riordan TG, Smaldone GC. Choice of Mechanical ventilator: influence on nebulizer performance. Respir Care. 1993;38(8):887–95.
65. Garner SS, Wiest DB, Bradley JW, Habib DM. Two administration methods for inhaled salbutamol in intubated patients. Arch Dis Child. 2002;87(1):49–53.
66. Ari A, Harwood R, Sheard M, Fink JB. An in-vitro evaluation of aerosol delivery through tracheostomy and endotracheal tubes using different interfaces. Respir Care. 2012;57(7):1066–70.
67. Berlinski A, Chavez A. Albuterol delivery via metered dose inhaler in a spontaneously breathing pediatric tracheostomy model. Pediatr Pulmonol. 2012;48(10):1026–34.
68. Chavez A, Holt S, Heulitt M, Berlinski A. Albuterol delivery Via MDI/spacer in a spontaneously breathing pediatric tracheostomy model: does bagging improve drug delivery? Am J Respir Crit Care Med. 2011;183:3383.
69. Piccuito CM, Hess DR. Albuterol delivery via tracheostomy tube. Respir Care. 2005;50(8):1071–6.
70. Chavez A, McCraken A, Berlinski A. Effect of face mask static dead volume, respiratory rate and tidal volume on inhaled albuterol delivery. Pediatr Pulmonol. 2010;45(3):224–9.
71. Berlinski A. In-vitro nebulized albuterol delivery in a model of spontaneously breathing children with tracheostomy. Respir Care. 2013;58(12):2076–86.
72. Pitance L, Vecellio L, Delval G, Reychler G, Reychler H, Liistro G. Aerosol delivery through tracheostomy tubes: an in vitro study. J Aerosol Med Pulm Drug Deliv. 2013;26(2):76–83.
73. DiBlasi RM, Coppolo DP, Nagel MW, Doyle CC, Avvakoumova VI, Ali RS, Mitchell JP. A novel, versatile valved holding chamber for delivering inhaled medications to neonates and small children: laboratory simulation of delivery options. Respir Care. 2010;55(4):419–26.
74. Branconnier MP, Hess DR. Albuterol delivery during noninvasive ventilation. Respir Care. 2005;50(12):1649–53.
75. Calvert LD, Jackson JM, White JA, Barry PW, Kinnear WJ, O'Callaghan C. Enhanced delivery of nebulised salbutamol during non-invasive ventilation. J Pharm Pharmacol. 2006;58(11):1553–7.
76. Chatmongkolchart S, Schettino GP, Dillman C, Kacmarek RM, Hess DR. In vitro evaluation of aerosol bronchodilator delivery during noninvasive positive pressure ventilation: effect of ventilator settings and nebulizer position. Crit Care Med. 2002;30(11):2515–9.
77. Abdelrahim ME, Plant P, Chrystyn H. In-vitro characterisation of the nebulized dose during non-invasive ventilation. J Pharm Pharmacol. 2010;62(8):966–72.
78. White CC, Crotwell DN, Shen S, Salyer J, Yung D, Diblasi RM. Bronchodilator delivery during simulated pediatric noninvasive ventilation. Respir Care. 2013;58(9):1459–66.
79. Dai B, Kang J, Sun LF, Tan W, Zhao HW. Influence of exhalation valve and nebulizer position on albuterol delivery during noninvasive positive pressure ventilation. J Aerosol Med Pulm Drug Deliv. 2014;27(2):125–32.

80. Michotte JB, Jossen E, Roeseler J, Liistro G, Reychler G. In vitro comparison of 5 nebulizers during noninvasive ventilation: analysis of inhaled and lost doses. J Aerosol Med Pulm Drug Deliv. 2014;27(6):430–40.
81. Chua HL, Collis GG, Newbury AM, Chan K, Bower GD, Sly PD, Le Souef PN. The influence of age on aerosol deposition in children with cystic fibrosis. Eur Respir J. 1994;7(12):185–91.
82. Parkes SN, Bersten AD. Aerosol kinetics and bronchodilator efficacy during continuous positive airway pressure delivered by face mask. Thorax. 1997;52(2):171–5.
83. Fauroux B, Itti E, Pigeot J, Isabey D, Meignan M, Ferry G, Lofaso F, Willemot JM, Clément A, Harf A. Optimization of aerosol deposition by pressure support in children with cystic fibrosis: an experimental and clinical study. Am J Respir Crit Care Med. 2000;162(6):2265–71.
84. França EE, Dornelas de Andrade AF, Cabral G, Almeida Filho P, Silva KC, Galindo Filho VC, Marinho PE, Lemos A, Parreira VF. Nebulization associated with bi-level noninvasive ventilation: analysis of pulmonary radioaerosol deposition. Respir Med. 2006;100(4):721–8.
85. Reychler G, Leal T, Roeseler J, Thys F, Delvau N, Liistro G. Effect of continuous positive airway pressure combined to nebulization on lung deposition measured by urinary excretion of amikacin. Respir Med. 2007;101(10):2051–5.
86. Brandao DC, Lima VM, Filho VG, Silva TS, Campos TF, Dean E, de Andrade AD. Reversal of bronchial obstruction with bi-level positive airway pressure and nebulization in patients with acute asthma. J Asthma. 2009;46(4):356–61.
87. Abdelrahim ME, Plant PK, Chrystyn H. The relative lung and systemic bioavailability of terbutaline following nebulisation in non-invasively ventilated patients. Int J Pharm. 2011; 420(2):313–8.
88. Galindo-Filho VC, Brandão DC, Ferreira Rde C, Menezes MJ, Almeida-Filho P, Parreira VF, Silva TN, Rodrigues-Machado Mda G, Dean E, Dornelas de Andrade A. Noninvasive ventilation coupled with nebulization during asthma crises: a randomized controlled trial. Respir Care. 2013;58(2):241–9.
89. Mouloudi E, Katsanoulas K, Anastasaki M, Hoing S, Georgopoulos D. Bronchodilator delivery by metered-dose inhaler in mechanically ventilated COPD patients: influence of tidal volume. Intensive Care Med. 1999;25(11):1215–21.
90. Amirav I, Newhouse MT. Review of optimal characteristics of face-masks for valved-holding chambers (VHCs). Pediatr Pulmonol. 2008;43(3):268–74.

Chapter 12
Adherence to Non-Invasive Ventilatory Support

Gillian M. Nixon

Introduction

Noninvasive respiratory support, including continuous positive airway pressure (CPAP) and bi-level noninvasive ventilation (NIV), is an important treatment option for children with sleep-disordered breathing. CPAP provides a continuous flow of air and is used to splint the upper airway in children with airway obstruction during sleep. Noninvasive ventilation usually refers to pressure-cycled ventilation, with or without volume-assured pressure support, and is used in cases of sleep-related hypoventilation. Both are delivered via an external interface (usually nasal mask or cannula or nasal-oral mask). Adherence to NIV in children has received virtually no attention in the medical literature. Where such evidence exists, it will be outlined in this review, but otherwise discussion is by necessity limited to CPAP. It is by no means assured however that the same findings would be found for NIV as for CPAP, and further studies are desperately needed in this area.

Obstructive Sleep Apnea and Continuous Positive Airway Pressure

Most children with obstructive sleep apnea (OSA) are treated with adenotonsillectomy [1]. However, a significant proportion of children have persisting OSA postoperatively, especially those who are obese [2, 3]. These children, plus those in

G.M. Nixon (✉)
The Ritchie Centre, Department of Paediatrics and The Hudson Institute of Medical Research, Monash University, Melbourne, VIC, Australia

Melbourne Children's Sleep Centre, Monash Children's Hospital, Melbourne, VIC, Australia
e-mail: gillian.nixon@monashhealth.org

© Springer Science+Business Media New York 2016
L.M. Sterni, J.L. Carroll (eds.), *Caring for the Ventilator Dependent Child*,
Respiratory Medicine, DOI 10.1007/978-1-4939-3749-3_12

Table 12.1 Summary of key aspects of reports of pediatric CPAP adherence

Study	Country	N	Obesity (%)	NDD (%)	Mean hours of use/night (number of patients with data)
Waters KA et al. Am J Resp Crit Care Med 1995 [11]	Australia	80	8	NA	NA
Marcus CL et al. J Pediatr 1995 [4]	Multi	94	18	27	NA
Massa F et al. Arch Dis Child 2002 [7]	UK	66	6	20	NA
O'Donnell A et al. Sleep 2006 [9]	Canada	79	15[a]	56[a]	4.7 (n=50)
Marcus CL et al. Pediatrics 2006 [6]	USA	29	66	3[b]	5.3 (n=21)
Uong EC et al. Pediatrics 2007 [10]	USA	46	67	35	7.0[c] (n=27)
Nixon GM et al. J Pediatr 2011 [8]	Australia	32	6	50	4.7 (n=30)
Marcus CL et al. Am J Resp Crit Care Med 2012 [5][d]	USA	52	69	19	2.8[e] (n=52)

[a]Details presented for 66 of 79 patients in the cohort studied
[b]Patients with Down syndrome excluded
[c]Only data from those using CPAP >4 h sleep available for analysis/night included
[d]Data from the same cohort is presented in two other publications [12, 13]
[e]Subjects who did not return for follow-up included with adherence of 0 h/night

whom upper airway obstruction is attributable to factors other than adenotonsillar hypertrophy (e.g., those with craniofacial disorders, neuromuscular disorders, or Down syndrome), form the majority of children who are prescribed continuous positive airway pressure (CPAP). They are spread throughout the pediatric age range, with the number on CPAP roughly distributed into equal thirds: 0–5 years, 6–12 years, and 13–19 years [4]. The range of patients included in studies of pediatric CPAP adherence highlight the heterogeneity of the populations treated, both within each center and between centers. For example, the proportion of children with significant neurodevelopmental disability such as Down syndrome or cerebral palsy ranges from 18 to 67 % and the proportion with obesity from 6 to 69 % [4–11] (Table 12.1).

Over time, CPAP has become a more commonly used therapy in pediatric practice [14]. This is likely to be due at least in part to the increasing number of children with obesity worldwide. In addition, there have been improvements in equipment, with a wider range of mask interfaces to fit children and an increasing recognition of the effectiveness of this treatment in young children who might otherwise be candidates for tracheostomy [15].

Noninvasive Ventilation

The majority of children prescribed NIV have sleep-related respiratory failure related to restrictive lung disease (e.g., neuromuscular disease, thoracic dystrophy), central hypoventilation (e.g., congenital central hypoventilation syndrome), or end-stage pulmonary disease (e.g., cystic fibrosis). NIV augments alveolar ventilation, thereby treating sleep-related hypoventilation. Similar to CPAP, the use of this therapy is increasing [14].

The Importance of Knowledge About Adherence to Respiratory Support

In a meta-analysis of studies of the relationship between adherence to medical treatment and treatment outcome in adults, DiMatteo et al. report that adherence (compared with nonadherence) reduces the risk for a null or poor treatment outcome by 26%, and the odds of a good outcome if the patient is adherent are almost three times higher than the odds of a good outcome if the patient is nonadherent [16]. In adults at least, this relationship between adherence and outcome is especially strong for sleep apnea compared to other medical conditions such as cancer and heart disease [16].

Thus, a significant influencing factor on the success of the treatment in modifying the consequences of the disease lies in the patient's ability to actually use the therapy as prescribed. Many potential barriers to use have been identified and are outlined below [17]. The use of the therapy may itself pose an additional burden to the child and family on top of the child's underlying condition, particularly in children with major comorbidity. While prescription of noninvasive respiratory support by a consulting physician takes little time, preparation and education of the family and choice of appropriate interfaces and treatment settings require considerable time and expertise. If the extent to which the child uses the treatment is not known, then measures to improve adherence and consequently improve medical outcomes are not likely to be instituted. It is therefore crucially important that individuals prescribed such therapy are closely followed clinically and their adherence monitored objectively. At the present time, we have limited data in children regarding the extent to which hours of use are related to benefit, such as improved concentration or daytime sleepiness. One would anticipate however that very poor adherence is unlikely to be of substantial clinical benefit.

Principles of Adherence in Children and Adolescents

Nonadherence occurs for a variety of reasons including doubt about the expected benefits and efficacy of treatment, real or perceived barriers including side effects and financial constraints, unique demands of the regimen itself, and lack of help and support from family members [16]. Adherence to ventilatory support in children and adolescents is clearly mediated by the role of the parents and caregivers, particularly in young children. Whereas studies in adults with OSA have found associations between personality types and poor adherence [18] and demonstrated the usefulness of cognitive behavioral therapy in improving adherence [19], the role of the parent needs to be taken into account when applying these findings to pediatric populations.

Adherence to CPAP in Children

A number of studies over the last decade have detailed adherence to CPAP in children [5, 6, 8–10, 12, 17]. Key features of these studies are outlined in Table 12.1. Mean hours of CPAP use per night varied from 3 [5, 12, 17] to 7 or 8 [10, 20], with several studies reporting around 5 h/night [6, 8, 9]. Some of this variability is related to the way data for inclusion was selected, with one study with the highest usage being confounded by only including children with usage over 4 h/night [10] and one of those with the lowest hours of use including a zero value for children who did not return for follow-up [5]. While these results are also comparable with adult studies, they fall well short of ideal when it is considered that children sleep longer than adults. Given that children sleep 9–12 h per night depending on age, the proportion of the sleep period spent using the therapy may be a much better way of judging adherence, especially when assessing the response to treatment in terms of daytime functioning.

The definition of any CPAP use on a given night also varies. Two pediatric studies have used a threshold of 1 h per night to define CPAP use on that night [8, 9]. This seems clinically reasonable given that young children may struggle as their parents attempt to apply CPAP, cry and try to remove the mask, or place the mask on their face with the machine running for a few moments without putting the headgear on, none of which could be construed as true therapeutic use during sleep that might confer clinical benefit. It is reasonable to assume that 1 h of CPAP at effective pressure is likely to include some time asleep, at least in younger children, although such a short period is unlikely to be of clinical benefit. Regular viewing of downloaded objective usage data for individual nights may therefore be helpful in assessing attempts to use CPAP and teasing out factors that may be interfering with good adherence [21].

Different definitions of good adherence clearly lead to different proportions of patient groups being classified as adherent. If good adherence is defined as at least 1 h per night on more than 50 % of nights, about three-quarters of children demonstrate good adherence [8, 9]. However, if more than 3 h sleep available for analysis/ night are used as the threshold, only a third of children meet that benchmark [6, 8].

Functional Correlates of Adherence to CPAP

The definition of good adherence with CPAP in adults is usually quoted as 4 or more hours of use per night. This threshold was supported by a study in 2007 which found that most adults with severe sleep apnea showed normalization of their subjective sleepiness (Epworth Sleepiness Scale) at 4 h/night of CPAP use [22]. However that study and several since have shown that more hours of use above that threshold equate to improved outcomes on other measures. For example, cognitive function, specifically memory and executive functioning, appears to be best if use is >6 h/night [23, 24].

Three studies have reported on the relationship between daytime functioning and CPAP use in children [5, 6, 25]. One divided the 13 adolescents studied at the median proportion of use (21 % of sleep) per night (assessed by parental report) and found that higher users had stable or improved attention, school grades, and school-related quality of life, while low users (<21 % of sleep) were more likely to show declining function in these areas [25]. An early paper found improvements in subjective parental assessment of sleepiness in children using PAP for treatment of obstructive sleep apnea, but no subjective improvement in behavior or school performance [6]. More recently, a study including children over a wider age range (2–16 years) showed a correlation between the change in the Epworth Sleepiness Scale modified for children and adherence as measured by both mean minutes of use/night and nights used [5]. Although highly significant improvements were seen in behavior problems and symptoms of attention deficit hyperactivity disorder compared to baseline in CPAP users (mean use 2.8 h/night), no relationship was seen between hours of CPAP use and the extent of improvement in these measures [5]. This study suggests that even a small amount of use may be associated with improvement in daytime functioning. The relationship between adherence to CPAP and outcomes is a complex one, however, and likely to be more so in children. Sleep requirements fall throughout childhood, and thus the hours of CPAP use that correspond to improvements in functioning may vary with age. To date, no studies have had sufficient power to tease out this relationship. It remains to clinicians to optimize adherence as far as possible, with the expectation that more is very likely to be better.

Patterns of Adherence to CPAP

Patterns of CPAP use in adults are established early after treatment initiation, with consistent users separating from the rest of the group by the fourth night of treatment [26] and use in the first month reliably predicting use in the third month [27, 28]. Similarly, consistent and intermittent pediatric CPAP users differ significantly in hours of CPAP use by the second night of therapy, and this difference is maintained over the first 3 months of therapy (Fig. 12.1) [8]. Skipping CPAP for one or more nights in the first weeks is also a marker of a group of patients that will likely go on to have poor CPAP hours of use even on nights the CPAP is worn [8]. Early review and reinforcement of treatment aims has been proposed as an important factor in promoting better adherence in adults [29]. Similar principles may be applied to children, with intensive follow-up and support in the first weeks of use highlighting the importance of consistent attempts to apply the mask from the very start of treatment.

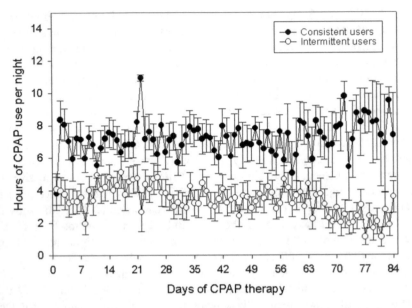

Fig. 12.1 Patterns of CPAP use over first 3 months. Reprinted from *Journal of Pediatrics* [8], Copyright (2011), with permission from Elsevier

Predictors of Adherence to CPAP

Age

The pediatric age range obviously includes children at a wide variety of developmental stages. The impact of age on successful treatment with noninvasive respiratory support may be separated into two issues with potentially different impacts, namely, initiation/acceptance of therapy and extent of actual use (days/week, hours/night, etc.). A study from the UK in which CPAP was initiated during an overnight sleep study showed lower rates of successful CPAP initiation in 1–5-year-old children compared to both infants and children aged over 5 years [7]. This fits with clinical experience of the difficulties with the preschool age group, although it might have been influenced by the fact that the study protocol included CPAP being initiated for the first time in the middle of the night. In that study, 30 % of those in whom the first attempt at initiation was not successful went on to use CPAP following home acclimatization [7]. Another study from Canada divided children by age in a different way but showed similarly that children aged 6–12 years were more likely to be successfully initiated on CPAP than those aged under 6 or over 12 years [9]. Thus preschool children, with the possible exception of infants, present the most challenging group for initial acceptance of CPAP.

The effect of age on hours of CPAP use has been reported by several groups. In a Canadian study, age was demonstrated to be negatively related to adherence, with percentage of days used and hours of use on days used being highest for children aged under 5 years and lowest for adolescents [9]. Conversely, several studies have found no effect of age on adherence [8, 10, 12]. One study reanalyzed this relationship including only those subjects without significant neurodevelopmental delay and confirmed an inverse relationship between days of use at 3 months and age, but no relationship was seen between age and hours of use per night [12]. Therefore, it could be concluded from these various studies that increasing age may adversely affect CPAP use in typically developing children, but the relationship is likely to be weak. In addition, older children have lower hours of sleep, and so lower hours of use in that age group may not actually represent a lower proportion of total sleep time.

Comorbidity

A high proportion of pediatric CPAP users have a major comorbid medical condition, including significant neurodevelopmental disabilities such as Down syndrome and cerebral palsy. These disorders have potential to impact on CPAP adherence in either a positive or negative sense. To date, studies assessing the impact of such comorbidities on adherence have been few and the results conflicting. Two studies found no difference in adherence between children with intellectual disability and typically developing children [8, 9], although O'Donnell et al. did find that children with intellectual disability may be more likely to take time to adapt to CPAP [9]. Conversely, DiFeo et al. found that subjects with developmental delay would be expected to use CPAP for about 2.4 h longer per night than typically developing children, using a regression analysis [12]. These differing results may be related to the very different and heterogeneous groups of patients studied.

Parent and Family Factors

Commitment of the child and family to the treatment contributes significantly to the likelihood of successful use, often adding a degree of complexity not present in the prescription of respiratory support to an adult patient. One study showed that the average number of nights/week on which CPAP was used for less than 1 h (skipped nights) was strongly correlated with duration of use on nights used [8]. This demonstrates that children (and hence their parents) who make consistent attempts to use the therapy every night from the initial education session are most likely to have long-term success in the establishment of therapeutic CPAP. This supports previously reported studies that have emphasized the importance of parental involvement and resolve in establishing CPAP therapy in children [4, 9, 30].

A recent study used qualitative techniques to establish that adherence to CPAP by adolescents was influenced by the degree of structure and routine in the home, social reactions (e.g., a desire on the part of the adolescent to alleviate the caregiver's anxiety by using CPAP), mode of communication among family members (reminders and explanation of reason for CPAP rather than threat and punishment), and perception of the benefits of treatment [31]. Family socioeconomic status has not been shown to be related to CPAP adherence [8], but maternal education is a relatively strong predictor of CPAP use [12].

Barriers to Use

Only one pediatric study has detailed barriers to CPAP use as perceived by patients (8–17 years) and parents, with poorer rates of adherence being associated with greater barriers [17]. Common barriers to CPAP use included not using CPAP when away from home (contributing to low overall usage), child not feeling well, forgetting to use the device, a negative emotional reaction to illness ("just want to forget about OSA"), and embarrassment about using CPAP. Illness-related knowledge was not an issue in this study, with no parents and less than a sixth of youths reporting difficulty in understanding OSA or CPAP. This study identifies several potentially modifiable factors influencing extent of CPAP use.

Side effects of CPAP are generally minor (local irritation, pressure effects) [4, 7, 11] and have not been reported to be associated with nonadherence [9], although this has not been extensively studied.

Disease Modification

Symptoms of OSA have not been shown to predict use of CPAP [6, 10]. Similarly, disease severity as defined by baseline obstructive apnea-hypopnea index (OAHI) has been consistently shown to be unrelated to adherence to CPAP in children [6, 8–10, 12, 25]. Conversely, the efficacy of treatment as defined by the residual OAHI on treatment has been shown to be related to adherence in adults [32]. One study in children found that the difference between the initially prescribed pressure and the treatment pressure defined by first titration polysomnogram predicted adherence [8], suggesting a similar relationship between undertreated OSA and poor adherence in children. This may be related to continued symptoms leading to perceived ineffectiveness of the treatment in the early days of therapy.

Technical Variables

Sub-analyses in two studies have not found a difference in adherence between treatment of OSA with CPAP and bi-level NIV [6, 10]. One study assessed the use of Bi-Flex technology (Philips Respironics), which results in pressure decrements during both late inspiration and expiration [13]. Adherence was comparable with both modes of therapy, and neither of these types of ventilatory support were shown to be superior to regular CPAP in terms of improvement in OAHI, hours of use, or improvements in subjective daytime sleepiness [5, 6].

Adherence to Noninvasive Ventilation

Few centers have reported experience with adherence to NIV. One review quoted local experience of nightly adherence at home in excess of 80 % [33]. Data from our own center are similar, with a series of 17 patients using NIV for an average of more than 4 h/night on 90 % of nights, with an average use per night of 9.3 (SD 1.4) hours [34]. This is substantially higher than that reported for CPAP in many centers and possibly reflects the way the treatment is perceived in the context of the patient's underlying condition. In contrast, a recent study from a single center found comparable adherence with CPAP (mean 8 h 22 min) and NIV (mean 7 h 54 min) in 62 patients with a mean age of 10 years [20], highlighting the likelihood that individual center factors that are as yet unidentified play a role in adherence. This center highlighted the possible influence of home visiting nurses in achieving their high levels of adherence [20].

Improving Adherence

While no single intervention strategy can improve the adherence of all patients, decades of research studies agree that successful attempts to improve patient adherence depend upon a set of key factors. These include realistic assessment of patients' knowledge and understanding of the regimen, clear and effective communication between health professionals and their patients, and the nurturance of trust in the therapeutic relationship. Taking into account each patient's (and family's) beliefs, attitudes, sociocultural context, and approach to medical care in general is essential [35].

Studies of the effectiveness of measures to improve adherence with noninvasive respiratory support in children are very limited but are likely to flow from recent studies of adherence predictors. Individually tailored behavioral interventions have been shown to lead to substantial improvement in hours of usage in a group of children who had been prescribed but were not consistently using CPAP treatment [30]. Involvement in clinic visits of a respiratory therapist skilled in the use of noninvasive respiratory support has also been shown to improve adherence in a group of children with poor adherence [21]. Admission to hospital for supported CPAP initiation, play therapy, cognitive behavioral therapy for older children, and further education and support of parents are other ways that clinicians can attempt to modify adherence patterns. These interventions need to be tailored to the needs of individual families. Further randomized studies are needed to establish which interventions help to reverse the pattern of low adherence in subsets of the pediatric age group and the best timing of these interventions.

Conclusions

CPAP and NIV are effective treatment strategies for sleep-disordered breathing in childhood. Adherence to CPAP treatment consistently falls well short of ideal, if the goal is treatment throughout the sleep period. Factors affecting adherence are similar to those found in adults, but the additional complexity in the therapeutic process of a parent and dependent child also has influences on treatment adherence. While data linking adherence and treatment outcomes such as improvements in daytime well-being and functioning are limited, studies to date suggest that this link exists. Clinicians caring for children on respiratory support should routinely assess adherence and institute vigorous efforts to improve hours of use, especially early in therapy when adherence patterns are established.

Acknowledgment This work was supported by the Victorian government's Operational Infrastructure Support Program.

References

1. Marcus CL, Brooks LJ, Draper KA, Gozal D, Halbower AC, Jones J, Schechter MS, Sheldon SH, Spruyt K, Ward SD, Lehmann C, Shiffman RN, American Academy of Pediatrics. Diagnosis and management of childhood obstructive sleep apnea syndrome. Pediatrics. 2012;130:576–84.
2. Bhattacharjee R, Kheirandish-Gozal L, Spruyt K, Mitchell RB, Promchiarak J, Simakajornboon N, Kaditis AG, Splaingard D, Splaingard M, Brooks LJ, Marcus CL, Sin S, Arens R, Verhulst SL, Gozal D. Adenotonsillectomy outcomes in treatment of obstructive sleep apnea in children: a multicenter retrospective study. Am J Respir Crit Care Med. 2010;182:676–83.
3. Friedman M, Wilson M, Lin HC, Chang HW. Updated systematic review of tonsillectomy and adenoidectomy for treatment of pediatric obstructive sleep apnea/hypopnea syndrome. Otolaryngol Head Neck Surg. 2009;140:800–8.
4. Marcus CL, Ward SL, Mallory GB, Rosen CL, Beckerman RC, Weese-Mayer DE, Brouillette RT, Trang HT, Brooks LJ. Use of nasal continuous positive airway pressure as treatment of childhood obstructive sleep apnea. J Pediatr. 1995;127:88–94.
5. Marcus CL, Radcliffe J, Konstantinopoulou S, Beck SE, Cornaglia MA, Traylor J, Difeo N, Karamessinis LR, Gallagher PR, Meltzer LJ. Effects of positive airway pressure therapy on neurobehavioral outcomes in children with obstructive sleep apnea. Am J Respir Crit Care Med. 2012;185:998–1003.
6. Marcus CL, Rosen G, Ward SLD, Halbower AC, Sterni L, Lutz J, Stading PJ, Bolduc D, Gordon N. Adherence to and effectiveness of positive airway pressure therapy in children with obstructive sleep apnea.[see comment]. Pediatrics. 2006;117:e442–51.
7. Massa F, Gonsalez S, Laverty A, Wallis C, Lane R. The use of nasal continuous positive airway pressure to treat obstructive sleep apnoea. Arch Dis Child. 2002;87:438–43.

8. Nixon GM, Mihai R, Verginis N, Davey MJ. Patterns of continuous positive airway pressure adherence during the first 3 months of treatment in children. J Pediatr. 2011;159:802–7.

9. O'Donnell AR, Bjornson CL, Bohn SG, Kirk VG. Compliance rates in children using nonin-vasive continuous positive airway pressure. Sleep. 2006;29:651–8.

10. Uong EC, Epperson M, Bathon SA, Jeffe DB. Adherence to nasal positive airway pressure therapy among school-aged children and adolescents with obstructive sleep apnea syndrome. Pediatrics. 2007;120:e1203–11.

11. Waters KA, Everett FM, Bruderer JW, Sullivan CE. Obstructive sleep apnea: the use of nasal CPAP in 80 children. Am J Respir Crit Care Med. 1995;152:780–5.

12. Difeo N, Meltzer LJ, Beck SE, Karamessinis LR, Cornaglia MA, Traylor J, Samuel J, Gallagher PR, Radcliffe J, Beris H, Menello MK, Marcus CL. Predictors of positive airway pressure ther-apy adherence in children: a prospective study. J Clin Sleep Med. 2012;8:279–86.

13. Marcus CL, Beck SE, Traylor J, Cornaglia MA, Meltzer LJ, Difeo N, Karamessinis LR, Samuel J, Falvo J, Dimaria M, Gallagher PR, Beris H, Menello MK. Randomized, double-blind clinical trial of two different modes of positive airway pressure therapy on adherence and efficacy in children. J Clin Sleep Med. 2012;8:37–42.

14. Edwards EA, Nixon GM, Australasian Paediatric Respiratory Group Working Party on Home, V. Paediatric home ventilatory support: changing milieu, proactive solutions. J Pediatr Child Health. 2013;49:13–8.

15. Guilleminault C, Nino-Murcia G, Heldt G, Baldwin R, Hutchinson D. Alternative treatment to tracheostomy in obstructive sleep apnea syndrome: nasal continuous positive airway pressure in young children. Pediatrics. 1986;78:797–802.

16. Dimatteo MR, Giordani PJ, Lepper HS, Croghan TW. Patient adherence and medical treatment outcomes: a meta-analysis. Med Care. 2002;40:794–811.

17. Simon SL, Duncan CL, Janicke DM, Wagner MH. Barriers to treatment of paediatric obstruc-tive sleep apnoea: Development of the adherence barriers to continuous positive airway pres-sure (CPAP) questionnaire. Sleep Med. 2012;13:172–7.

18. Brostrom A, Stromberg A, Martensson J, Ulander M, Harder L, Svanborg E. Association of type D personality to perceived side effects and adherence in CPAP-treated patients with OSAS. J Sleep Res. 2007;16:439–47.

19. Richards D, Bartlett DJ, Wong K, Malouff J, Grunstein RR. Increased adherence to CPAP with a group cognitive behavioral treatment intervention: a randomized trial. Sleep. 2007;30:635–40.

20. Ramirez A, Khirani S, Aloui S, Delord V, Borel JC, Pépin JL, Fauroux B. Continuous positive airway pressure and noninvasive ventilation adherence in children. Sleep Med. 2013;14:1290–4.

21. Jambhekar SK, Com G, Tang X, Pruss KK, Jackson R, Bower C, Carroll JL, Ward W. Role of a respiratory therapist in improving adherence to positive airway pressure treatment in a pedi-atric sleep apnea clinic. Respir Care. 2013;58:2038–44.

22. Weaver TE, Maislin G, Dinges DF, Bloxham T, George CFP, Greenberg H, Kader G, Mahowald M, Younger J, Pack AI. Relationship between hours of CPAP use and achieving normal levels of sleepiness and daily functioning. Sleep. 2007;30:711–9.

23. Antic NA, Catcheside P, Buchan C, Hensley M, Naughton MT, Rowland S, Williamson B, Windler S, McEvoy RD. The effect of CPAP in normalizing daytime sleepiness, quality of life, and neurocognitive function in patients with moderate to severe OSA. Sleep. 2011;34:111–9.

24. Zimmerman ME, Arnedt JT, Stanchina M, Millman RP, Aloia MS. Normalization of memory performance and positive airway pressure adherence in memory-impaired patients with obstructive sleep apnea. Chest. 2006;130:1772–8.

25. Beebe DW, Byars KC. Adolescents with obstructive sleep apnea adhere poorly to positive airway pressure (PAP), but PAP users show improved attention and school performance. PLoS One. 2011;6, e16924.

26. Weaver TE, Kribbs NB, Pack AI, Kline LR, Chugh DK, Maislin G, Smith PL, Schwartz AR, Schubert NM, Gillen KA, Dinges DF. Night-to-night variability in CPAP use over the first three months of treatment. Sleep. 1997;20:278–83.

27. Kribbs NB, Pack AI, Kline LR, Smith PL, Schwartz AR, Schubert NM, Redline S, Henry JN, Getsy JE, Dinges DF. Objective measurement of patterns of nasal CPAP use by patients with obstructive sleep apnea.[see comment]. Am Rev Respir Dis. 1993;147:887–95.
28. Pepin JL, Krieger J, Rodenstein D, Cornette A, Sforza E, Delguste P, Deschaux C, Grillier V, Levy P. Effective compliance during the first 3 months of continuous positive airway pressure. A European prospective study of 121 patients.[see comment]. Am J Respir Crit Care Med. 1999;160:1124–9.
29. Weaver TE, Grunstein RR. Adherence to continuous positive airway pressure therapy: the challenge to effective treatment. Proc Am Thorac Soc. 2008;5:173–8.
30. Koontz KL, Slifer KJ, Cataldo MD, Marcus CL. Improving pediatric compliance with positive airway pressure therapy: the impact of behavioral intervention. Sleep. 2003;26:1010–5.
31. Prashad PS, Marcus CL, Maggs J, Stettler N, Cornaglia MA, Costa P, Puzino K, Xanthopoulos M, Bradford R, Barg FK. Investigating reasons for CPAP adherence in adolescents: a qualitative approach. J Clin Sleep Med. 2013;9:1303–13.
32. Ye L, Pack AI, Maislin G, Dinges D, Hurley S, McCloskey S, Weaver TE. Predictors of continuous positive airway pressure use during the first week of treatment. J Sleep Res. 2012;21:419–26.
33. Teague WG. Non-invasive positive pressure ventilation: current status in paediatric patients. Paediatr Respir Rev. 2005;6:52–60.
34. Widger JA, Davey MJ, Nixon GM. Sleep studies in children on long-term non-invasive respiratory support. Sleep Breathing. 2014;18:885–9.
35. Martin LR, Williams SL, Haskard KB, Dimatteo MR. The challenge of patient adherence. J Ther Clin Risk Manage. 2005;1:189–99.

Chapter 13
Ventilator Support in Children with Obstructive Sleep Apnea Syndrome

Kiran Nandalike and Raanan Arens

Introduction

Obstructive sleep apnea syndrome (OSAS) in children is defined as recurrent events of partial or complete upper airway obstruction during sleep resulting in disruption of normal ventilation and normal sleep architecture [1]. OSAS may present in mild, moderate, or severe forms according to the number of respiratory events, severity of gas exchange abnormalities, and the degree of sleep disruption. In children, these can produce long-term adverse effects in behavior and cognition and in the regulation of the cardiovascular, autonomic, and metabolic systems.

The estimated prevalence of OSAS in children ranges from 1.2 to 5.7 %. It peaks between 2 and 8 years of age and is usually associated with the phenotype of adenotonsillar hypertrophy. However, OSAS can occur in children of all ages, even those having normal size adenoid and tonsils, or those that have undergone adenotonsillectomy (AT). During infancy, underlying conditions such as craniofacial anomalies affecting upper airway structure and neurological disorders affecting upper airway motor tone may manifest as other phenotypes of OSAS. In addition, obesity, particularly in late childhood and during adolescent years, is also a known risk factor and may contribute to a higher incidence of OSAS that may exceed 50 % [2, 3].

Understanding the physiological mechanisms leading to OSAS in the different phenotypes is important in order to direct the most effective care for such children. The process of diagnosis and treatment of childhood OSAS continues to evolve as more morbidities are recognized and more evolved diagnostic and treatment modalities become available [4].

K. Nandalike, M.D. • R. Arens, M.D. (✉)
Division of Pediatric Respiratory and Sleep Medicine, The Children's Hospital at Montefiore,
Albert Einstein College of Medicine, 3415 Bainbridge Ave, Bronx, NY 10467, USA
e-mail: rarens@montefiore.org

© Springer Science+Business Media New York 2016
L.M. Sterni, J.L. Carroll (eds.), *Caring for the Ventilator Dependent Child*,
Respiratory Medicine, DOI 10.1007/978-1-4939-3749-3_13

We would like to emphasize that the current recommendation set by the American Academy of Pediatrics (AAP) is to consider initially the need for AT as the first line of care for children with OSAS [5, 6]. However, when AT fails to resolve the disorder or when it is not indicated, and particularly when nonanatomical causes perpetuate the disorder, other treatments are available. Ventilatory support during sleep by positive airway pressure (PAP) is the most common and effective nonsurgical modality to treat OSAS in both adults and children with OSAS. Thus, this chapter will focus on this form of therapy as it relates to OSAS and will expand on its mechanical mechanism of support, the various forms of PAP, indications, adherence, and adverse effects of such treatment in children.

Pathophysiological Mechanisms of OSAS

The upper airway in humans is a collapsible structure. Its particular shape is defined by its surrounding tissues and its neuromuscular and functional properties. The upper airway has three main functions: respiration, deglutition, and speech. Each function has differing requirements—speech and deglutition benefit from the pliable nature of the airway. But respiration, particularly during sleep, is better served by a stiffer airway preserving patency. Thus, it is these attributes that make the upper airway prone to collapse during sleep in humans.

Functional Considerations

There are several arguments that suggest that functional attributes have an important role in the causation of OSAS in children. First, airway obstruction occurs only during sleep and not during wakefulness, suggesting that neuromotor activation keeps the upper airway open while awake but not always during sleep when activation is diminished. Second, a significant number of children with OSAS who undergo AT continue to have the disorder after surgery. This suggests that other anatomical or functional factors persist. Finally, many children with OSAS do not have adenotonsillar hypertrophy or other apparent anatomical risk factors such as obesity or craniofacial disorders. This suggests that functional factors contributing to a more collapsible airway exist during sleep and perpetuate the disorder.

In order to measure the functional properties of the upper airway, the pharynx has been commonly modeled as a Starling resistor representing a collapsible segment bounded by two more rigid segments: upstream (nasal cavity) and downstream (trachea) [7]. The Starling resistor model predicts that, in the condition of flow limitation, inspiratory airflow is determined by the pressure upstream (nasal) to the collapsible portion of the upper airway and is independent of the downstream (tracheal) negative pressure generated by the diaphragm. Collapse occurs when the pressure surrounding the collapsible segment of the upper airway, known as critical tissue pressure (Pcrit), becomes greater than the pressure within the collapsible segment of the airway and when upstream pressure is lower than Pcrit. Upstream pressure can drop sufficiently enough during inspiration to allow collapse when nasal resistance is increased as in craniofacial abnormalities. Of note, Pcrit depends on neuromuscular activation in addition to the passive tissue properties of the airway because the pharynx is not merely a passive tube; it contains active musculature [7].

Ventilatory and Chemical Drive

The central ventilatory drive changes with age from infancy to adulthood. Methodological limitations in measuring ventilatory drive and mechanical and anatomical differences across the age spectrum do not allow precise comparisons throughout the life span. Overall, it appears that ventilatory drive gradually declines from childhood to old age, possibly because of declining basal metabolic rate with age. Adults with OSAS can have high-gain ventilatory control systems that modeling system predicts will predispose these individuals to irregular or periodic breathing, ventilatory instability, and apnea. However, other studies have shown normal or even reduced ventilatory responses in the same age group. These discrepancies could suggest various OSAS phenotypes based on their respiratory response to various respiratory perturbations [8]. In comparison, nonobese children with OSAS have normal ventilatory responses to hypoxia and hypercapnia [7]. This could be due to the shorter lifetime exposure to OSAS effects, fewer associated comorbidities, or due to an intrinsic difference in pathophysiology of OSAS in children as compared to adults. However, subtle changes such as lack of a consistent ventilatory response to hypercapnia in the early morning and association with airway collapsibility with reduced ventilatory drive during sleep may be seen in children [7]. In obese adolescents, a recent study reported a reduced ventilatory response to hypercapnia during sleep, but this has not been confirmed by other studies [9].

Ventilatory Response to Inspiratory Loading

During wakefulness, addition of an external resistive load leads to an immediate compensatory increase in ventilatory effort that maintains gas exchange. In sleep, this compensatory response is not normally seen unless there is a complete airway occlusion. With partial occlusion during sleep, a decrease in minute ventilation ensues, and compensatory increase of ventilation is delayed; the eventual correction is believed to be in response to gas exchange abnormalities. In normal children, this compensation can be limited and delayed by 3 min or more as compared to adults [10]. Children with OSAS have reduced arousal responses to inspiratory resistive loads during sleep that together with the aforementioned inadequate compensation of ventilation may explain the prolonged periods of obstructive hypoventilation observed in childhood OSAS [7].

Arousal

Arousal is a normal phenomenon of sleep and is defined as sudden shifts in EEG frequency toward the awake state lasting for 3 s. However, if arousals occur too often, they produce sleep disruption and interfere with the restorative nature of sleep. It should also be pointed out that arousals may be considered protective to subjects with OSAS since they coincide with increased dilator muscle activity, reduced upper airway resistance, and restoration of normal ventilation.

Studies in children and adults have clearly shown that frequent arousal and sleep fragmentation often lead to decreased vigilance, sleepiness, and other neurocognitive impairments. Interestingly, children are much less prone to arousals due to respiratory events than adults and typically are less sleepy compared to adults with OSAS. The major stimuli for arousals from OSAS are thought to be mechanical stimulation of the lung and chest wall stretch receptors due to increased respiratory effort. However, hypercapnia is also considered a potent arousal stimulus. The majority of obstructive events in adults are associated with arousals from non-REM sleep. In children the majority of obstructive events occur during REM sleep, and associated arousals are less frequent than in adults. Normal children have a higher arousal threshold than adults; children with OSAS seem to have an even loftier threshold for arousal in response to inspiratory loading [10] and hypercapnia [11] compared to children without OSAS.

Neuromotor Tone and Its Evaluation

Patency allows flow through the upper airway and depends not only on mechanical and anatomic factors but also the active dilation of the airway by neuromotor tone. Pressure-flow relationships based on the Starling model provide an understanding of airway stability in the "active" state with neuromotor activation and in the "passive state" when neuromotor tone is reduced or absent and can be measured in subjects and patients. In the Pcrit test, plotting a range of continuous positive airway pressure (CPAP) and continuous negative airway pressure (CNAP) applied airway pressures, against the resulting maximal inspiratory flows of breaths, generates a flow versus pressure graph with the critical closing pressure or Pcrit being represented by the intercept on the pressure axis (where flow effectively becomes zero, equivalent to complete airway obstruction). Airway pressure is applied by a nasal mask with the subject in a supine position, and airflow is measured by a pneumotach; the pressures applied range from positive pressures to negative (subatmospheric) pressures. The derived Pcrit value is considered a measure and index of airway collapsibility for the subject.

The Pcrit is typically lower for the neuronally active airway as compared to the passive airway. In children especially, the Pcrit intercept value tends to be very negative (i.e., motor tone is very high) due to unreliable extrapolation of the graphed pressure flow line; in such cases the slope of the pressure flow line is taken as the next best estimate of upper airway collapsibility. Developing the Pcrit technique further can provide additional information: airflow in the first few breaths following a suddenly applied drop in pressure to the subject, before neuromotor responses can occur, represents the "passive airway"; this passive Pcrit can be used to estimate mechanical and structural properties of the airway.

A passive airway closing pressure can also be estimated by measuring the pressure cross-sectional area relationship observed endoscopically in anesthetized subjects (in whom neuromotor activation is suppressed). This method is analogous to the pressure-airflow relationship evaluated by the Pcrit method. Neuromotor activation can also be directly quantified by measuring the EMG activity of the genioglossus muscle which is the major pharyngeal dilator.

The pediatric airway is very resistant to collapse compared to the adult airway; airway collapsibility increases with age during adolescence but is not a function of pubertal development. In children and adolescents with OSAS, the Pcrit is much higher (i.e., indicating more propensity for airway collapse) than in non-OSAS children [7, 12]. Childhood OSAS is most prominent in REM sleep which is associated with reduced pharyngeal tone and wide fluctuations of airflow, both of which probably contribute to OSAS. While Pcrit is difficult to measure in REM sleep for practical reasons, reduced airway tone can be demonstrated by EMG studies of the tongue muscles. Awake children with OSAS have higher baseline EMG tone than normal children most probably to compensate for their narrower airways resulting from anatomical and/or functional causes. However, with sleep onset these children have a rapid decline in EMG tone [13] with yet further decline in the REM stage, predisposing them to airway obstruction during sleep [14].

It is important to recognize that there can be various contributory factors to OSAS in children either independent of or coincident with anatomical factors. Moreover, several physiometric methods are available to evaluate alterations in upper airway function. In conclusion and, importantly, for children with OSAS, the finding of high Pcrit or diminished ventilatory or chemical drive in the absence of anatomical abnormality restricting the upper airway would favor ventilatory support during sleep rather than surgical management.

Anatomical Considerations

Anatomical factors are commonly important contributors to childhood OSAS. A structural abnormality may be congenital, acquired, simple, or complex. They can be solely responsible for OSAS but can coincide with functional abnormalities discussed above. Often, simple diagnostic procedures such as physical examination and lateral neck x-ray will suffice to identify the cause of OSAS, and correcting the primary abnormality will resolve or improve the disorder. However, in more complex conditions as with children with craniofacial abnormalities, identifying the precise structural and/or functional abnormality may require more involved methods such as computerized tomography, magnetic resonance imaging, or sleep endoscopy, as well as functional studies like Pcrit. In addition, clinical assessment by a multidisciplinary team to ascertain the most proper treatment course is very helpful. Since anatomical abnormalities usually present different phenotypes of OSAS, these will be discussed according to stage of development.

Infancy

OSAS can occur in preterm and term infants in the first year of life. Infants are predisposed to obstructive events and desaturation during sleep because of high nasal resistance, reduced airway stiffness, and a highly compliant chest wall with reduced functional residual capacity [7, 15]. Spontaneous neck flexion can also result in airway obstruction in premature infants [16]. Nasal occlusion results in a switch to oral breathing only in a minority of infants [17], and therefore obstruction of the nasal passages from respiratory infection, craniofacial syndromes, or choanal stenosis can result in significant OSAS. Upper airway obstruction may also occur as a result of airway edema, laryngospasm, and airway edema from gastroesophageal reflux disease (GERD). The high laryngeal compliance of laryngomalacia in infants has been demonstrated to be associated with obstructive sleep apnea with improvement after supraglottoplasty [18].

OSAS in infancy is notable for its association with craniofacial anomalies, soft tissue enlargement, and neuromuscular abnormalities. Craniofacial abnormalities are present in single gene disorders such as Crouzon and Apert syndrome and chromosomal abnormalities such as Down syndrome. Mechanisms for airway obstruction with craniofacial abnormalities include increased upper airway resistance with maxillary hypoplasia, choanal stenosis, or compromised pharyngeal space with mandibular hypoplasia as in the Pierre Robin sequence. Soft tissue enlargement is present in disorders such as Down syndrome and Beckwith-Wiedemann syndrome including relative or absolute enlargement of the tongue that predisposes to sleep-related airway obstruction. In infants older than 6 months of age, adenotonsillar hypertrophy and particularly adenoidal hypertrophy can result in severe OSAS with failure to thrive that resolves after adenotonsillectomy. Conditions such as cerebral palsy and Moebius syndrome can result in lower airway tone in the upper airway with OSAS in infants because of their intrinsic airway collapsibility. Interestingly, Down syndrome predisposes to OSAS with a confluence of smaller bony structure, larger soft tissues, and lower airway tone. Overall, OSAS in infancy has not been extensively studied, and the incidence of OSAS is not known. Limited information is available regarding the physiological effects of OSAS in infants except for the observation of extreme morbidities such as failure to thrive or cor pulmonale [19].

Childhood

Anatomical factors contributing to OSAS in childhood can be discussed in terms of location of obstruction, soft tissue enlargement, and craniofacial structure. The location of maximal upper airway narrowing in children is usually at the level of the adenoid and soft palate based on endoscopic and MRI data [7]. The airway is narrowest at the level of the "overlap region" where the adenoid overlaps the palatine tonsils in the upper two thirds of the pharynx [20]. Adenotonsillar tissues grow commensurate with age in children without OSAS maintaining a constant proportionality with the pharyngeal airway [7]. It has been speculated that disproportional overgrowth of the adenoid and tonsils in children with OSAS results from inflammation and/or infections, but the mechanisms leading to this process have not been elucidated. Adenotonsillar size is only weakly correlated with OSAS severity, and position and orientation of these tissues may be important to causation of airway obstruction. Removal of adenoid and tonsils results in improvement of OSAS in approximately 85 % of children with OSAS and adenotonsillar hypertrophy, but the rest continue to have some degree of obstruction indicating the importance of other factors in the causation of childhood OSAS.

Other soft tissues have not been implicated in the causation of OSAS in childhood. The tongue, the largest soft tissue structure around the pharynx, has been reported to be similar in size in children with OSAS and in controls. The soft palate is increased in size with OSAS, but the difference in size is not large enough to contribute significantly to OSAS, and the enlargement is probably secondary to inflammation from snoring [21].

The evidence regarding craniofacial structures causing OSAS in childhood is mixed, except in cases of distinct craniofacial syndromes. Studies using cephalometrics suggest that minor differences in anatomy such as retrognathic mandibles and increased craniomandibular, intermaxillary, and mandibular plane angles which indicate a divergent growth pattern may promote OSAS. However, other investigators have reported mild changes and reversibility in these measurements after adenotonsillectomy suggesting these are effects of OSAS rather than causations. MRI evaluation of the mandibular, maxillary, and palatal dimensions has not revealed smaller dimensions in children with OSAS suggesting that these do not contribute to OSAS in children without craniofacial syndromes [7].

Obesity in childhood has now become a recognizable contributor to pediatric OSAS; national estimates of obesity are 12 % and 18 % in children aged 2–5 years and 6–11 years, respectively [22]. Epidemiologic evidence suggests that obesity increases the odds of OSAS by 4.5 [23], and children with obesity have smaller adenotonsillar tissue size for a similar degree of OSAS [24], even though adenotonsillar hypertrophy continues to be a significant factor in obese children with OSAS [25]. The factors that potentially lead to OSAS in children with obesity include deposition of adipose tissue in fat pads and soft tissue around the pharynx resulting in limitation of airway size, increased airway tissue pressure, altered chest wall mechanics, and reduction of functional residual capacity that reduces oxygen reserves and predisposes to hypoxemia and reduced ventilator drive [7, 24].

Adolescence

The prevalence of OSAS in adolescents has not been widely reported, but the prevalence of OSAS in obese adolescents is high ranging from 19 to 32 % [26, 27]. Obesity is seen in 18.4 % of adolescents in the USA (12–19 years) [22] and is a major contributor to OSAS in this age group. Adenotonsillar hypertrophy is associated with OSAS in older children and adolescents [26, 27], but the response of OSAS to adenotonsillectomy in obese children is limited [28] suggesting the role of other contributors such as obesity and functional factors. Comparison of obese adolescents with and without OSAS in a recent study showed larger adenoid, tonsils, and retropharyngeal lymph nodes in the OSAS group but no difference in tongue or mandible size. Neck parapharyngeal fat and visceral adiposity were greater in OSAS adolescents but did not correlate with degree of OSAS, perhaps due to the small sample size or because these may be associated only with severe OSAS. Interestingly, lymphoid tissue did not correlate with BMI z-score suggesting that lymphoid hypertrophy was not secondary to obesity-induced inflammation and occurs due to a separate etiological process [25].

Ventilatory Support in Children with OSAS

OSAS in children carries significant long-term effects such as cardiovascular morbidities in the form of hypertension and left ventricular dysfunction, behavior and cognitive deficits, autonomic dysregulation, and metabolic derangements such as insulin resistance and the metabolic syndrome. Thus, the need for early diagnosis and intervention is essential to prevent the long-term consequences of the untreated disorder. As mentioned above, the AAP recommends AT as the treatment of choice for children with OSAS. However, when AT or other upper airway surgeries are not effective or indicated, and particularly when functional attributes are considered, PAP therapy during sleep has been shown to be an effective treatment.

The first publication to demonstrate the efficacy of PAP was in adult patients with OSAS and was reported by Sullivan et al. in 1981 [29]. This treatment was approved in 1985 by the FDA for adults with the disorder [29]. Soon after, PAP was successfully introduced by Guilleminault et al. as an alternative modality to tracheotomy for children with OSAS due to severe underlying craniofacial disorders [30]. Since the above reports, many forms of PAP devices have been developed for children with sleep-disordered breathing and OSAS and are now available for the pediatric population all over the world.

Mechanism of PAP Ventilation in OSAS

The mechanical effect of PAP therapy is by maintaining a pneumatic splint between the upper airway and surrounding tissues by maintaining the intraluminal pressure above the Pcrit pressure. Schwab at al. have studied the effects of PAP on upper airway in normal adult subjects using magnetic resonance imaging studies [31, 32]. Effective PAP increases the mean and minimal cross-sectional upper airway area and overall upper airway volume and particularly provides an increase in the lateral airway diameter that tends to be reduced in adults with OSAS. PAP also reduces the lateral pharyngeal wall thickness and reduces upper airway edema resulting from chronic vibration and occlusion of the airway. PAP has also shown to increase the end expiratory volume, thereby exerting a tracheal tug and stiffening the upper airway [33]. Airway resistance is inversely proportional to the fourth power of airway radius. Even a small increase in airway diameter can significantly decrease the airway resistance and therefore decrease the work of breathing. PAP therapy has been documented to be effective in eliminating both obstructive and mixed apneas as well as some central apneas that are observed in patients with predominant obstructive apnea. Thus, PAP can alleviate both the short-term impact of OSAS by improving ventilation and sleep efficiency as well as reducing their long-term consequences.

Forms of PAP Ventilation and Technical Considerations

Various forms of PAP therapy exist to treat sleep-disordered breathing and OSAS (Table 13.1). PAP can be administered invasively through a tracheotomy site or noninvasively using interfaces applied to the nose or mouth and nose combined. In most instances PAP is administered noninvasively for OSAS subjects. The most common form of PAP ventilation is continuous PAP (CPAP). This form of therapy provides a constant positive air pressure throughout the respiratory cycle and is

Table 13.1 Forms of PAP ventilation

Form	Mechanism of action	Indications
Continuous positive airway pressure (CPAP)	Continuous pressure during both inspiration and expiration	OSAS secondary to isolated upper airway obstruction
	Mechanical splint effect	
	Increase the lung volume and exerts tracheal tug	
Bilevel positive airway pressure (BLPAP): available in spontaneous (S), spontaneous timed (S/T), or timed (T) modes	Two-level pressures, inspiratory (IPAP) and expiratory (EPAP); the difference in pressure (PS) delivers the tidal volume and the backup rate that can be timed to patient's breathing, ensures adequate ventilation	OSAS with obstructive hypoventilation, obesity hypoventilation and neuromuscular diseases, and nonobstructive hypoventilation, CCHS
Automatic positive airway pressure (auto PAP)	Pressure adjusted with patient's breathing cycle	Subjects with sleep stage dependent or positional sleep apnea (role not well studied in children)
Adaptive servo-ventilation (ASV)	Analyzes breath to breath ventilation and delivers set ventilation by adjusting the pressure with each respiratory cycle	Complex sleep apnea or central sleep apnea (role not well studied in children)

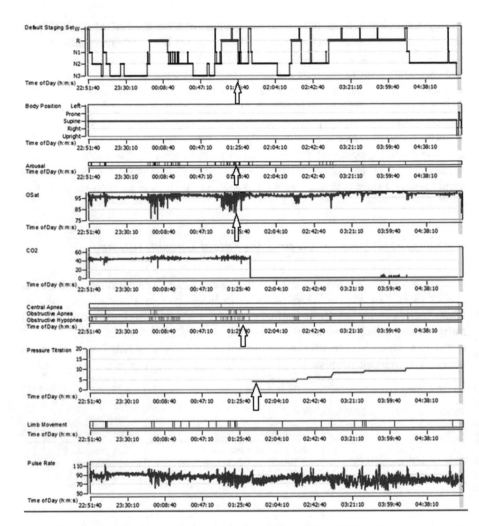

Fig. 13.1 A split-night PSG in an 18-year-old male with severe OSAS. The red arrows point to the improvement in sleep architecture (*upper panel*), arousals (*brown bars*), and oxygen saturation (O₂ sat, red trace, and obstructive events (*green bars*) with introduction of PAP therapy (green tracing of pressure measured by cm H2O, in *lower panel*))

usually sufficient to overcome both obstructive and/or hypopnea events while correcting any gas exchange abnormalities and restoring sleep patterns. Pressure adjustments are performed during an overnight sleep study, and the goals are to eliminate all respiratory events while restoring normal ventilation and oxygenation and sleep architecture and while ensuring patient tolerability. Figure 13.1 exhibits a CPAP titration study in a child with OSAS.

In addition to CPAP therapy for OSAS, other devices are available for the use of children today (Table 13.1). Bilevel positive airway pressure (BLPAP) provides two adjustable levels of pressures: inspiratory positive airway pressure (IPAP) and the expiratory positive airway pressure (EPAP). In addition this device is capable of providing a backup rate of ventilation. BLPAP is useful to treat children with OSAS as well as other forms of sleep-disordered breathing including chronic alveolar hypoventilation that will be discussed below and more extensively in other chapters in this book. Briefly, chronic alveolar hypoventilation could be isolated as seen in congenital central hypoventilation syndrome (CCHS) or could be part of sleep-disordered breathing as seen in children with neuromuscular diseases. Both IPAP and EPAP help maintain the airway patency, and the pressure support (IPAP-EPAP) augments the ventilation. The BLPAP respiratory rate can be set at spontaneous mode (S), spontaneous/time mode (S/T) mode, or as timed mode (T), to ensure adequate ventilation. There are no specific criteria for use of BLPAP in children with isolated OSAS. BLPAP is better tolerated in some individuals with severe OSAS because of the pressure relief during exhalation and lower mean airway pressure during the respiratory cycle [34].

Auto PAP (auto-titrating PAP/self-adjusting PAP) senses the subtle changes in users' breathing and delivers only the amount of pressure needed to keep the airway open. The variable pressure response of auto-CPAP may better suit the children under different conditions such as upper airway infections, different sleeping positions, and abrupt changes in weight. Although auto PAP has shown to improve the acceptance and compliance in older individuals with OSAS, its use has not been well studied in children [35]. Adaptive servo-ventilation (ASV) is indicated in subjects with central sleep apnea of any form (heart failure, complex sleep apnea, or drug induced). ASV adapts to patient's ventilator needs on breath by breath basis, automatically calculates the target ventilation, and adjusts the pressure support to achieve this. ASV use has shown to improve the survival in some adult patients with heart failure [36]. The use of ASV in children is not well studied.

A PAP device has a flow generator, a hose that connects the flow generator to the interface, and an interface that connects the hose to the patient. PAP device technology has improved significantly in recent years in order to increase patient tolerance and therapy compliance [37]. The newer devices are less noisy and less bulky. They are equipped with inbuilt humidifiers which provide heated humidification and reduce naso-oral dryness. The newer devices also have optional heated tubings, mask liners to reduce facial irritation, options for ramp time (pressure gradually increases to the set pressure over a set time), flexible chin straps to decrease the air leak through the mouth, expiratory pressure relief (Cflex), as well as data logging records (compliance chips) which allow the physicians to monitor compliance and effectiveness of the treatment either locally or remotely.

Similarly, interface technology has improved significantly in recent years, and this is critical because establishing a comfortable but effective interface is key to the success of PAP acceptance and adherence. A poor fitting mask can lead to air leak that results in ineffective pressure and frequent arousals, discomfort, and facial injury. There are different varieties of interfaces including nasal, nasal pillow,

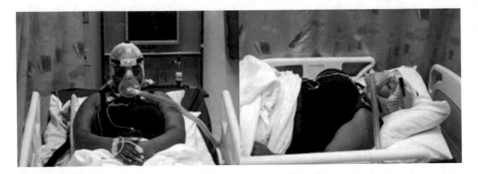

Fig. 13.2 A 17-year-old girl with OSAS receiving PAP titration trial in our lab

oronasal, and full-face masks. The comparative studies in terms of acceptance and adherence between different interfaces are limited in children. It is frequently difficult to find a correctly fitting mask in young children especially those with craniofacial anomalies. Different interfaces need to be trialed during the introduction of the PAP therapy to find the best interface. Also, the interfaces need to be frequently reevaluated and adjusted for a growing child. Custom-made interfaces have shown promise in terms of easy adaptability and less facial complications [38]. However, currently the custom-made masks are not available in the USA. Also, FDA has not approved any PAP devices or interfaces for children with weight less than 10 kgs, mostly, due to the lack of data on efficacy and compliance in this age group.

PAP therapy for children should be initiated under appropriate supervision, ideally in an accredited sleep laboratory or in the hospital while monitoring respiratory and sleep parameters by expert technicians or respiratory therapist trained in the care of children. Figure 13.2 shows a picture of a child receiving PAP titration therapy in our lab. The children and the families should receive appropriate education, hands-on demonstration, careful mask fitting, and acclimatization prior to initiating full-time therapy. On the night of titration, the optimal PAP pressure, that which eliminates all apneas, hypopneas, and respiratory flow-related arousals both in supine and lateral positions, needs to be determined. PAP titration can be done on the night the OSAS is diagnosed (split night) or on a second full-night study. However, in children two night studies are preferred over a split-night study in order to improve PAP acceptance. The technical details on the PAP titration are available from the American Academy of Sleep Medicine guidelines (AASM) from 2008 [39].

Invasive PAP is rarely indicated in children with OSAS; however, it may be required in children with severe OSAS who have a tracheotomy or those who cannot tolerate any form of mask interface. Tracheotomy alone relives the obstruction in majority of these children without the need for further PAP via tracheotomy. However, invasive PAP may be required in some children, for example, those with neuromuscular weakness or when there is significant daytime hypoventilation. Please refer to the chapter on home ventilation in children with neuromuscular diseases for further details. Invasive ventilation/PAP may also be required in some children with obesity hypoventilation syndrome.

Indications for PAP Ventilation

PAP is clinically indicated for children with OSAS and other forms of sleep-disordered breathing resulting from a wide spectrum of clinical disorders. In general, these can be stratified into four main categories as illustrated in Table 13.2: OSAS in otherwise healthy children, OSAS associated with craniofacial malformations and genetic disorders, OSAS associated with altered CNS function, and OSAS associated with miscellaneous conditions. In this section we will review the most common medical conditions in which PAP has been shown to be an effective therapy.

OSAS in Otherwise Healthy Children

OSAS Associated with Obesity

Obesity is reaching epidemic proportions across all age groups including children. OSAS is a common comorbid condition in obese children. Presence of obesity has been shown to increase the risk of OSAS by more than fourfold [40]. Adenotonsillar hypertrophy is frequently seen in obese children, and some studies have reported OSAS prevalence as high as 45% in obese children [25]. AAP recommends AT as the first-line treatment for OSAS, even in obese children, because of such high prevalence of adenotonsillar hypertrophy and low compliance with PAP therapy in these children [5, 6]. AT significantly improves the symptoms and polysomnography parameters in obese children with OSAS, but the cure rate is low and ranges between 26 and 46% [41]. The reasons for such high failure rate are not well understood but include anatomical risk factors such as increased parapharyngeal fat pad size and visceral adiposity that may further reduce upper airway size and stability during sleep, independently of tonsillar and adenoidal tissue [2, 3]. PAP is a good treatment alternative for these children who have failed AT or who for those who do not have evidence of adenotonsillar hypertrophy.

Residual OSAS After AT

A common indication for PAP therapy is for otherwise healthy nonobese children without apparent craniofacial or neurological disorders who present with residual OSAS after AT. In addition to the recurrence of clinical symptoms, a diagnosis of OSAS should be confirmed by polysomnography in these children. The success rate of AT varies between studies but is usually reported to be between 71 and 87%, though some studies suggest a much lower cure rate [5, 6]. Several studies identify risk factors for residual OSAS including older age group, presurgical severity of OSAS, obesity, asthma, and family history of OSAS [42].

Table 13.2 Indications for PAP ventilation in children with OSAS

OSAS in otherwise healthy children
OSAS associated with obesity
Residual OSAS after AT
Isolated upper airway deformities/anomalies
Choanal atresia
Choanal stenosis
Laryngomalacia
Subglottic stenosis
Laryngeal cyst
Laryngeal stenosis
Laryngeal web
Subglottic stenosis
Tracheomalacia
OSAS associated with craniofacial malformations and genetic disorders
Craniofacial anomalies:
Apert syndrome
Crouzon syndrome
Pfeiffer syndrome
Treacher Collins syndrome
Robin sequence
Stickler syndrome
Nager syndrome
Hallermann-Streiff syndrome
Goldenhar syndrome
Rubinstein-Taybi syndrome
Down syndrome
Beckwith-Wiedemann syndrome
Achondroplasia
Klippel-Feil syndrome
Marfan syndrome
Prader-Willi syndrome
Mucopolysaccharidoses (Hurler, Hunter)
Craniosynostosis
OSAS associated with altered CNS function (Stratification according to level of involvement)
Upper motor neuron
Cerebral palsy
Brain stem
Congenital central hypoventilation syndrome (CCHS), Arnold Chiari type I and II
Spinal cord injury
C1–C5
Motor neuron
Spinal muscular atrophy, poliomyelitis

(continued)

Table 13.2 (continued)

Peripheral nerve
Vocal cord paralysis, phrenic nerve injury, hereditary motor and sensory neuropathies (Charcot-Marie-Tooth), hereditary sensory autonomic neuropathy, leukodystrophies, Guillain-Barre, polyneuropathy
Neuromuscular junction
Myasthenia gravis, congenital myasthenia
Muscle (types)
Dystrophinopathies
Duchenne muscular dystrophy, Becker muscular dystrophy
Non-dystrophinopathies
Facioscapulohumeral, merosin deficient, merosin positive
Myotonic dystrophy
Myotonic dystrophy, congenital myotonic dystrophy
Congenital myopathies
Nemaline, central core, centronuclear, multicore, minicore
Mitochondrial myopathies
Mitochondrial myopathy with ophthalmoplegia, MELAS
Inflammatory myopathies
SLE, polymyositis
OSAS associated with miscellaneous conditions
Metabolic disorders
Lysosomal storage diseases (mucopolysaccharidoses)
Glycogenoses (glycogen storage diseases)
Sickle cell disease
Face and neck burns

OSAS Associated with Laryngomalacia

In otherwise healthy nonsyndromic children, several medical conditions including deformities or anomalies along the upper airway could lead to flow limitation and OSAS (Table 13.2). However, the most common condition is laryngomalacia. This condition is defined as the collapse of the supraglottic structures in to the laryngeal inlet during inspiration. Laryngomalacia is the most common cause of stridor and OSAS in infants with a reported prevalence between 8 and 50 %. Laryngomalacia is also common in children with neuromuscular disorders (NMD) and especially in children with Down syndrome. Late-onset laryngomalacia has been reported in a significant number of older children with OSAS (3.5 %).

In 80 % of children with infant laryngomalacia, symptoms resolve within 6–9 months of life. However, severe laryngomalacia with secondary consequences is seen in the remaining 20 %. Though symptoms may appear throughout the day, they are most prominent in the supine position during sleep and are associated with severe upper airway obstruction, alterations of gas exchange, increased work of breathing, poor feeding, and poor weight gain. In some severe cases pulmonary hypertension and cor pulmonale have been reported [43]. Polysomnography is an important tool to assess the severity of laryngomalacia as well as treatment follow-up; however, most centers do not routinely perform polysomnography for these children. Supraglottoplasty is the treatment of choice in severe cases of laryngomalacia [44]. This surgery has shown to significantly improve the symptoms as well as PSG findings both in infants and children [45]. However, supraglottoplasty is not always successful in children with associated comorbid conditions. PAP therapy is the preferred mode of treatment for children with laryngomalacia with significant comorbid conditions as well as in those who fail surgery. Efficacy of such treatment in young infants with laryngomalacia has been established by several studies [46–49].

OSAS Associated with Craniofacial Malformations and Genetic Disorders

Craniosynostosis

Children with syndromic craniosynostosis are reported to have high prevalence of OSAS. Craniosynostosis, characterized by premature closure of cranial sutures, is an autosomal dominant condition but can be an isolated disorder or coincide with several genetic syndromes such as Crouzon, Apert, and Pfeiffer. Cranial malformations, particularly when associated with a smaller anterior cranial base, midface hypoplasia, mandibular hypoplasia, choanal atresia cleft palate, and excessive pharyngeal collapsibility, increase the risk of OSAS [50]. In addition, such individuals may have increased intracranial pressure and decreased brain growth; the further presence of OSAS can increase the risk for central apnea, neurocognitive deficits, risk of heart failure, and sudden death [51].

Monitoring of sleep-disordered breathing is essential in these patients; the treatment of their OSAS may be difficult. Treatment approaches depend on the type of sleep-disordered breathing and OSAS and severity of upper airway obstruction and as they relate to underlying anatomical and functional causes. In regard to surgical management, these could include some of the following: adenotonsillectomy [52], facial advancement surgery [53], and mandibular advancement. However, these are not always successful in reducing the severity of OSAS in these children. PAP therapy can be a useful treatment alternative in some of the milder cases who are either waiting for the surgery or who have responded only partially to surgery. PAP therapy should also be attempted in at least some of these children before tracheotomy, to determine if it would be an adequate alternative. It should be mentioned that a significant obstacle for treatment success and adherence with PAP is matching the appropriate mask or nasal prong interface for such children, since custom masks are not usually available. However, PAP has been tried and shown to be effective in reducing the severity of OSAS in many of these disorders [50].

Pierre Robin Sequence

OSAS is a common comorbid condition in a majority of children with Pierre Robin sequence. Pierre Robin sequence, first described in 1928, is characterized by retrognathia and glossoptosis with and without cleft palate. This sequence could be a part of genetic syndrome or could be an isolated finding not related to any genetic syndrome. A small mandible seems to be the main culprit in this sequence with resulting glossoptosis and impaired palate development. Presence of micrognathia with glossoptosis significantly increases the risks of developing OSAS, and studies have reported high prevalence of OSAS in (46–83 %) these children [54]. Often times, OSAS in these children can be suspected from feeding difficulties or failure to gain weight rather than typical symptoms of OSAS such as snoring or difficulty breathing [55]. Several oral appliances and mandibular distraction techniques have been shown to improve the OSAS symptoms in these children. Upper airway dimensions can improve over time, making PAP therapy a good alternative therapy to consider before mandibular surgeries [56].

Achondroplasia

OSAS is common in children with achondroplasia. This autosomal dominant genetic condition is characterized by short-limb dwarfism. OSAS is highly prevalent (~75 %) [57] and starts to manifest early in life. Several risk factors including smaller cranium, small midface, relative adenotonsillar hypertrophy, hydrocephalus, and stenotic foramen magnum with brain stem compression increase the risk of OSAS in these children [58]. AT improves OSAS, but residual OSAS is seen in a high proportion of these children. Upper airway surgeries, including facial advancement, are shown to improve OSAS. PAP has been tried and is shown to be beneficial in majority of these children with OSAS [57].

Down Syndrome

Down syndrome is the most common genetic cause of intellectual impairment with the incidence of about 1:670 live births. Children with Down syndrome suffer from significant comorbid conditions including congenital heart disease, hearing and vision impairment, thyroid disease, certain hematological malignancies, and some bone disease. The prevalence of sleep-disordered breathing and OSAS among children with Down syndrome is reported to be between 30 and 100 % [59–61]. The reasons for such high variation in prevalence is likely due to different definitions used to define these disorders in various studies, lack of normative data of these populations, different age groups, and different sources of recruitment.

Nevertheless, the reasons for such high prevalence of OSAS in this population is explained by the anatomical differences including smaller midface, small mandible, relative macroglossia, decreased airway tone with easy collapsibility of hypopharyngeal space, and enlarged lingual tonsils, as well as a significantly high proportion of laryngomalacia, especially in infants [62–66]. The prevalence of obesity is also high in children with Down syndrome adding to their overall risk for OSAS. Children with Down syndrome also have a high prevalence of hypothyroidism (20–30%) which starts manifesting as early as infancy and increases their risks of OSAS [67].

It is important to mention that due to the high prevalence of sleep-disordered breathing in these children, the American Academy of Pediatrics recommends screening for SDB/OSAS in these children during early and late childhood and adolescent years. The consequences of OSAS in this population are especially serious given their underlying heart disease and low intellectual capacity. Unrecognized and untreated OSAS puts these children at high risk for additional neurocognitive impairment, disruptive behavior, systemic hypertension, pulmonary hypertension, and cor pulmonale [68–71].

Adenotonsillectomy has a success rate of only about ~20 % in these children [72]. This is not surprising given their multifaceted airway obstruction risks. PAP is shown to be an effective mode of treatment in these children. Adherence to PAP is shown to be improved by avoiding split-night polysomnography studies, gradual introduction of mask use, and close clinical follow-up and tracking the therapy compliance data.

Prader-Willi Syndrome

Sleep-disordered breathing including OSAS, central sleep apnea, and obstructive hypoventilation is commonly seen in children with Prader-Willi syndrome (PWS). PWS is a genetic condition resulting from deletions on chromosome 15. Several phenotypic characteristics of PWS children increase their risks for OSAS including hypotonia, obesity, and hypothalamic dysfunction [73]. Growth hormone has shown to significantly decrease the body mass index and body fat distribution in children with PWS. Long-term treatment with growth hormone can reasonably be expected to decrease the risk of OSAS in these children. However, studies have shown that there is a risk of sudden death secondary to worsening OSAS in children with PWS within the first 6–8 weeks of starting growth hormone therapy [74]. Even with optimal treatment of OSAS, some PWS children exhibit excessive daytime sleepiness or daytime hyperactivity. These could be related to their inherent hypothalamic dysfunction. Despite this, PAP therapy is still a good treatment option for OSAS in these children [75].

OSAS Associated with Altered CNS Function

Neuromuscular Disorders

Sleep-disordered breathing (SDB), with or without OSAS, is well recognized in children with neuromuscular disorders. Several risk factors including reduced ventilatory responses, reduced activity of respiratory muscles during sleep, reduced upper airway dilator tone, and poor lung mechanics due to the underlying neuromuscular disorder predispose these children to develop SDB. In addition, the presence of adenotonsillar hypertrophy and obesity may exaggerate the underlying SDB. SDB can be present as OSAS, nocturnal obstructive hypoventilation, or diurnal hypoventilation. Untreated SDB may contribute to significant cardiovascular morbidities, neurocognitive deficits, and premature death. PAP therapy for these children includes CPAP, BLPAP or invasive ventilation depending on the severity of SDB [2, 3].

Congenital Central Hypoventilation Syndrome

Congenital central hypoventilation syndrome (CCHS) is a rare autosomal dominant, lifelong condition caused by PHOX2B mutation, wherein control of breathing is abnormal and patients present with hypoventilation. Adequate ventilation during wakefulness and sleep is the key to the overall well-being and good quality of life for these children. CCHS patients who are on diaphragm pacing at night are at risk for OSAS during sleep. Both invasive and noninvasive ventilators have been successfully used in these children [76, 77]. Please refer to the chapter on CCHS in this book for further details.

Chiari Malformation

Sleep-disordered breathing, more commonly a central sleep apnea and occasionally obstructive sleep apnea, has been reported in children with type 1 Chiari malformation. Decompression surgery with resulting decrease in intracranial pressure has shown to improve SDB symptoms in a majority of these children [78]. There are some reports of successful PAP therapy including adaptive servo-ventilation in some children with residual SDB post decompression [79].

Cerebral Palsy

OSAS is frequently seen in children with cerebral palsy. The presence of poor medullary control of breathing, inadequate neuromuscular tone, seizure, gastroesophageal reflux, increased oral secretions, and inability to change the posture and protect the airway at night increases their risk of obstructive hypoventilation and obstructive apneas during sleep [80]. The tonsils and adenoid, if only mildly enlarged, can increase the risk of OSA in these children, and adenotonsillectomy has shown to significantly improve OSA in these children [81]. Uvulopalatopharyngoplasty and tongue base suspension, in addition to adenotonsillectomy, may benefit some children. PAP therapy is successfully implemented in some children with residual OSAS post surgery as well as in children who are not considered surgical candidates. Tracheotomy is needed is some children with severe OSAS.

Miscellaneous

Mucopolysaccharidosis (MPS)

Sleep-disordered breathing is noted in more than 80 % of patients with MPS [82]. Several factors including mucopolysaccharide deposition in the upper airway and trachea, abnormalities of the skeletal structure, alteration of thoracic cage, restrictive lung disease with reduced lung capacity, and reduced diaphragmatic activity increase the risk of OSA and obstructive hypoventilation in these children. OSA and nocturnal hypoventilation can result in pulmonary hypertension, cor pulmonale, respiratory failure, and early death in these children. PAP therapy has shown to be beneficial in this population even though compliance remains a major issue. Tracheotomy may be required if PAP therapy fails, and tracheotomy with PAP therapy may be required when there is daytime hypoventilation [83]. However, tracheotomy carries certain specific risks in these children including stomal narrowing, granulation formation, infrastomal tracheal stenosis, wound infection, and tracheomalacia [83–85].

OSAS in Children That Are Not Candidates for AT

PAP, instead of AT, can be considered a first-line therapy for those children who do not meet the criteria or suitability for AT. Absence of tonsils and adenoids, lack of AT hypertrophy, surgical comorbidities like bleeding disorders, or in children whose parents decline AT are examples.

Efficacy of PAP Ventilation

PAP therapy has shown to be effective in improving both respiratory parameters and sleep architecture in children with OSAS [86]. PAP therapy has also shown to improve neurobehavioral aspects of OSAS such as attention span, hyperactivity, and daytime sleepiness, as well as school performance [86, 87]. The data regarding neurocognitive, metabolic, inflammatory, and cardiovascular outcomes in children are limited, however. For adults, a number of studies have shown significant improvement in nocturnal sleep, daytime sleepiness, and improvement in quality of life, improvement in mood, a short-term improvement in blood pressure, improvement in glycemic control, as well as an improvement in cognitive function [88–92].

Adherence to PAP Ventilation

PAP therapy is shown to be an effective treatment modality for OSAS across all age groups of children with different underlying pathophysiological mechanisms. However, effectiveness of PAP is limited by poor adherence. Information on barriers to effective PAP therapy and techniques to overcome those barriers are limited.

Studies have shown that older children (late teens), lower maternal education, lower socioeconomic status, African American race, oronasal interface, lesser body mass index, and lesser severity of OSAS predict poor compliance with PAP therapy [93]. The side effects/complications from PAP therapy including oronasal irritation, dryness, facial abrasion, facial pain, epistaxis, and the feeling of claustrophobia from interface are also important barriers to PAP therapy. Marcus et al., in their prospective study on compliance in a small group of children with OSAS, have noted a high dropout rate (35%), overall low average nightly use (5.3 h/night), and frequent overreporting of the adherence by parents compared to the objective compliance data [86]. Uong et al. have shown that PAP compliance can be significantly improved (85%) with intensive PAP education and close clinical follow-up [94]. It is also reported that children with more severe OSAS were more adherent with the PAP treatment [87]. O'Donnell et al. have reported that the gradual introduction of PAP mask and close follow-up is helpful in PAP acceptance and long-term adherence in children with OSA across all age groups with different underlying comorbid conditions [95]. Behavioral analysis and therapy for the children and the families who are noncompliant with PAP therapy has also shown to improve the adherence [96]. The specific measures to improve the adherence are lacking in adults as well. However, a multilayered approach in both adults and children which includes intense education and support, cognitive behavioral therapy, and occasional hypnotic therapy has been shown to improve adherence to therapy [37].

Adverse Effects of PAP Ventilation

The common reported side effects from PAP therapy include nasal congestion, oronasal dryness, epistaxis, eye irritation from air leak, facial pain, and skin abrasion [97]. Oronasal dryness is the most commonly experienced side effect from PAP therapy and hinders the adherence with PAP therapy. The newer devices with heated humidification are shown to improve the oronasal dryness and improve adherence in some subjects. Claustrophobia about the interface is also one of the commonly experienced symptoms in children and adults at the initiation of PAP therapy.

Continued use of the PAP and a trial of different interfaces are shown to overcome this barrier [98]. Skin necrosis and ulceration at the pressure points, mostly glabella, have been reported in some cases [99]. Facial deformity secondary to long-term PAP use has also been an issue. Guilleminault et al. first reported a case of severe maxillary hypoplasia secondary to long-term PAP use in a 15-year-old obese, African American male child [100]. The second case of midface hypoplasia secondary to long-term mechanical ventilation in a child with CCHS is reported by Maria Villa et al., and the authors have also shown reversal of this deformity using the custom-made mask [101, 102]. Furoux et al. have studied a larger group of children on long-term PAP use and noted global facial flattening in up to 68 % of the children and maxillary retrusion in 38 % of the subjects. These deformities were directly linked to the amount of daily PAP use. The authors also reported significant skin injury in 48 % of their patient population including skin necrosis in 8 %. The study was limited by lack of radiological studies to confirm the findings and then lack of long-term follow-up to look for resolution of the anatomical defects in their study group [103]. Data is still not conclusive on the long-term effects of PAP on growing skeleton. However, routine follow-up with special attention to midface growth is essential in children especially in young children in whom long-term PAP is anticipated.

Alternative Treatments to PAP Ventilation

Alternative treatments for PAP ventilation should be considered in children who cannot tolerate PAP or show low compliance. Several alternative therapies should be considered and are discussed here briefly.

Medications

Intranasal steroids and leukotriene receptor antagonists have shown to improve subjective symptoms as well as polysomnography parameters in children with mild and moderate OSAS with or without adenotonsillar hypertrophy [104–106]

Treatment with Nasal Insufflation

High-flow warm, humidified air, through nasal cannula, has shown to improve the sleep architecture and respiratory parameters in a small group of children with mild and moderate OSA [107]. Even though it is not as effective as PAP therapy, the acceptability and compliance with high-flow oxygen also seems to better compared to PAP therapy.

Nasal Expiratory Positive Airway Pressure (EPAP) Device

Nasal expiratory positive airway pressure (nEPAP) delivered with a disposable device (**Provent**, Ventus Medical) has been shown to improve OSAS in some adults with mild to moderate OSAS [108]. This device has not been studied in children yet.

Oral Appliances

Oral appliances including tongue devices and mandibular advancement devices move the tongue and mandible forward and away from posterior pharynx and improve upper airway patency. Oral appliances have been studied in a small group of children with OSA. In children with mild OSA and dental malocclusion/mandibular malposition/micrognathia, oral appliances are shown to reduce AHI, improve nocturnal sleep, and improve daytime sleepiness [101, 109].

Rapid Maxillary Expansion

Rapid maxillary expansion is an orthodontic procedure used in children with maxillary restriction and dental malocclusion. In this procedure the transverse diameter of the hard palate is gradually increased over months by a fixed dental device which has an expansion screw. Two studies have shown that rapid maxillary expansion normalizes polysomnography parameters and symptoms of OSAS in a small group of children with dental malocclusion and narrow palate [110, 111].

Complex Upper Airway Surgery

Upper airway surgeries such as maxillomandibular expansion and mandibular distraction osteogenesis are shown to improve OSA in some children with either isolated or syndromic midface and or mandibular hypoplasia [112, 113].

Tracheotomy

Tracheotomy is the most extreme surgical treatment to treat OSAS and is highly effective. Tracheotomy should be considered in children with severe craniofacial malformation who have severe OSAS or children who present with other significant comorbid conditions that hinder the use of the PAP ventilation or other upper airway surgeries or in cases where the other surgical modalities fail. Tracheotomy can also be used as temporary measure in some children with severe OSAS awaiting surgery.

Future Directions

Despite the wide use of PAP therapy in children with OSAS, there is still a great need for information regarding its clinical efficacy. Most studies addressing efficacy of PAP ventilation in respect to neurocognitive, behavioral, cardiovascular, and metabolic outcomes are derived from adults. Thus, similar studies need to be conducted in children. However, there are several barriers to such studies in children, particularly in respect to performing randomized control studies requiring use of sham PAP therapy, the fact that AT is the historical default treatment of choice, and the fact that there are various phenotypes of OSAS in children. All of these need to be accounted in the design of good efficacy studies.

Finally, there is a need for the development of new PAP modalities and especially masks and other delivery interfaces for infants and young children with OSAS, for phenotypes of OSAS associated with craniofacial disorders, and for children who are neurologically impaired.

References

1. American Academy of Sleep Medicine. International classification of sleep disorders: diagnostic and coding manual. Westchester, IL: American Academy of Sleep Medicine; 2005.
2. Arens R, Muzumdar H. Childhood obesity and obstructive sleep apnea syndrome. J Appl Physiol. 2010;108(2):436–44.
3. Arens R, Muzumdar H. Sleep, sleep disordered breathing, and nocturnal hypoventilation in children with neuromuscular diseases. Paediatr Respir Rev. 2010;11(1):24–30.
4. Muzumdar H, Arens R. Diagnostic issues in pediatric obstructive sleep apnea. Proc Am Thorac Soc. 2008;5(2):263–73.
5. Marcus CL, Brooks LJ, et al. Diagnosis and management of childhood obstructive sleep apnea syndrome. Pediatrics. 2012;130(3):576–84.
6. Marcus CL, Brooks LJ, et al. Diagnosis and management of childhood obstructive sleep apnea syndrome. Pediatrics. 2012;130(3):e714–55.
7. Arens R, Marcus CL. Pathophysiology of upper airway obstruction: a developmental perspective. Sleep. 2004;27(5):997–1019.
8. Eckert DJ, White DP, et al. Defining phenotypic causes of obstructive sleep apnea. Identification of novel therapeutic targets. Am J Respir Crit Care Med. 2013;188(8):996–1004.
9. Yuan H, Pinto SJ, et al. Ventilatory responses to hypercapnia during wakefulness and sleep in obese adolescents with and without obstructive sleep apnea syndrome. Sleep. 2012;35(9):1257–67.
10. Marcus CL, Moreira GA, et al. Response to inspiratory resistive loading during sleep in normal children and children with obstructive apnea. J Appl Physiol. 1999;87(4):1448–54.

11. Marcus CL, Lutz J, et al. Arousal and ventilatory responses during sleep in children with obstructive sleep apnea. J Appl Physiol. 1998;84(6):1926–36.
12. Huang J, Pinto SJ, et al. Upper airway collapsibility and genioglossus activity in adolescents during sleep. Sleep. 2012;35(10):1345–52.
13. Katz ES, White DP. Genioglossus activity in children with obstructive sleep apnea during wakefulness and sleep onset. Am J Respir Crit Care Med. 2003;168(6):664–70.
14. Katz ES, White DP. Genioglossus activity during sleep in normal control subjects and children with obstructive sleep apnea. Am J Respir Crit Care Med. 2004;170(5):553–60.
15. Katz ES, Mitchell RB, et al. Obstructive sleep apnea in infants. Am J Respir Crit Care Med. 2012;185(8):805–16.
16. Thach BT, Stark AR. Spontaneous neck flexion and airway obstruction during apneic spells in preterm infants. J Pediatr. 1979;94(2):275–81.
17. Swift PG, Emery JL. Clinical observations on response to nasal occlusion in infancy. Arch Dis Child. 1973;48(12):947–51.
18. Zafereo ME, Taylor RJ, et al. Supraglottoplasty for laryngomalacia with obstructive sleep apnea. Laryngoscope. 2008;118(10):1873–7.
19. Brouillette RT, Fernbach SK, et al. Obstructive sleep apnea in infants and children. J Pediatr. 1982;100(1):31–40.
20. Arens R, McDonough JM, et al. Upper airway size analysis by magnetic resonance imaging of children with obstructive sleep apnea syndrome. Am J Respir Crit Care Med. 2003; 167(1):65–70.
21. Arens R, McDonough JM, et al. Magnetic resonance imaging of the upper airway structure of children with obstructive sleep apnea syndrome. Am J Respir Crit Care Med. 2001; 164(4):698–703.
22. Ogden CL, Carroll MD, et al. Prevalence of obesity and trends in body mass index among US children and adolescents, 1999-2010. JAMA. 2012;307(5):483–90.
23. Redline S, Tishler PV, et al. Risk factors for sleep-disordered breathing in children. Associations with obesity, race, and respiratory problems. Am J Respir Crit Care Med. 1999;159 (5 Pt 1):1527–32.
24. Dayyat E, Kheirandish-Gozal L, et al. Obstructive sleep apnea in children: relative contributions of body mass index and adenotonsillar hypertrophy. Chest. 2009;136(1):137–44.
25. Arens R, Sin S, et al. Upper airway structure and body fat composition in obese children with obstructive sleep apnea syndrome. Am J Respir Crit Care Med. 2011;183(6):782–7.
26. Verhulst SL, Schrauwen N, et al. Sleep-disordered breathing in overweight and obese children and adolescents: prevalence, characteristics and the role of fat distribution. Arch Dis Child. 2007;92(3):205–8.
27. Wing YK, Hui SH, et al. A controlled study of sleep related disordered breathing in obese children. Arch Dis Child. 2003;88(12):1043–7.
28. Mitchell RB, Kelly J. Adenotonsillectomy for obstructive sleep apnea in obese children. Otolaryngol Head Neck Surg. 2004;131(1):104–8.
29. Sullivan CE, Issa FG, et al. Reversal of obstructive sleep apnoea by continuous positive airway pressure applied through the nares. Lancet. 1981;1(8225):862–5.
30. Guilleminault C, Nino-Murcia G, et al. Alternative treatment to tracheostomy in obstructive sleep apnea syndrome: nasal continuous positive airway pressure in young children. Pediatrics. 1986;78(5):797–802.
31. Schwab RJ, Gupta KB, et al. Upper airway and soft tissue anatomy in normal subjects and patients with sleep-disordered breathing. Significance of the lateral pharyngeal walls. Am J Respir Crit Care Med. 1995;152(5 Pt 1):1673–89.
32. Schwab RJ, Pack AI, et al. Upper airway and soft tissue structural changes induced by CPAP in normal subjects. Am J Respir Crit Care Med. 1996;154(4 Pt 1):1106–16.
33. Heinzer RC, Stanchina ML, et al. Lung volume and continuous positive airway pressure requirements in obstructive sleep apnea. Am J Respir Crit Care Med. 2005;172(1):114–7.

34. Kushida CA, Chediak A, et al. Clinical guidelines for the manual titration of positive airway pressure in patients with obstructive sleep apnea. J Clin Sleep Med. 2008;4(2):157–71.
35. Palombini L, Pelayo R, et al. Efficacy of automated continuous positive airway pressure in children with sleep-related breathing disorders in an attended setting. Pediatrics. 2004;113(5):e412–7.
36. Oldenburg O. Cheyne-stokes respiration in chronic heart failure. Treatment with adaptive servoventilation therapy. Circ J. 2012;76(10):2305–17.
37. Sawyer AM, Gooneratne NS, et al. A systematic review of CPAP adherence across age groups: clinical and empiric insights for developing CPAP adherence interventions. Sleep Med Rev. 2011;15(6):343–56.
38. Ramirez A, Delord V, et al. Interfaces for long-term noninvasive positive pressure ventilation in children. Intensive Care Med. 2012;38(4):655–62.
39. Berry RB, Chediak A, et al. Best clinical practices for the sleep center adjustment of noninvasive positive pressure ventilation (NPPV) in stable chronic alveolar hypoventilation syndromes. J Clin Sleep Med. 2010;6(5):491–509.
40. Redline S, Kirchner HL, et al. The effects of age, sex, ethnicity, and sleep-disordered breathing on sleep architecture. Arch Intern Med. 2004;164(4):406–18.
41. Costa DJ, Mitchell R. Adenotonsillectomy for obstructive sleep apnea in obese children: a meta-analysis. Otolaryngol Head Neck Surg. 2009;140(4):455–60.
42. Bhattacharjee R, Kheirandish-Gozal L, et al. Adenotonsillectomy outcomes in treatment of obstructive sleep apnea in children: a multicenter retrospective study. Am J Respir Crit Care Med. 2010;182(5):676–83.
43. Jacobs IN, Teague WG, et al. Pulmonary vascular complications of chronic airway obstruction in children. Arch Otolaryngol Head Neck Surg. 1997;123(7):700–4.
44. Marcus CL, Crockett DM, et al. Evaluation of epiglottoplasty as treatment for severe laryngomalacia. J Pediatr. 1990;117(5):706–10.
45. Chan DK, Truong MT, et al. Supraglottoplasty for occult laryngomalacia to improve obstructive sleep apnea syndrome. Arch Otolaryngol Head Neck Surg. 2012;138(1):50–4.
46. Guilleminault C, Pelayo R, et al. Home nasal continuous positive airway pressure in infants with sleep-disordered breathing. J Pediatr. 1995;127(6):905–12.
47. Waters KA, Everett F, et al. The use of nasal CPAP in children. Pediatr Pulmonol Suppl. 1995;11:91–3.
48. Essouri S, Nicot F, et al. Noninvasive positive pressure ventilation in infants with upper airway obstruction: comparison of continuous and bilevel positive pressure. Intensive Care Med. 2005;31(4):574–80.
49. Fauroux B, Pigeot J, et al. Chronic stridor caused by laryngomalacia in children: work of breathing and effects of noninvasive ventilatory assistance. Am J Respir Crit Care Med. 2001;164(10 Pt 1):1874–8.
50. Al-Saleh S, Riekstins A, et al. Sleep-related disordered breathing in children with syndromic craniosynostosis. J Craniomaxillofac Surg. 2011;39(3):153–7.
51. Mitsukawa N, Satoh K, et al. A reflectable case of obstructive sleep apnea in an infant with Crouzon syndrome. J Craniofac Surg. 2004;15(5):874–8. discussion 878-879.
52. Willington AJ, Ramsden JD. Adenotonsillectomy for the management of obstructive sleep apnea in children with congenital craniosynostosis syndromes. J Craniofac Surg. 2012;23(4):1020–2.
53. Bannink N, Nout E, et al. Obstructive sleep apnea in children with syndromic craniosynostosis: long-term respiratory outcome of midface advancement. Int J Oral Maxillofac Surg. 2010;39(2):115–21.
54. Mackay DR. Controversies in the diagnosis and management of the Robin sequence. J Craniofac Surg. 2011;22(2):415–20.
55. Anderson IC, Sedaghat AR, et al. Prevalence and severity of obstructive sleep apnea and snoring in infants with pierre robin sequence. Cleft Palate Craniofac J. 2011;48(5):614–8.

56. Staudt CB, Gnoinski WM, et al. Upper airway changes in Pierre Robin sequence from childhood to adulthood. Orthod Craniofac Res. 2013;16(4):202–13.

57. Afsharpaiman S, Sillence DO, et al. Respiratory events and obstructive sleep apnea in children with achondroplasia: investigation and treatment outcomes. Sleep Breath. 2011;15(4): 755–61.

58. Julliand S, Boule M, et al. Lung function, diagnosis, and treatment of sleep-disordered breathing in children with achondroplasia. Am J Med Genet A. 2012;158A(8):1987–93.

59. Dyken ME, Lin-Dyken DC, et al. Prospective polysomnographic analysis of obstructive sleep apnea in down syndrome. Arch Pediatr Adolesc Med. 2003;157(7):655–60.

60. Marcus CL, Keens TG, et al. Obstructive sleep apnea in children with Down syndrome. Pediatrics. 1991;88(1):132–9.

61. Ng DK, Hui HN, et al. Obstructive sleep apnoea in children with Down syndrome. Singapore Med J. 2006;47(9):774–9.

62. Donnelly LF, Shott SR, et al. Causes of persistent obstructive sleep apnea despite previous tonsillectomy and adenoidectomy in children with down syndrome as depicted on static and dynamic cine MRI. AJR Am J Roentgenol. 2004;183(1):175–81.

63. Guimaraes CV, Donnelly LF, et al. Relative rather than absolute macroglossia in patients with Down syndrome: implications for treatment of obstructive sleep apnea. Pediatr Radiol. 2008;38(10):1062–7.

64. Guimaraes CV, Kalra M, et al. The frequency of lingual tonsil enlargement in obese children. AJR Am J Roentgenol. 2008;190(4):973–5.

65. Shott SR, Donnelly LF. Cine magnetic resonance imaging: evaluation of persistent airway obstruction after tonsil and adenoidectomy in children with Down syndrome. Laryngoscope. 2004;114(10):1724–9.

66. Uong EC, McDonough JM, et al. Magnetic resonance imaging of the upper airway in children with Down syndrome. Am J Respir Crit Care Med. 2001;163(3 Pt 1):731–6.

67. Bull MJ. Health supervision for children with Down syndrome. Pediatrics. 2011;128(2): 393–406.

68. Andreou G, Galanopoulou C, et al. Cognitive status in Down syndrome individuals with sleep disordered breathing deficits (SDB). Brain Cogn. 2002;50(1):145–9.

69. Carskadon MA, Pueschel SM, et al. Sleep-disordered breathing and behavior in three risk groups: preliminary findings from parental reports. Childs Nerv Syst. 1993;9(8):452–7.

70. Hawkins A, Langton-Hewer S, et al. Management of pulmonary hypertension in Down syndrome. Eur J Pediatr. 2011;170(7):915–21.

71. Levine OR, Simpser M. Alveolar hypoventilation and cor pulmonale associated with chronic airway obstruction in infants with Down syndrome. Clin Pediatr (Phila). 1982;21(1): 25–9.

72. Rosen D. Management of obstructive sleep apnea associated with Down syndrome and other craniofacial dysmorphologies. Curr Opin Pulm Med. 2011;17(6):431–6.

73. Cassidy SB, Schwartz S, et al. Prader-Willi syndrome. Genet Med. 2012;14(1):10–26.

74. Al-Saleh S, Al-Naimi A, et al. Longitudinal evaluation of sleep-disordered breathing in children with Prader-Willi Syndrome during 2 years of growth hormone therapy. J Pediatr. 2013;162(2):263–8. e261.

75. Clift S, Dahlitz M, et al. Sleep apnoea in the Prader-Willi syndrome. J Sleep Res. 1994; 3(2):121–6.

76. Healy F, Marcus CL. Congenital central hypoventilation syndrome in children. Paediatr Respir Rev. 2011;12(4):253–63.

77. Patwari PP, Carroll MS, et al. Congenital central hypoventilation syndrome and the PHOX2B gene: a model of respiratory and autonomic dysregulation. Respir Physiol Neurobiol. 2010;173(3):322–35.

78. Losurdo A, Dittoni S, et al. Sleep disordered breathing in children and adolescents with Chiari malformation type I. J Clin Sleep Med. 2013;9(4):371–7.

79. Fahim A, Johnson AO. Chiari malformation and central sleep apnoea: successful therapy with adaptive pressure support servo-ventilation following surgical treatment. BMJ Case Rep. 2012. doi:10.1136/bcr-2012-007143.
80. Fitzgerald DA, Follett J, et al. Assessing and managing lung disease and sleep disordered breathing in children with cerebral palsy. Paediatr Respir Rev. 2009;10(1):18–24.
81. Magardino TM, Tom LW. Surgical management of obstructive sleep apnea in children with cerebral palsy. Laryngoscope. 1999;109(10):1611–5.
82. Berger KI, Fagondes SC, et al. Respiratory and sleep disorders in mucopolysaccharidosis. J Inherit Metab Dis. 2013;36(2):201–10.
83. Muhlebach MS, Wooten W, et al. Respiratory manifestations in mucopolysaccharidoses. Paediatr Respir Rev. 2011;12(2):133–8.
84. Jeong HS, Cho DY, et al. Complications of tracheotomy in patients with mucopolysaccharidoses type II (Hunter syndrome). Int J Pediatr Otorhinolaryngol. 2006;70(10):1765–9.
85. Pelley CJ, Kwo J, et al. Tracheomalacia in an adult with respiratory failure and Morquio syndrome. Respir Care. 2007;52(3):278–82.
86. Marcus CL, Rosen G, et al. Adherence to and effectiveness of positive airway pressure therapy in children with obstructive sleep apnea. Pediatrics. 2006;117(3):e442–51.
87. Uong EC, Epperson M, et al. Adherence to nasal positive airway pressure therapy among school-aged children and adolescents with obstructive sleep apnea syndrome. Pediatrics. 2007;120(5):e1203–11.
88. Faccenda JF, Mackay TW, et al. Randomized placebo-controlled trial of continuous positive airway pressure on blood pressure in the sleep apnea-hypopnea syndrome. Am J Respir Crit Care Med. 2001;163(2):344–8.
89. Giles TL, Lasserson TJ, et al. Continuous positive airways pressure for obstructive sleep apnoea in adults. Cochrane Database Syst Rev. 2006;3, CD001106.
90. Haentjens P, Van Meerhaeghe A, et al. The impact of continuous positive airway pressure on blood pressure in patients with obstructive sleep apnea syndrome: evidence from a meta-analysis of placebo-controlled randomized trials. Arch Intern Med. 2007;167(8):757–64.
91. Pepperell JC, Ramdassingh-Dow S, et al. Ambulatory blood pressure after therapeutic and subtherapeutic nasal continuous positive airway pressure for obstructive sleep apnoea: a randomised parallel trial. Lancet. 2002;359(9302):204–10.
92. Simon S, Collop N. Latest advances in sleep medicine: obstructive sleep apnea. Chest. 2012;142(6):1645–51.
93. DiFeo N, Meltzer LJ, et al. Predictors of positive airway pressure therapy adherence in children: a prospective study. J Clin Sleep Med. 2012;8(3):279–86.
94. Jambhekar SK, Com G, et al. Role of a respiratory therapist in improving adherence to positive airway pressure treatment in a pediatric sleep apnea clinic. Respir Care. 2013;58(12):2038–44.
95. Kirk VG, O'Donnell AR. Continuous positive airway pressure for children: a discussion on how to maximize compliance. Sleep Med Rev. 2006;10(2):119–27.
96. Koontz KL, Slifer KJ, et al. Improving pediatric compliance with positive airway pressure therapy: the impact of behavioral intervention. Sleep. 2003;26(8):1010–5.
97. Pepin JL, Leger P, et al. Side effects of nasal continuous positive airway pressure in sleep apnea syndrome. Study of 193 patients in two French sleep centers. Chest. 1995;107(2):375–81.
98. Chasens ER, Pack AI, et al. Claustrophobia and adherence to CPAP treatment. West J Nurs Res. 2005;27(3):307–21.
99. Ahmad Z, Venus M, et al. A case series of skin necrosis following use of non invasive ventilation pressure masks. Int Wound J. 2013;10(1):87–90.
100. Li KK, Riley RW, et al. An unreported risk in the use of home nasal continuous positive airway pressure and home nasal ventilation in children: mid-face hypoplasia. Chest. 2000;117(3):916–8.

101. Villa MP, Bernkopf E, et al. Randomized controlled study of an oral jaw-positioning appliance for the treatment of obstructive sleep apnea in children with malocclusion. Am J Respir Crit Care Med. 2002;165(1):123–7.
102. Villa MP, Pagani J, et al. Mid-face hypoplasia after long-term nasal ventilation. Am J Respir Crit Care Med. 2002;166(8):1142–3.
103. Fauroux B, Lavis JF, et al. Facial side effects during noninvasive positive pressure ventilation in children. Intensive Care Med. 2005;31(7):965–9.
104. Kheirandish-Gozal L, Gozal D. Intranasal budesonide treatment for children with mild obstructive sleep apnea syndrome. Pediatrics. 2008;122(1):e149–55.
105. Kheirandish L, Goldbart AD, et al. Intranasal steroids and oral leukotriene modifier therapy in residual sleep-disordered breathing after tonsillectomy and adenoidectomy in children. Pediatrics. 2006;117(1):e61–6.
106. Goldbart AD, Greenberg-Dotan S, et al. Montelukast for children with obstructive sleep apnea: a double-blind, placebo-controlled study. Pediatrics. 2012;130(3):e575–80.
107. McGinley B, Halbower A, et al. Effect of a high-flow open nasal cannula system on obstructive sleep apnea in children. Pediatrics. 2009;124(1):179–88.
108. Braga CW, Chen Q, et al. Changes in lung volume and upper airway using MRI during application of nasal expiratory positive airway pressure in patients with sleep-disordered breathing. J Appl Physiol. 2011;111(5):1400–9.
109. Carvalho FR, Lentini-Oliveira D, et al. Oral appliances and functional orthopaedic appliances for obstructive sleep apnoea in children. Cochrane Database Syst Rev. 2007;2, CD005520.
110. Pirelli P, Saponara M, et al. Rapid maxillary expansion in children with obstructive sleep apnea syndrome. Sleep. 2004;27(4):761–6.
111. Villa MP, Malagola C, et al. Rapid maxillary expansion in children with obstructive sleep apnea syndrome: 12-month follow-up. Sleep Med. 2007;8(2):128–34.
112. Rachmiel A, Emodi O, et al. Management of obstructive sleep apnea in pediatric craniofacial anomalies. Ann Maxillofac Surg. 2012;2(2):111–5.
113. Rachmiel A, Srouji S, et al. Distraction osteogenesis for tracheostomy dependent children with severe micrognathia. J Craniofac Surg. 2012;23(2):459–63.

Chapter 14
Ventilator Support in Children with Neuromuscular Disorders

Anita K. Simonds

Introduction

Children with neuromuscular disease involving the respiratory muscles have a restrictive ventilatory defect which results from a combination of inspiratory muscle weakness, the presence of a thoracic scoliosis and decreased chest wall and pulmonary compliance. Reduced cough efficacy and bronchial secretion clearance occur due to expiratory muscle weakness together with inspiratory muscle weakness. In many neuromuscular conditions, e.g. Duchenne muscular dystrophy (DMD) and congenital myopathies, inspiratory and expiratory muscle strengths decline in tandem; in others, e.g. spinal muscular atrophy (SMA), relative preservation of diaphragm strength and early involvement of expiratory muscles mean that secretion clearance problems predate the development of ventilatory decompensation during sleep. This has implications for clinical management which are discussed below.

The main questions to address regarding timely and appropriate introduction of ventilatory support in patients with neuromuscular disease are as follows:

- What is the natural history of the disorder?
- What is the probability of respiratory failure and at what age?
- What is the likelihood of problems with secretion clearance/recurrent chest infections?
- What other complications will impact on these decisions?
- What is the expected outcome of ventilatory support?
- What are the consequences of not providing ventilatory support?

Table 14.1 shows the probability of respiratory complications across a range of conditions. These data have become clearer over the last 10–15 years. Much has been

A.K. Simonds, M.D., F.R.C.P. (✉)
NIHR Respiratory Biomedical Research Unit, Royal Brompton & Harefield NHS Foundation Trust, Sydney Street, London SW3 6NP, UK
e-mail: A.Simonds@rbht.nhs.uk

© Springer Science+Business Media New York 2016
L.M. Sterni, J.L. Carroll (eds.), *Caring for the Ventilator Dependent Child*, Respiratory Medicine, DOI 10.1007/978-1-4939-3749-3_14

learnt from paediatric neurology and neuroscience colleagues in understanding the molecular basis of the disorders and the link between genotype and phenotype. For example, it is evident that limb-girdle muscular dystrophy consists of a range of different disorders, and this is true of congenital muscular dystrophies (CMDs) and congenital myasthenia. The application of this knowledge in forecasting the outlook for each case and personalising interventions and care plans is explored below. However, in broad terms, there are groups in which early ventilatory failure is inevitable, e.g. type 1 SMA, SMARD (spinal muscular atrophy with respiratory distress) and X-linked myotubular myopathy; diagnoses where ventilatory failure develops gradually over time, e.g. DMD and congenital muscular dystrophy; and others where respiratory failure is rare, e.g. facioscapulohumeral muscular dystrophy [1]. Further, there are some disorders in which respiratory complications are hugely heterogeneous, e.g. nemaline myopathy—here we simply do not yet understand differences in genotype and other genetic and epigenetic variables which influence the expression of the disease.

Pathophysiology

The natural history of decline in many neuromuscular disorders is indicated in Fig. 14.1. In slowly progressive conditions such as DMD, pulmonary function may develop along normal expected growth vectors until the early teenage years when ambulation is lost. At this point, a plateau in vital capacity is seen followed by a decline in vital capacity as inspiratory muscle weakness becomes severe and complications, such as scoliosis, develop [2]. The peak vital capacity (VC) obtained in the plateau phase in the absence of ventilatory support is a prognostic factor, in that a peak VC of less than 1.2 L was associated with an average age of death of 17 years and those with a peak VC in excess of 1.7 L often had a life expectancy greater than 30 years of age. With the advent of routine ventilatory support, individuals with DMD survive for many years, but peak vital capacity is still likely to be a prognostic factor. The use of steroid therapy has tended to increase duration of time that Duchenne boys remain ambulant. Wheelchair dependency at an older age allows more normal growth of the lungs and spine and reduces the tendency of scoliosis, hence preserving vital capacity further. For example, in a non-randomised study that matched boys with DMD for age and pulmonary function at baseline, a scoliosis of >20° occurred in 67 % of the control group but only 17 % of the steroid (deflazacort)-treated group [3]. It is likely that this decrease in scoliosis severity and gain in lung function lead to a survival advantage, but there have been no definitive long-term randomised controlled trials of steroid therapy in DMD to test this hypothesis.

Sleep-disordered breathing tends to occur when VC is less than 60 % predicted and inspiratory muscle strength less than around 30–40% predicted [4]. Ragette et al. [4] found that vital capacity was a more sensitive and specific predictor of sleep-disordered breathing than measures of inspiratory muscle strength. In some conditions, e.g. DMD, obstructive apnoeas and hypopnoeas may be the initial predominant

Table 14.1 Neuromuscular conditions and associated respiratory features (from [1] with permission)

Condition	Respiratory failure	Secretion clearance difficulty	Recurrent pneumonia	Progression	Disease-specific features
SMA					
Type 1	All by 2 years	Marked	All	Rapid	All require full-time respiratory support
Type 2	~40 % in childhood	Early	~25 % in first 5 years	Slow	
Type 3	Rare in childhood	Rare in childhood	Rare in childhood	Slow	
SMA with respiratory distress type 1	All by 6 months	Marked	All	Rapid in first year, then slows.	All require full-time respiratory support
DMD/severe childhood onset limb-girdle muscular dystrophy	After loss of ambulation	After loss of ambulation	Late		Cardiomyopathy usually occurs after respiratory problems but may precede them
Facioscapulohumeral muscular dystrophy	When onset <20 years	With infantile onset	With infantile onset	Slow	Severe infantile onset type is frequently associated with sensorineural deafness
Congenital muscular dystrophy					
All types	Any age depending on severity	Any age depending on severity	Any age depending on severity	Slow	
Ullrich	70 % in adolescence	Mild	Infrequent		Proximal contractures with marked distal laxity
Rigid spine muscular dystrophy	Early while ambulation preserved	Mild	Infrequent		Hypoventilation may occur in ambulant children with relatively preserved vital capacity

(continued)

Table 14.1 (continued)

Condition	Respiratory failure	Secretion clearance difficulty	Recurrent pneumonia	Progression	Disease-specific features
Congenital myopathy					
Central core	Uncommon except in severe recessive type	Uncommon	Uncommon	Slow	Susceptible to malignant hyperthermia
Minicore	Early while ambulation preserved				
Nemaline	Early in severe neonatal form, mild later onset form may develop early while ambulation preserved	In severe form	In severe form	Slow	
Myotubular	85 % in severe X-linked form	In severe form	In severe form	Slow	Ophthalmoplegia, rare coagulopathy and liver haemorrhage
Fibre type disproportion	Depends on genotype	Uncommon	Uncommon		
Myotonic dystrophy					
Myotonic dystrophy 1	Common in severe congenital onset, usually improves	Common in severe congenital onset	Common in severe congenital onset	Initial improvement, later slow deterioration	Prominent learning difficulty, somnolence, central hypoventilation
Myotonic dystrophy 2	Uncommon	Uncommon	Uncommon		
Congenital myasthenic syndromes	Often in neonatal period, may occur during inter-current illnesses	Especially during inter-current illnesses	Possible if weakness severe and persistent		Weakness may fluctuate, episodic apnoea in some. Congenital stridor in those with DOK7 mutations.

	Common	Possible	Possible	Acute deterioration possible	
Mitochondrial myopathy					
Charcot-Marie-Tooth	With severe early onset, especially with GDAP1 mutation	With severe early onset	With severe early onset		Stridor, especially with GDAP1 mutation
Pompe	Infantile onset, may be early in later onset while ambulation preserved	Infantile onset	Infantile onset	Infantile rapid, late onset slow	Variable relationship between motor and respiratory progression

DMD Duchenne muscular dystrophy, *SMA* spinal muscular atrophy

Fig. 14.1 Natural history
of respiratory
decompensation in
neuromuscular disease

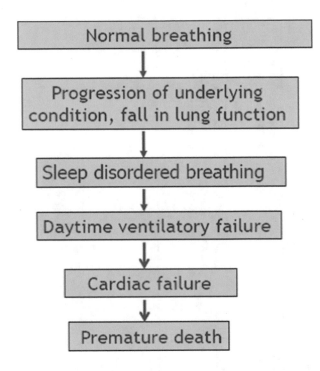

problem, which then evolves into nocturnal hypoventilation. The latter first occurs in rapid eye movement (REM) sleep due to loss in intercostal and upper airway muscle tone and the decrease in chemosensitivity and arousal response which occurs during this stage and then progressing to non-rapid eye movement (NREM) sleep (which occupies the majority of sleep time) once vital capacity is <40 % predicted. If nocturnal hypoventilation is unaddressed, daytime ventilatory failure ensures when vital capacity is less than 30 % predicted (Fig. 14.1).

The clinical course is often punctuated by chest infections which become protracted as cough efficiency deteriorates. Cough can be assessed by peak cough flow measurements and in younger children by qualitative assessment of the sound volume of cough and of descriptions of difficulty with secretions at the time of respiratory tract infections.

Bulbar muscle weakness is common in type 1 SMA and myotubular myopathy and may occur in some variants of CMD but is a late feature in DMD. Severe bulbar weakness with recurrent aspiration is a contraindication to non-invasive ventilation, although mild to moderate levels of swallowing impairment may be successfully managed with a combination of non-invasive ventilation, cough assistance and percutaneous gastrostomy feeding. It should be noted that swallowing function may deteriorate at the time of a chest infection even in patients who had not had prior difficulty with aspiration. Assessment of swallowing is therefore best carried out after a chest infection has resolved, where possible, unless the evidence for marked bulbar weakness is overwhelming, for example, choking when eating meals.

Assessment of Respiratory Function in Neuromuscular Disorders

Clinical assessment of symptoms, examination and measurement of lung function, measurement of cough peak flow and evaluation for the presence of sleep-disordered breathing are key in children with neuromuscular disease [1]. Symptoms of nocturnal hypoventilation are typically non-specific and can include restlessness and sweating at night, snuffly or very quiet breathing, a requirement for extra turning in bed at night, vivid dreams, sudden wakening from sleep, anorexia for breakfast, poor concentration at school/college especially in the morning, daytime lassitude and failure to thrive.

A restrictive pattern of spirometry can be seen on pulmonary function testing with reductions in forced vital capacity, FEV1, residual volume and total lung capacity. Diffusing capacity of the lung for carbon monoxide (DLCO) is reduced, but the DLCO adjusted for accessible alveolar volume is normal or supranormal. This is caused by various permutations of reduced inspiratory muscle strength, the presence of a thoracic scoliosis and reduced chest wall and pulmonary compliance—the latter caused by micro- or macro-atelectasis. Inspiratory and expiratory muscle strengths usually decrease in tandem, but when diaphragm strength is preserved, expiratory muscle weakness may predominate such as in SMA. Expiratory muscle weakness combined with inspiratory muscle weakness leads to poor cough efficacy and reduced secretion clearance and can be measured by cough peak flow— values less than 270 L/min in children of approximately 10 years and above suggest reduced cough power, and value of less than 160 L/min is associated with an increased frequency of chest infections.

A vital capacity of less than 60 % predicted is predictive of the presence of sleep-disordered breathing which initially occurs in REM sleep and then progresses to all sleep stages [3]. Usually this manifests as nocturnal hypoventilation, but obstructive hypoventilation can be seen in some conditions, e.g. DMD. Sleep studies are indicated routinely in these children or in any with sleep-related symptoms, recurrent chest infections (or those requiring hospitalisation for chest infections) or failure to thrive.

Scoliosis is common and will occur in virtually all those with SMA types 1 and 2 and in 70–90% of those with DMD. Scoliosis almost inevitably progresses with the adolescent growth spurt and requirement of permanent wheelchair use. The use of steroid therapy and preservation of standing using frames may reduce scoliosis severity, as discussed. Scoliosis surgery is performed to prevent progression of the curvature and achieve comfort rather than to increase lung volumes.

Assessment of swallowing function is a key part of respiratory management in any child with neuromuscular weakness as suggested by slow feeding, choking, aspiration and recurrent chest infections. Nutritional assessment is also crucial, and if adequate nutrition cannot be achieved safely orally, then percutaneous gastrostomy placement may significantly improve quality of life and reduce respiratory complications. This may be safely performed in children receiving NIV [5].

Sleep Studies

Overnight oximetry is often used to screen for sleep-disordered breathing in children with neuromuscular disease. A normal trace in a child who has slept well normally excludes a significant problem, but values of arterial oxygen saturation within the normal range can be seen occasionally in children with mild obstructive sleep apnoea/hypopnea accompanied by mild hypercapnia. If there is a high suspicion of sleep-disordered breathing, multichannel monitoring including a measure of overnight carbon dioxide tension, e.g. transcutaneous CO_2, is preferred.

Guidelines for respiratory and sleep study assessment are given in British Thoracic Society recommendations and other consensus documents [1, 6, 7].

Aims of Ventilatory Support

The range of goals of ventilatory support are listed in Table 14.2. There is no evidence that prophylactic use of ventilator support in asymptomatic individuals without sleep-disordered breathing is beneficial; however, in some centres, children are familiarised with NIV so that it can be used intermittently during acute chest infections or in the perioperative period during intercurrent surgery (e.g. correction of scoliosis). NIV may also reduce the work of breathing during physiotherapy [8] and allow the child to complete longer periods of secretion clearance and may be valuable for acute use in children with apnoeic crises secondary to some congenital myasthenia genotypes [9]. Use of NIV for short periods during the day may improve chest wall compliance and reduce some chest wall deformities such as bell-shaped chest in type 1–2 SMA.

Table 14.2 Aims when considering introduction of non-invasive ventilation

Goals of non-invasive ventilation
1. Control of nocturnal hypoventilation
2. Control of diurnal ventilator failure
3. Treatment of chest infections
4. Use perioperatively during intercurrent procedures, e.g. scoliosis surgery, insertion of percutaneous gastrostomy
5. Use to aid chest wall development and reduce chest wall deformity
6. Application to palliate symptoms, e.g. breathlessness in end-stage disease

Timing of Initiation of Nocturnal NIV

While previously daytime hypercapnia was used as an indication for nocturnal NIV, most authorities now suggest the introduction of NIV once symptomatic nocturnal hypoventilation has developed. This is based on one randomised controlled trial [10] in which patients, including young patients, with a variety of neuromuscular disorders and nocturnal hypoventilation but normal daytime $PaCO_2$ received either nocturnal NIV or follow-up without NIV. Ninety percent of those in the control follow-up group developed preset criteria for initiation of NIV (e.g. daytime hypercapnia, recurrent chest infections, symptomatic nocturnal hypoventilation), and 70 % fulfilled these criteria within 1 year. This suggests that once individuals develop nocturnal hypoventilation, daytime ventilatory decompensation is likely to ensue in the next 12–24 months, and so NIV can be introduced in a planned and timely manner, rather than precipitously during acute chest infection. The findings of this study are also supported by clinical experience. In a series of 30 children (mean age of 12.3 years and SD of 4.1 years) with inherited neuromuscular disease, NIV normalised nocturnal PCO_2 and SaO_2 (which reduced arousals from sleep), the respiratory disturbance index and the heart rate and improved sleep architecture [11]. In a subgroup in which NIV was then withdrawn for three nights, a rapid deterioration in nocturnal gas exchange occurred which was corrected once NIV was restarted. Around half the children in this study had nocturnal hypoventilation alone, and the remainder had daytime ventilatory failure. Improvements occurred in both groups. In other observational studies, improvements in quality of life and nocturnal symptoms are reported [12, 13].

Choice of Ventilator and Mode

There are still limited numbers of ventilators designed for long-term home use in children with neuromuscular disease. The choice will depend on the age and size of child, tracheostomy or non-invasive ventilation, degree of ventilator dependency and pathophysiology. The challenge for manufacturers is to create a ventilator that can deliver small tidal volumes at high frequency. The device should also be capable in spontaneous mode of being able to detect the onset of the child's inspiratory effort and deliver in response a preset pressure or volume with a time delay in keeping with the child's respiratory rate. Trigger delays of >100 ms are inadequate as patients will have completed inspiration before the delivery of the preset pressure or volume.

Continuous positive pressure airway therapy (CPAP) may be sufficient in children with obstructive apnoeas, upper airway obstruction due to laryngomalacia and/ or mild nocturnal gas exchange problems due to SMA, but NIV will be required in children with significant nocturnal hypoventilation and obstructive hypopnoeas. In essence therefore, CPAP is indicated to maintain airway patency and will reduce the work of breathing to some degree, but where there is significant hypoventilation, NIV is the correct choice.

During pressure support ventilation (PSV), each breath is triggered and terminated by the patient, so the patient determines the respiratory rate, inspiratory duration and tidal volume. Tidal volume is not predetermined as it will depend on the inspiratory positive airway pressure (IPAP) set, the inspiratory effort and respiratory rate of the patient and mechanical properties of their lungs and chest wall. In practice, a back-up respiratory rate is added to prevent hypoventilation during sleep when respiratory rate falls. Bi-level positive airway pressure (BiPAP) ventilation supplies IPAP together with positive pressure in expiration (EPAP). The presence of EPAP may help splint the upper airway open through the expiratory part of the cycle, increase functional residual capacity by recruiting alveoli, reduce work of breathing and allow easier triggering of the NIV when intrinsic positive end-expiratory pressure (PEEP) exists. By contrast, volume-targeted ventilators deliver a preset tidal volume, but the airway pressure generated by this volume is not predictable, and leaks are less well compensated for than with pressure preset ventilators. Some ventilator models now offer a combination of modes (hybrid device) in which bi-level positive pressure is delivered with an assured tidal volume or minute volume back-up. The place of these hybrid modes in children is not clear, as studies comparing their advantages and disadvantages with standard modes have not been carried out. One trial [14] in young and older neuromuscular patients has, however, shown that stage 1 sleep was reduced using hybrid mode compared to standard bi-level mode, suggesting that patients fell asleep quicker, although control of nocturnal hypoventilation by the hybrid machine was comparable to that achieved with the conventional bi-level ventilator.

Fauroux et al. [15] have carried out a bench study simulating six different paediatric ventilatory profiles which included neuromuscular disease, upper airway obstruction, cystic fibrosis and central apnoeas. When using 17 different ventilators recommended for long-term use in children, the results showed significant variability in performance, which depended on whether flow or pressure trigger sensing was used, the patient profile and the type of circuit. Differences were observed between the preset and measured airway pressure and tidal volume as assessed by ventilator or external bench monitoring. Leaks resulted in failure to trigger or auto-triggering. This work therefore highlights the need for ventilators to be carefully assessed when applied to each individual. Clearly trigger problems can be ameliorated by setting a high back-up rate, but improvements in ventilators are being made with some models capable of providing continuing feedback on triggering in the presence of leak and detection of weak patient effort versus detection of regular patient effort, in an attempt to smooth these problems.

Interface

As with ventilators, specifically designed masks suitable for children have only recently been introduced into the market. These are designated as nasal mask, oronasal (facial) mask, nasal pillows, oral interface or helmet.

Nasal masks are more frequently used. In some children, an oronasal mask is required to overcome mouth leak—here there is a risk of vomiting and aspiration so great care should be exercised. True aspiration resulting from use of an oronasal mask is however rare. Vented masks are used with CPAP therapy; non-vented masks are used for NIV circuits where there is an exhalation valve.

Short- and long-term major complications from interfaces include facial pressure sores which most frequently occur over the bridge of the nose and forehead where there is little subcutaneous tissue. The incidence of pressure sores can be reduced by using customised masks [16], careful placement of mask and attention to mask strap pressure, and rotating interfaces such that each impinges on different areas of the face.

Mid-facial hypoplasia has been reported in children using NIV or CPAP at night for long term. Risk factors appear to be age at first use of NIV (with younger children having the worse outlook), duration of use and facial muscle weakness. Fauroux and colleagues [16] found that substitution of a customised mask could help this problem too. Careful follow-up with yearly lateral cephalic X-ray may be helpful in establishing the development of mid-facial hypoplasia.

Titrating Settings

In all situations, NIV should be titrated to optimise the control of alveolar hypoventilation during sleep such that values of arterial oxygen saturation and PCO_2 by night and during the day are normal. Best practice guidelines for NIV setting adjustments have been drawn up [17]. These can only set out broad principles as therapy must be adapted to the individual. In general, a minimum expiratory positive airway pressure level of 4 cm H_2O in bi-level devices is required to flush out interface dead space, and in children less than 12 years, a maximum inspiratory positive airway pressure of <30 cm H_2O or pressure support of <20 cm H_2O is indicated. Starting at a low IPAP level, e.g. around 8 cm H_2O, and titrating upwards helps. Adjusting IPAP to central apnoeas and hypoventilation and EPAP to obstructive events during polysomnography or respiratory polygraphy, is recommended. Additionally adjusting IPAP to PCO_2 overnight measurement, e.g. transcutaneous CO_2 ($TcCO_2$), can be very useful, provided that the $TcCO_2$ monitor has been validated against arterial PCO_2 measurements and the time course of response is understood. End tidal CO_2 ($EtCO_2$) is difficult to use in patients receiving NIV as delivered flow within the mask limits accuracy of readings. Ventilators should be used in spontaneous/timed mode (i.e. with a timed back-up rate) in all patients with nocturnal hypoventilation or central apnoeas. A back-up rate of one to two breaths below spontaneous breathing rate while awake is usually helpful. Ventilator set-up is usually done during a hospital stay, but in children with stable nocturnal hypoventilation, outpatient set-up with home monitoring may be feasible, equally efficacious and acceptable to child and parents [18].

Supplemental oxygen therapy is rarely required in children with pure alveolar hypoventilation; however in a clinical scenario of atelectasis or pulmonary hypoplasia in which SaO_2 remains less than 93 % with optimal control of PCO_2 and adjustment of EPAP, O_2 should be added to normalise SaO_2. It should be entrained proximally into the ventilator circuit or through the ventilator itself if an O_2 mixer is present. Adjustment of O_2 therapy should always be accompanied by PCO_2 monitoring.

Monitoring Efficacy of Ventilator Support

As indicated above, respiratory polygraphy together with $TcCO_2$ measurements will indicate whether alveolar ventilation has been controlled. Information downloaded from ventilator software provides important additional information on mask leak, number of residual apnoeas and hypopnoeas and adherence to therapy. It should be borne in mind that the software which calculates apnoeas and hypopnoeas in patients receiving NIV is not the same as that calculating respiratory events during diagnostic studies; therefore although comparison on and off treatment is important, the results are not completely comparable. Janssens et al. [19] have provided a helpful algorithm to diagnose problems related to ventilator efficacy. Home telemonitoring is now available with some ventilator systems and may be helpful in the initial period of therapy as the child adjusts to the device and provides feedback to parents and also long term in heavily ventilator-dependent children.

Acute Chest Infections

While there is evidence that the use of NIV reduces the frequency of chest infections in neuromuscular disorders, these remain one of the commonest complications. Infections may be triggered by aspiration from bulbar weakness, and even in those in whom aspiration has not occurred, it is likely that swallowing efficacy is reduced during acute infections. There is also good supportive evidence that cough peak flow falls during an acute infection. It should also be remembered that cardiomyopathy is common in some conditions (e.g. DMD, Emery-Dreifuss MD, sarcoglycanopathies) and pulmonary shadowing may be due to pulmonary oedema or a combination of pulmonary consolidation and oedema. Measurement of brain natriuretic peptide (BNP), echocardiography and chest X-ray are helpful in distinguishing these conditions. Creatine phosphokinase (CPK) may be raised and there may also be chronically mildly elevated troponin levels—although not at a level to suggest cardiac ischaemia. NIV should be used more intensively during a chest infection and especially during physiotherapy. Supplemental O_2 therapy may need to be entrained to normalise SaO_2. As described below, if cough is inefficient, cough assistance with insufflation-exsufflation may improve secretion clearance markedly. Considerations for dealing with established ventilator users when admitted with a chest infection are shown in Fig. 14.2.

• Use NIV intensively
• Carry out physiotherapy while patient uses NIV as cough enhanced and patient less likely to tire
• Use cough in-exsufflator
• Add supplememtal oxygen therapy to NIV to maintain SaO2 >93%
• It may help to increase IPAP by 2-5 cmH2O incrementally according to PCO2 level and EPAP by 1-2 cmH2O to a maximum of say, 7 cmH2O. Increasing back-up rate to just below spontaneous breathing rate will improve CO2 control
• If patient becomes near 24 hour NIV dependent during an acute episode consider alternating masks to prevent pressure sores and alternate day and night between 2 ventilators of the same model, so as not to run ventilator continuously for days
• Optimise humidfication to help mobilise secretions
• Consider bronchodilator therapy if evidence of asthma, bronchial hyper-reactivity or wheezy bronchitis
• Consider steroid therapy if evidence of asthma, bronchial hyper-reactvity or wheezy bronchitis
• Ensure hydration and nutrition maintained.

Fig. 14.2 Clinical considerations to optimise NIV during an acute chest infection in neuromuscular disease patient

Clearly all other sensible standard respiratory measures should be carried out including use of broad-spectrum antibiotics, hydration and attention to nutrition. Nebulised bronchodilator is helpful in wheezy children and those with asthma, but there is no evidence to support routine use in the absence of evidence of reversible airflow obstruction. Humidification of the ventilator is often helpful in reducing sputum viscosity.

Cough Assistance

Assistance with secretion clearance can be provided by the physiotherapy techniques of secretion mobilisation, postural drainage and manual techniques such as chest percussion and shaking. Cough can also be augmented by breath stacking using an ambu bag-type device with one-way valve. If these are not sufficient, then the cough insufflator-exsufflator (of which there are several models now on the market) can be effectively combined with NIV or used alone in children with marked expiratory muscle weakness but who do not yet fulfil indications for NIV [20].

Cough efficacy can be assessed by cough peak flow and maximum inspiratory and expiratory pressures. The insufflator-exsufflator provides a large positive pressure breath to augment inspiration and then cycles manually or automatically to negative pressure to augment cough and suck secretions into upper airway and mouth. Setting up the cough machine is well described in references [20, 21].

Progression to Tracheostomy Ventilation

The indications for tracheostomy ventilation are given in Table 14.3. The most common indication is bulbar weakness resulting in aspiration or 24-h ventilatory dependency in a younger child. Children in the group requiring long-term tracheostomy ventilation are more likely to have a diagnosis of type 1 SMA, myotubular myopathy or other severe myopathies such as nemaline or a high cervical cord lesion. Progression from NIV to tracheostomy ventilation is relatively uncommon in childhood but is more frequent in Duchenne muscular dystrophy patients and those with other progressive conditions.

An advance care plan detailing choices regarding tracheostomy ventilation and resuscitation preferences of the family is vital and should be discussed regularly and updated according to progress.

Table 14.3 Indications for tracheotomy ventilation	Indications for tracheotomy ventilation
	• Severe bulbar weakness leading to aspiration
	• Upper airway problems limiting delivery of NIV
	• Failure to control ventilation with non-invasive mode
	• Intractable interface problems
	• Near 24-h ventilator dependency, especially in early infancy
	• Patient/family preference

Palliative NIV/Ethics

Palliative care is discussed in Chap. 5. NIV may be used to palliate symptoms and facilitate discharge to home in some children with a very poor prognosis. In a series of these children with type 1 SMA, NIV was used not to extend prognosis but to allow transfer from hospital to home so the child could spend the last months with the family [22]. Careful discussion with the family on the goals and realistic possibilities of therapy and expectations is key. It is important that continuing assessment is carried out as if NIV is not achieving those goals, e.g. reducing breathlessness, it can be withdrawn and the management directed to other methods of palliative care, such as opiates, when appropriate.

References

1. Hull J, Aniapravan R, Chan E, Chatwin M, Forton J, Gallagher J, et al. British Thoracic Society guideline for respiratory management of children with neuromuscular weakness. Thorax. 2012;67(i):1–40.
2. Rideau Y, Jankowski W, Grellet J. Respiratory function in the muscular dystrophies. Muscle Nerve. 1981;4:155–64.
3. Alman BA, Raza SN, Biggar WDB. Steroid treatment and the development of scoliosis in males with Duchenne muscular dystrophy. J Bone Joint Surg Am. 2004;86:519–24.
4. Ragette R, Mellies U, Schwake C, Voit T, Teschler H. Patterns and predictors of sleep disordered breathing in primary myopathies. Thorax. 2002;57:724–8.
5. Chatwin M, Bush AB, Macrae DJ, Clarke SA, Simonds AK. Risk management protocol for gastrostomy and jejunostomy insertion in ventilator dependent infants. Neuromusc Disord. 2013;23:289–97.
6. Finder J, Birnkrant D, Carl J, Farber HJ, Gozal D, Iannaconne ST, et al. ATS consensus statement: respiratory care of the patient with Duchenne muscular dystrophy. Am J Respir Crit Care Med. 2004;170:456–65.
7. Wang CH, Finkel RS, Bertini E, Schroth M, Simonds A, Wong B, et al. Consensus statement for standard of care in spinal muscular atrophy. J Child Neurol. 2007;22:1027–49.
8. Fauroux B, Boule M, Lofaso F, Zerah F, Clement A, Harf A, et al. Chest physiotherapy in cystic fibrosis: improved tolerance with nasal pressure support ventilation. Pediatrics. 1999;103, E32.
9. Robb SA, Muntoni F, Simonds AK. Respiratory management of congenital myasthenic syndromes in childhood. Neuromusc Disord. 2010;20(12):833–8.
10. Ward SA, Chatwin M, Heather S, Simonds AK. Randomised controlled trial of non-invasive ventilation (NIV) for nocturnal hypoventilation in neuromuscular and chest wall disease patients with daytime normocapnia. Thorax. 2005;60:1019–24.
11. Mellies U, Ragette R, Schwake C, Boehm H, Voit T, Teschler H. Long-term noninvasive ventilation in children and adolescents with neuromuscular disorders. Eur Respir J. 2003;22:631–6.
12. Wallgren-Pettersen C, Bushby K, Mellies U, Simonds AK. Ventilatory support in congenital neuromuscular disorders—ongenital myopathies, congenital muscular dystrophies, congenital myotonic dystrophy and SMA II. Neuromusc Disord. 2004;14:56–69.
13. Mellies U, Dohna-Schwake C, Stehling F, Voit T. Sleep disordered breathing in spinal muscular atrophy. Neuromusc Disord. 2004;14:797–803.
14. Jaye J, Chatwin M, Dayer M, Morrell MJ, Simonds AK. Autotitrating versus standard noninvasive ventilation: a randomised crossover trial. Eur Respir J. 2009;33:566–71.

15. Fauroux B, Leroux K, Desmarais G, Isabey D, Clement A, Lofaso F, et al. Performance of ventilators for noninvasive positive pressure ventilation in children. Eur Respir J. 2008;31:1300–7.
16. Fauroux B, Lavis J-F, Nicot F, Picard A, Boelle P-Y, Clement A, et al. Facial side effects during noninvasive ventilation in children. Int Care Med. 2005;31:965–9.
17. Berry RB, Chediak A, Brown LK, Finder J, Gozal D, Iber C, et al. Best clinical practices for the sleep center adjustment of noninvasive positive pressure ventilation in stable chronic alveolar hypoventilation syndromes. J Clin Sleep Med. 2010;6:491–509.
18. Chatwin M, Ward S, Nickol AH, Polkey MI, Simonds AK. A randomised trial of outpatient versus inpatient initiation of non-invasive ventilation (NIV) in nocturnal hypoventilation due to neuromuscular and chest wall disease. Eur Respir J. 2004;24:476s.
19. Janssens JP, Borel J-C, Pepin J-L, on behalf of SomnoNIV Group. Nocturnal monitoring of home non-invasive ventilation: the contribution of simpl tools such as pulse oximetry, capnography, built-in ventilator software and autonomic markers of sleep fragmentation. Thorax. 2011;66(5):438–45.
20. Chatwin M. How to use a mechanical insufflator-exsufflator 'cough assist machine'. Breathe. 2008;4:320–9.
21. Chatwin M, Ross E, Hart N, Nickol A, Polkey MI, Simonds AK. Cough augmentation with mechanical insufflation/exsufflation in patients with neuromuscular weakness. Eur Respir J. 2003;21:502–8.
22. Chatwin M, Bush A, Simonds AK. Outcome of goal-directed non-invasive ventilation and mechanical insufflation/exsufflation in spinal muscular atrophy type I. Arch Dis Child. 2011;96:426–32.

Chapter 15
Long-Term Ventilator Support in Bronchopulmonary Dysplasia

Sharon A. McGrath-Morrow and J. Michael Collaco

Epidemiology of Bronchopulmonary Dysplasia

Definition and Risk Factors: Bronchopulmonary dysplasia (BPD) is a common cause of chronic lung disease in infants born prematurely (<37 weeks gestation) and is associated with high morbidity, particularly during the first 2 years of life [1]. The diagnosis of BPD is given to preterm infants who require supplemental oxygen for at least the first 28 days of life [2]. Infants who are diagnosed with severe BPD have an oxygen requirement of greater than 30 % and/or the need for positive pressure ventilation at 36 weeks post-conceptual age or at discharge [2]. Infants with severe BPD are most likely to have persistent respiratory failure requiring home invasive ventilation. Although BPD is more likely to occur in infants born at very early gestational age, other factors have been shown to independently predict the development of BPD in infants born between 22 and 30 weeks gestation. These factors include birth weight, race/ethnicity, sex, and the need for ventilatory support or elevated FiO_2 within the first 28 days of life [3].

Prevalence: Preterm birth is a common occurrence in the United States with 11.72 % of live births being premature in 2011. Although this is the lowest rate in more than a decade, it remains higher than in prior decades [4]. In addition, 1.44 % of infants in 2011 were born at very low birth weight (VLBW <1500 g) compared to 1.27 % in 1990, and it is VLBW infants who are at highest risk of developing BPD. More of these high-risk infants are surviving with ongoing advances in neonatology with infant mortality rates reaching an all time low of 6.05 deaths per

S.A. McGrath-Morrow, M.D., M.B.A. • J.M. Collaco, M.D., M.P.H. (✉)
Eudowood Division of Pediatric Respiratory Sciences, Johns Hopkins University School of Medicine, 200 N. Wolfe St., David M. Rubenstein Building, Baltimore, MD 21287, USA
e-mail: mcollac1@jhmi.edu

© Springer Science+Business Media New York 2016
L.M. Sterni, J.L. Carroll (eds.), *Caring for the Ventilator Dependent Child*,
Respiratory Medicine, DOI 10.1007/978-1-4939-3749-3_15

1000 live births in 2011 [4]. The decrease in infant mortality in VLBW infants is associated with an increase in the number of technology-dependent children in the home environment.

Tracheostomy Placement and Home Ventilator Support in Infants and Children with BPD: There are limited data regarding rates of home ventilatory support in infants and children with BPD, and certainly VLBW infants are at highest risk. In retrospective studies examining a NICU cohort ($n=10,428$), it was reported that 0.7% of the NICU cohort had tracheostomies, with a 2.8% tracheostomy placement rate in the subset of VLBW infants ($n=636$) [5, 6]. Estimates of the incidence of infants/children with BPD requiring positive pressure ventilation vary. For example, a recent study from Riley Children's Hospital estimated the incidence to be 4.77 per 100,000 live births in 2010 with a median age of liberation from home ventilator support of 24 months of age [7]. Given approximately 4 million live births in the United States in 2010, it can be extrapolated that there are approximately 400 infants/children with BPD on home ventilation at any given time. However, other studies suggest a higher incidence. The Healthcare Cost and Utilization Project reported that 1500 infants, mostly preterm, received tracheostomies in 2008 [8]. In another study, Boroughs and Dougherty reported that an estimated 8000 children in the United States are receiving home invasive ventilation [9]. Based on their 2011 data from the Ventilator Assisted Children's Home Program in Pennsylvania, they reported that 36% of ventilator-dependent children in their program were diagnosed with chronic lung disease and that 77% of these children had the diagnosis of BPD [9]. Extrapolating from the Pennsylvania data, it can be estimated that approximately 2000 infants and children with BPD may be receiving home invasive ventilation at any given time in the United States.

In the BPD population, there are also limited data regarding risk factors associated with the requirement for home ventilatory support. One study examined risk factors associated with tracheostomy placement in the NICU. They found that longer mean duration of intubation (128.8 days vs. 44.5 days), a higher median number of intubation events (11.5 vs. 6.0), and a longer initial hospitalization (156.9 days vs. 88.9 days) were associated with tracheostomy placement in 18 VLBW infants compared to 36 VLBW control infants who did not require tracheostomy [6]. As all children who require home invasive ventilation have tracheostomies, the risk factors for home ventilator support may be similar to risk factors for tracheostomy placement in the BPD population.

Mortality: Risk of death in children on home mechanical ventilation is high despite current monitoring technology, with a mortality rate of 18.6% among infants and children with BPD at one institution [7]. Avoidable causes for this high mortality may include poor training of caregiver and home support staff leading to inadequate responses in emergency situations, particularly with tracheostomy management. In a retrospective study of 228 children on home mechanical ventilation, Edwards et al. reported 47 deaths (21% mortality rate) with 49% being unexpected deaths including 19% of deaths related to tracheostomy complications [10].

Respiratory Phenotypes in the Preterm Child with BPD

BPD is formally defined on the basis of oxygen requirement at specific post-conceptual time points, but this measure does not capture the spectrum of respiratory phenotypes that encompass BPD. Infants and children may have varying combinations of parenchymal, vascular, small airway and large airway disease. The contributions of these disease components are often difficult to assess. Furthermore, the combination of the disease components may change with time and lung growth. The protean manifestations of BPD frequently require tailoring of ventilator management and other respiratory care on the individual level. For these reasons frequent assessment of respiratory support requirements should be done in infants and children on home ventilator support with appropriate changes as warranted. These changes may be done in the home setting in children who are relatively stable and in an acute or subacute setting in children who are less stable. Nevertheless, during acute respiratory illnesses, changes in ventilatory support should always be done in an acute care setting due to the diversity of lung phenotypes and complexity of ventilating these patients when sick.

Parenchymal Disease: The lung parenchymal disease found in children with BPD often manifests as a paucity of alveoli due to severe prematurity and impaired postnatal alveolar growth. Unlike children with neuromuscular disease and respiratory failure, children with severe BPD and respiratory failure can often be weaned off mechanical ventilation if postnatal lung growth takes place. Since the majority of postnatal alveolar lung growth occurs during the first 2 years of life, it is imperative that lung injury be minimized during this critical period of lung development [11].

Impaired alveolar growth often occurs due to barotrauma from mechanical ventilation, exposure to hyperoxia, and respiratory/systemic infections. Poor nutrition in the neonatal period may also be associated with the development of BPD [12]. In addition, the severity of BPD may significantly worsen in children who aspirate due to impaired swallowing and gastroesophageal reflux [13]. To maximize alveolar growth during the first years of life, attention to preventing ongoing lung insults and maintaining good nutrition is critical. In addition to impaired alveolar growth, many infants and children with severe BPD may have significant cystic airspace disease. The presence of cystic disease may lead to regional heterogeneity of time constants for ventilation, which can manifest as areas of hyperinflation and atelectasis simultaneously within different regions of the lung.

Vascular Disease: The recognition of vascular disease in preterm infants with BPD, manifested as pulmonary hypertension (PH), is an emerging phenomenon. Thebault and Abman were among the first to describe alveolar hypoplasia in extremely preterm infants with chronic lung disease [14]. This "new BPD" pathology was felt to be due to a variety of factors, including decreased vascular endothelial growth factor (VEGF) and other molecular pathways involved in alveolar growth [15, 16]. Abman and colleagues also recognized that a subset of infants with severe BPD were at increased risk for the development of PH and associated higher mortality [17].

Risk factors for the development of PH in children with BPD include very early gestational age, oligohydramnios, and infants who are small for gestational age [18]. There may also be genetic and epigenetic factors that contribute to the development of PH in infants with severe BPD.

Infants and children with BPD and PH may have a fixed and reactive component to their PH. The fixed component is a function of an underdeveloped vascular bed with limited volume. Ideally, with optimal lung growth, this fixed component improves with time. The reactive component may be responsive to vasodilator therapies such as oxygen, nitric oxide, and sildenafil but also may be subject to vasoconstriction by relative hypoxic events, such as respiratory infections or anesthesia induction [19, 20]. The clinical manifestations of pulmonary hypertension may range from subtle evidence of right heart strain or increased respiratory effort/oxygen requirements to more severe presentations with cardiorespiratory failure. Although cardiac catheterization is the gold standard for assessing for PH, in practice echocardiograms are frequently used along with non-approved biomarkers, such as brain natriuretic peptide (BNP) and its precursor, pro-BNP [21]. Guidelines for the use of pharmacological agents in pediatric pulmonary hypertension were published in 2015 with limited evidence in BPD [22]. Improving lung growth, minimizing ventilation perfusion mismatch, and reducing episodes of hypoxia and hypercarbia may improve outcomes [18, 23]. In children with PH including those receiving home invasive ventilation, attention to higher oxygen saturations should be given as oxygen is a pulmonary vasodilator. It has been recommended that children with BPD and PH should maintain oxygen saturations above at least 92 % to minimize pulmonary vasoconstriction [21, 22, 24–26].

Small Airway Disease: Infants with severe BPD commonly have small airway disease as demonstrated by pulmonary function testing (PFT) [27], and it has been reported that these pulmonary function abnormalities frequently persist into later childhood and adult life [28]. In clinical practice, infant PFTs are infrequently utilized owing to limited availability at tertiary care centers as well as the sedation risks associated with conducting these tests.

Children with BPD on chronic mechanical ventilation often have evidence of severe air trapping on chest radiographs (Fig. 15.1). Inflammation is believed to play a major role in the development of BPD [29] and may lead to reduced small airway flows. However, optimal regimens of anti-inflammatory treatments to minimize BPD development have not been well established. In the NICU, the use of systemic anti-inflammatory medications has been controversial due in part to a reported association between cerebral palsy and early use of dexamethasone in preterm infants with respiratory failure [30]. In the BPD child on home ventilation, intermittent and limited use of systemic glucocorticoids may improve mucous plugging and inflammation during acute pulmonary exacerbations. Although use of inhaled steroids has not been found to reduce prevalence of BPD or the risk of short-term acute respiratory outcomes in the NICU [31], inhaled corticosteroids as a maintenance medication may be useful in BPD children with significant small airway pathology. The adequacy of inhaled particle deposition into the small airways of infants with BPD is unknown.

Fig. 15.1 Chest
radiograph of a toddler
with severe
bronchopulmonary
dysplasia demonstrating
hyperinflation and
significant chronic changes

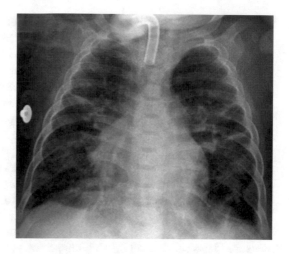

Children with BPD may also have fixed airway obstruction based on dysnaptic airway growth [32]. This fixed airway obstruction may account for the component of nonreversible airway obstruction frequently seen in children with severe BPD and may not be amenable to bronchodilator therapy [33].

Large Airway Disease: A subset of children with severe BPD may have a component of large airway disease due to malacia of the trachea and bronchi. This is more commonly seen in children who required high-pressure support while in the NICU. Preterm infants with vascular rings may also have significant compression of the large airways even after surgical correction. Besides wheezing unresponsive to beta-agonist therapy, infants and children with significant malacia may experience sudden, profound desaturations that may require resuscitation in severe cases. The use of higher positive end-expiratory pressure (PEEP) may be beneficial in these children with large airway compromise and respiratory failure but also carries the risks of hyperinflation and pneumothoraces.

Ventilator Management in the Preterm Child with Bronchopulmonary Dysplasia

Noninvasive Ventilation: The role of noninvasive ventilation for BPD outside of an inpatient setting is extremely limited owing to the paucity of FDA-approved medical devices for outpatient use for infants.

Invasive Ventilation: The following sections will primarily focus on issues unique to BPD as general requirements for home invasive ventilation will be covered in more detail in other chapters.

Ventilator Strategies: Typically in the home setting, most infants with BPD on home ventilators are either on (i) SIMV mode with pressure control/pressure support,

(ii) CPAP mode with pressure support, or (iii) CPAP only. Unlike children with neuromuscular disease and chronic ventilatory failure, volume modes of ventilation are infrequently used in children with BPD owing to the perceived risk of barotrauma. Although there are no BPD-specific guidelines regarding home ventilation, clinical practice guidelines regarding pediatric chronic home invasive ventilation were published in 2016 and focus on discharge criteria, training, and equipment necessary for safe ventilation in the home [34]. The strategies used to ventilate a child in chronic respiratory failure with BPD will likely need to be modulated based on the presenting combination of respiratory phenotypes. In general, it is advisable to stabilize ventilator settings in the NICU setting or subacute inpatient setting prior to initial discharge to home.

In contrast to the treatment of acute respiratory failure in the neonatal intensive care unit, children with BPD and chronic respiratory failure may require larger tidal volumes, longer inspiratory and expiratory times, and slower respiratory rates due to the alveolar and airway abnormalities that are common in these children. For instance, these children often exhibit hyperinflation due to small airway disease and may require longer expiratory times (Fig. 15.1). Children with a component of large airway malacia often require a higher PEEP to maintain airway patency. Assessment of malacia may require evaluation by an otolaryngologist or pulmonologist using flexible bronchoscopy to titrate airway pressures under direct visualization. Dynamic computed tomography can also be helpful in assessing malacia where this technology is available [35]. With regard to parenchymal disease, children with alveolar disease often require higher FiO_2. Children with cystic changes and regional airspace heterogeneity may also require longer inspiratory and expiratory times. Patients with pulmonary hypertension may require increased ventilator and oxygen support during pulmonary hypertensive crises [18], which may be triggered by aspiration, respiratory infections [19], or anesthesia [20].

Supplemental Oxygen Therapy: There are no specific guidelines regarding what FiO_2 setting is acceptable for hospital discharge, but in practice FiO_2 >30–40 % is difficult to maintain in the home setting due to the large amounts of oxygen required owing to ventilator flow. Furthermore, patients requiring an FiO_2 >30–40 % are likely not stable enough for discharge. There are no specific guidelines for goal oxygen saturations for preterm infants in the outpatient setting. At sea level, it may be beneficial to maintain saturations ≥92 % to promote neurodevelopment and lung/somatic growth. For preterm infants with pulmonary hypertension, it has been suggested to maintain saturations ≥95 % once the retinal vasculature has matured [21, 24–26].

Ventilator Weaning: In contrast to many of the other pediatric respiratory or neuromuscular diseases that require home invasive ventilation, many infants and children with BPD are able to be weaned from invasive ventilation over the first several years of life. The core principle of weaning an infant or toddler from home mechanical ventilation is close monitoring. This involves pulse oximetry, end-tidal carbon dioxide measurements, and clinical observation of the patient for increased work of breathing, tachypnea, fatigue, and central apneas. Given the mortality associated with pulmonary hypertension (12–38 %) [26, 36–40], it may be strongly preferable to postpone ventilator weaning until the patient's pulmonary hypertension is resolved or stable.

Inpatient Weaning: There are no published guidelines for ventilator weaning for infants and children with BPD. Most commonly ventilator weaning occurs during the day with weaning for short periods of time (15–60 min) at first, and these time periods are gradually increased. Weaning strategies may include taking patients off the ventilator completely, placing patients on CPAP, or a more gradual approach with reduced settings depending on the patient's tolerance. One approach to more gradual ventilator weaning is to wean the rate first. Once a rate of 2–4 breaths per minute is achieved, the patient can be transitioned to CPAP plus pressure-supported breaths; care must be taken during this phase to monitor the patient for central apneas as infants and children with neurological issues may be more prone to prolonged central apneas. Following this, the pressure support is gradually weaned until the patient is solely on CPAP. Once this is accomplished, the patient may be able to transition to tracheostomy collar with humidified air or oxygen, again for short trials at first, then gradually increasing during the day while awake. Some patients may be able to be successfully weaned from ventilator support during the day, but may experience increased fatigue, atelectasis, poor growth, and/or central apneas when ventilation is weaned at night, thus necessitating the use of a ventilator at night and possibly with naps as well.

Outpatient Weaning: As opposed to weaning of supplemental oxygen, which is typically weaned in the outpatient setting, the default location for ventilator weaning for infants with BPD is the inpatient setting, either acute or subacute. However, ventilator weaning can be successfully performed in the outpatient setting with the appropriate family dynamics, the presence of home nursing, frequent in-office assessments, and home end-tidal carbon dioxide monitoring. Because of the absence of continuous clinical observation, ventilator parameter weaning in an outpatient setting typically occurs more gradually than in an inpatient setting.

The Role of Polysomnography: For outpatient management, overnight polysomnography can be very useful in assessing the adequacy of ventilator settings or safety off of a ventilator, specifically with respect to gas exchange and monitoring for central apneas. For weaning purposes, it may be appropriate to obtain studies after weaning is accomplished during the day but prior to instituting reduced parameters at night and with sleep. Obtaining studies should be considered with significant ventilator parameter weans, with discontinuation of the ventilator, and with capping of the tracheostomy tube. In patients with stable ventilator parameters, routine studies should be considered every 12–24 months to reassess requirements due to changes in respiratory disease and growth. It should be recognized that not all pediatric sleep laboratories are able to accommodate and appropriately assess ventilated patients, particularly if titration during the study is desired.

Decannulation: Decannulation should ideally take place under the supervision of an otolaryngologist. Typically, once the patient is weaned from the ventilator and the patient is judged to be a candidate for eventual decannulation, tracheostomy capping can be considered. Frequently, the otolaryngologist may decrease the tracheostomy size prior to capping to allow for more airflow around the tracheostomy. The first trial of capping is usually performed in an outpatient office visit under medical observation to assess tolerance. Duration of capping while the patient is awake is increased gradually. In our center, once the patient is tolerating capping all day, overnight polysomnography is conducted with the tracheostomy capped to assess for obstruction, hypoxemia, and/or hypoventilation. Although the tracheostomy may have been placed for ventilation and not upper airway obstruction, providers should be aware that significant obstructive sleep apnea may be more prevalent in the preterm population and thus may be diagnosed on studies performed for decannulation purposes [41].

Other Home Ventilation Management Issues

Home Monitoring Equipment: Monitoring devices for preterm infants with home ventilation are essential with a pulse oximeter at a minimum as supported by recent pediatric ventilation guidelines [34]. Recent data for the State of Massachusetts suggest that most (75 %; $n=97$) pediatric patients on home invasive ventilation are meeting this requirement [42]. A preparedness plan for electrical outages and/or other emergencies is needed for caregivers of children who are technology dependent. This includes, among other things, battery backup for essential equipment such as the ventilator, oxygen concentrator, and pulse oximeter. Sakashita et al. reported poor preparedness in many families with technology-dependent children in the event of a power outage [43]. Beside the ventilator itself, a non-recording pulse-oximeter and batteries, other guideline-recommended equipment includes a back-up ventilator, a self-inflating bag and mask, suctioning equipment (portable), heated humidifier, supplemental oxygen for emergency use, and a nebulizer [34].

Tracheostomies: Edwards and colleagues reported that 19 % of deaths in their pediatric patients ventilated at home were tracheostomy related and likely all preventable [10]. Infants with BPD may be at higher risk for tracheostomy-related complications owing to a higher risk of mucous plugging with a small tracheostomy tube and ineffective clearance coughs. The use of secretory drying agents, such as glycopyrrolate, may lead to tracheostomy plugging, and their use should be avoided if possible or closely monitored if their use is required. For frequent mucous plugging, pulmonary clearance techniques, such as chest physiotherapy, and the use of scheduled inhaled beta-agonists may be very helpful. Lastly, the presence of an artificial, potentially unstable airway in an infant or small child warrants the presence of an awake and alert caregiver at all times as recommended by pediatric home ventilation guidelines [34].

Training: Training for at least two family members is recommended including tracheostomy changes/cares and ventilator management [34]. Asking caregivers to demonstrate all cares at bedside and extended in-house stays (12–24 h) where caregivers perform all cares are highly recommended. However, standardized education, or professional training as is the case for home nurses, does not necessarily translate into appropriate knowledge for emergency situations for children on home ventilators [44].

Caregivers: Given the risk of acute life-threatening events with tracheostomies, we would strongly recommend that infants and toddlers with BPD with tracheostomies with or without mechanical ventilation have an awake and alert caregiver at all times. In practice, this requires licensed professional home care (e.g., registered nurses (RN) or licensed practical nurses (LPN)) at a minimum for nights and when family members work. All caregivers, family and professional, must be proficient with tracheostomy management and the specific ventilator being utilized.

Medical Home: Owing to the multisystem consequences of prematurity, any infant or child with BPD requiring home ventilation should be managed using a medical home approach including close collaboration with the appropriate subspecialists. Based on data from the State of Massachusetts, Graham et al. reported that pediatric pulmonologists manage ventilators for the majority of children on home ventilators and demonstrated a higher admission rate in the past 6 months for patients with ventilator management by general pediatricians (47 %) vs. pediatric pulmonologists (24 %) [42]. However, based on data from Children's Hospital of Los Angeles, Kun et al. reported that the frequency of pediatric pulmonary visits was not associated with readmission [45]. It is also recommended that routine otolaryngology follow-up should occur with any patient with a tracheostomy.

Comorbidities Affecting Ventilator Management

Aspiration: Any type of persistent aspiration, whether related to gastroesophageal reflux, dysphagia, or the patient's own oral secretions, can result in ongoing lung injury leading to difficulty weaning ventilator support [13]. During ventilator weaning, it may be preferable to avoid compressing gastrostomy tube feed duration or advancing oral intake to maximize chances of success.

Gastrointestinal motility is frequently impaired in the preterm infant with BPD and can worsen with any pulmonary exacerbation. This may result in gastric distention leading to impaired ventilation via altered respiratory mechanics. Intravenous hydration or the use of enteral rehydration solutions may decrease gastric distention during a pulmonary exacerbation.

Pulmonary Exacerbations: Rates of readmission are high among premature infants on home ventilation; a recent study by Kun et al. performed at a pediatric tertiary care center found that 39 % of patients with a history of prematurity on home mechanical ventilation were nonelectively readmitted within 12 months of initial discharge on ventilation ($n = 51$) [45]. Among the total home ventilated population in this study, 64 % of readmissions were associated with respiratory causes. Pneumonia, tracheitis, and even upper respiratory viral infections may result in increased ventilator or oxygen support in infants with BPD. Typically with supportive care, increased pulmonary toilet, and use of antibiotics if appropriate, ventilator parameters return to baseline. Owing to the need for frequent ventilator setting adjustment, episodes requiring increased support are frequently managed in an inpatient setting.

Respiratory viruses commonly cause pulmonary exacerbation in children with severe BPD [46]. Rhinovirus which generally is considered an upper airway pathogen can lead to severe lower respiratory tract disease in children with BPD [47]. Children with small airway disease and pulmonary hypertension may be at highest for pulmonary decompensation from respiratory viruses through small airway obstruction and elevated pulmonary vascular pressures, respectively. Palivizumab should be used for the first 2 years of life in the ventilated BPD child to reduce morbidity and death from respiratory syncytial virus (RSV) [48].

Children with tracheostomies are at higher risk for bacterial infections and bacterial colonization of the lower airways due to the bypassing of natural defenses of the upper airway. The pneumococcal polysaccharide vaccine (PPSV23) should be considered in older BPD children on home mechanical ventilation since PCV7 vaccine failures have been reported in children with lower airway conditions such as asthma [49]. Colonization with respiratory pathogens, such as *Pseudomonas aeruginosa*, may increase the risk of tracheitis following viral infections. Suppressive inhaled or oral antibiotic treatment in children with chronic tracheitis may be considered but may lead to antibiotic resistance.

Conclusions

Chronic lung disease of prematurity is a frequent indication for home invasive ventilation in the pediatric population. Although the heterogeneity of lung disease and its various components of parenchymal, vascular, small airway and large airway disease make it challenging to manage, infants with BPD can be ventilated in the home setting effectively. Successful ventilation is dependent on caregiver training, appropriate resources, and availability of subspecialty care. Unlike many other pediatric respiratory diseases that may require home invasive ventilation, infants and children with BPD have a higher likelihood of being weaned from support with good lung growth.

References

1. Greenough A. Long-term pulmonary outcome in the preterm infant. Neonatology. 2008;93(4):324–7.
2. Jobe AH, Bancalari E. Bronchopulmonary dysplasia. Am J Respir Crit Care Med. 2001;163(7):1723–9.
3. Laughon MM, Langer JC, Bose CL, Smith PB, Ambalavanan N, Kennedy KA, et al. Prediction of bronchopulmonary dysplasia by postnatal age in extremely premature infants. Am J Respir Crit Care Med. 2011;183(12):1715–22. Pubmed Central PMCID: 3136997.
4. Hamilton BE, Hoyert DL, Martin JA, Strobino DM, Guyer B. Annual summary of vital statistics: 2010-2011. Pediatrics. 2013;131(3):548–58.

5. Sidman JD, Jaguan A, Couser RJ. Tracheotomy and decannulation rates in a level 3 neonatal intensive care unit: a 12-year study. Laryngoscope. 2006;116(1):136–9.

6. Sisk EA, Kim TB, Schumacher R, Dechert R, Driver L, Ramsey AM, et al. Tracheotomy in very low birth weight neonates: indications and outcomes. Laryngoscope. 2006;116(6):928–33.

7. Cristea AI, Carroll AE, Davis SD, Swigonski NL, Ackerman VL. Outcomes of children with severe bronchopulmonary dysplasia who were ventilator dependent at home. Pediatrics. 2013;132(3):e727–34. Pubmed Central PMCID: 3876749.

8. Joseph RA. Tracheostomy in infants: parent education for home care. Neonatal Network. 2011;30(4):231–42.

9. Boroughs D, Dougherty JA. Decreasing accidental mortality of ventilator-dependent children at home: a call to action. Home Healthc Nurse. 2012;30(2):103–11; quiz 12–3.

10. Edwards JD, Kun SS, Keens TG. Outcomes and causes of death in children on home mechanical ventilation via tracheostomy: an institutional and literature review. J Pediatr. 2010;157(6):955–9. e2.

11. Thurlbeck WM. Postnatal human lung growth. Thorax. 1982;37(8):564–71. Pubmed Central PMCID: 459376.

12. Frank L, Sosenko IR. Undernutrition as a major contributing factor in the pathogenesis of bronchopulmonary dysplasia. Am Rev Respir Dis. 1988;138(3):725–9.

13. Lefton-Greif MA, McGrath-Morrow SA. Deglutition and respiration: development, coordination, and practical implications. Semin Speech Lang. 2007;28(3):166–79.

14. Thebaud B, Abman SH. Bronchopulmonary dysplasia: where have all the vessels gone? Roles of angiogenic growth factors in chronic lung disease. Am J Respir Crit Care Med. 2007;175(10):978–85. Pubmed Central PMCID: 2176086.

15. Hadchouel A, Franco-Montoya ML, Delacourt C. Altered lung development in bronchopulmonary dysplasia. Birth Defects Res A Clin Mol Teratol. 2014;100(3):158–67.

16. Abman SH. Impaired vascular endothelial growth factor signaling in the pathogenesis of neonatal pulmonary vascular disease. Adv Exp Med Biol. 2010;661:323–35.

17. Mourani PM, Abman SH. Pulmonary vascular disease in bronchopulmonary dysplasia: pulmonary hypertension and beyond. Curr Opin Pediatr. 2013;25(3):329–37.

18. Collaco JM, Romer LH, Stuart BD, Coulson JD, Everett AD, Lawson EE, et al. Frontiers in pulmonary hypertension in infants and children with bronchopulmonary dysplasia. Pediatr Pulmonol. 2012;47(11):1042–53. Pubmed Central PMCID: 3963167.

19. Farquhar M, Fitzgerald DA. Pulmonary hypertension in chronic neonatal lung disease. Paediatr Respir Rev. 2010;11(3):149–53.

20. Carmosino MJ, Friesen RH, Doran A, Ivy DD. Perioperative complications in children with pulmonary hypertension undergoing noncardiac surgery or cardiac catheterization. Anesth Analg. 2007;104(3):521–7. Pubmed Central PMCID: 1934984.

21. Kim GB. Pulmonary hypertension in infants with bronchopulmonary dysplasia. Korean J Pediatr. 2010;53(6):688–93. Pubmed Central PMCID: 2994133.

22. Abman SH et al. Pediatric pulmonary hypertension: Guidelines from the American Heart Association and American Thoracic Society. Circulation. 2015 Nov 24;132(21):2037–99.

23. Mourani P, Mullen M, Abman SH. Pulmonary hypertension in bronchopulmonary dysplasia. Prog Pediatr Cardiol. 2009;27(1–2):43–8.

24. Abman SH. Monitoring cardiovascular function in infants with chronic lung disease of prematurity. Arch Dis Child Fetal Neonatal Ed. 2002;87(1):F15–8. Pubmed Central PMCID: 1721426.

25. Dhillon R. The management of neonatal pulmonary hypertension. Arch Dis Child Fetal Neonatal Ed. 2012;97(3):F223–8.

26. Khemani E, McElhinney DB, Rhein L, Andrade O, Lacro RV, Thomas KC, et al. Pulmonary artery hypertension in formerly premature infants with bronchopulmonary dysplasia: clinical features and outcomes in the surfactant era. Pediatrics. 2007;120(6):1260–9.

27. Vrijlandt EJ, Gerritsen J, Boezen HM, Grevink RG, Duiverman EJ. Lung function and exercise capacity in young adults born prematurely. Am J Respir Crit Care Med. 2006;173(8):890–6.

28. Landry JS, Chan T, Lands L, Menzies D. Long-term impact of bronchopulmonary dysplasia on pulmonary function. Canad Respir J. 2011;18(5):265–70. Pubmed Central PMCID: 3267603.

29. Wright CJ, Kirpalani H. Targeting inflammation to prevent bronchopulmonary dysplasia: can new insights be translated into therapies? Pediatrics. 2011;128(1):111–26. Pubmed Central PMCID: 3124103.
30. Doyle LW, Ehrenkranz RA, Halliday HL. Postnatal hydrocortisone for preventing or treating bronchopulmonary dysplasia in preterm infants: a systematic review. Neonatology. 2010;98(2):111–7.
31. Onland W, Offringa M, van Kaam A. Late (>/= 7 days) inhalation corticosteroids to reduce bronchopulmonary dysplasia in preterm infants. Cochrane Database Syst Rev. 2012;4, CD002311.
32. ad hoc Statement Committee ATS. Mechanisms and limits of induced postnatal lung growth. Am J Respir Crit Care Med. 2004;170(3):319–43.
33. Baraldi E, Filippone M. Chronic lung disease after premature birth. N Engl J Med. 2007;357(19):1946–55.
34. Sterni LM et al. An official American Thoracic Society clinical practice guideline: Pediatric chronic home invasive ventilation. Am J Respir Crit Care Med. 2016 Apr 15;193(8):e16–35.
35. Lee KS, Sun MR, Ernst A, Feller-Kopman D, Majid A, Boiselle PM. Comparison of dynamic expiratory CT with bronchoscopy for diagnosing airway malacia: a pilot evaluation. Chest. 2007;131(3):758–64.
36. Kim DH, Kim HS, Choi CW, Kim EK, Kim BI, Choi JH. Risk factors for pulmonary artery hypertension in preterm infants with moderate or severe bronchopulmonary dysplasia. Neonatology. 2012;101(1):40–6.
37. An HS, Bae EJ, Kim GB, Kwon BS, Beak JS, Kim EK, et al. Pulmonary hypertension in preterm infants with bronchopulmonary dysplasia. Korean Circ J. 2010;40(3):131–6. Pubmed Central PMCID: 2844979.
38. Slaughter JL, Pakrashi T, Jones DE, South AP, Shah TA. Echocardiographic detection of pulmonary hypertension in extremely low birth weight infants with bronchopulmonary dysplasia requiring prolonged positive pressure ventilation. J Perinatol. 2011;31(10):635–40.
39. Bhat R, Salas AA, Foster C, Carlo WA, Ambalavanan N. Prospective analysis of pulmonary hypertension in extremely low birth weight infants. Pediatrics. 2012;129(3):e682–9. Pubmed Central PMCID: 3289526.
40. Kumar VH, Hutchison AA, Lakshminrusimha S, Morin 3rd FC, Wynn RJ, Ryan RM. Characteristics of pulmonary hypertension in preterm neonates. J Perinatol. 2007;27(4):214–9.
41. Sharma PB, Baroody F, Gozal D, Lester LA. Obstructive sleep apnea in the formerly preterm infant: an overlooked diagnosis. Front Neurol. 2011;2:73. Pubmed Central PMCID: 3226060.
42. Graham RJ, Fleegler EW, Robinson WM. Chronic ventilator need in the community: a 2005 pediatric census of Massachusetts. Pediatrics. 2007;119(6):e1280–7.
43. Sakashita K, Matthews WJ, Yamamoto LG. Disaster preparedness for technology and electricity-dependent children and youth with special health care needs. Clin Pediatr. 2013;52(6):549–56.
44. Kun SS, Davidson-Ward SL, Hulse LM, Keens TG. How much do primary care givers know about tracheostomy and home ventilator emergency care? Pediatr Pulmonol. 2010;45(3):270–4.
45. Kun SS, Edwards JD, Ward SL, Keens TG. Hospital readmissions for newly discharged pediatric home mechanical ventilation patients. Pediatr Pulmonol. 2012;47(4):409–14. Pubmed Central PMCID: 3694986.
46. Panitch HB. Viral respiratory infections in children with technology dependence and neuromuscular disorders. Pediatr Infect Dis J. 2004;23(11 Suppl):S222–7.
47. Chidekel AS, Rosen CL, Bazzy AR. Rhinovirus infection associated with serious lower respiratory illness in patients with bronchopulmonary dysplasia. Pediatr Infect Dis J. 1997;16(1):43–7.
48. American Academy of Pediatrics Committee on Infectious Diseases, American Academy of Pediatrics Bronchiolitis Guidelines C. Updated guidance for palivizumab prophylaxis among infants and young children at increased risk of hospitalization for respiratory syncytial virus infection. Pediatrics. 2014;134(2):415–20.
49. Hsu KK, Shea KM, Stevenson AE, Pelton SI, Members of the Massachusetts Department of Public H. Underlying conditions in children with invasive pneumococcal disease in the conjugate vaccine era. Pediatr Infect Dis J. 2011;30(3):251–3.

Chapter 16
Chronic Ventilatory Support for Children Following Trauma or Severe Neurologic Injury

Iris A. Perez, Sally L. Davidson Ward, Sheila Kun, and Thomas G. Keens

Introduction

Trauma is a leading cause of death in children and can result in significant morbidity in survivors. The most common causes of traumatic injuries in childhood are falls, motor vehicle accidents (MVA), sports, and inflicted injuries. With advances in resuscitation and acute care, the majority of children now survive ([1, 2]. However, those who survive can suffer from long-term disabilities and are at high risk of pulmonary complications including acute and chronic respiratory failure, sleep-related breathing disorders, dysphagia leading to recurrent aspiration, and ventilator-associated pneumonia, atelectasis, and pneumothorax. Other complications associated with trauma include pulmonary embolism, cardiopulmonary arrest not resulting in death, central nervous system (CNS) infection, progression of original neurologic insult, and seizure [3]. All of these conditions can lead to chronic respiratory failure and the need for prolonged ventilatory support. In this chapter, we review the pulmonary complications of trauma, the pathophysiology of respiratory failure, and the long-term care of trauma survivors needing chronic assisted ventilation and respiratory care.

Many pediatric trauma victims do well and can be discharged to home, but some cannot and may require extended care. In one pediatric series, 8 of 14 patients were readmitted to a rehabilitation center because of the consequences of severe cerebral injuries or injuries to extremities. One patient had to be transferred to a nursing home due to prolonged coma, and the remaining five children were admitted to an acute care facility [4].

I.A. Perez, M.D. (✉) • S.L.D. Ward, M.D. • S. Kun, R.N., M.S. • T.G. Keens, M.D.
Division of Pediatric Pulmonology and Sleep Medicine, Children's Hospital Los Angeles,
Keck School of Medicine of the University of Southern California,
4650 Sunset Blvd, Box #83, Los Angeles, CA 90027, USA
e-mail: iaperez@chla.usc.edu; sward@chla.usc.edu; skun@chla.usc.edu; tkeens@chla.usc.edu

© Springer Science+Business Media New York 2016   311
L.M. Sterni, J.L. Carroll (eds.), *Caring for the Ventilator Dependent Child*,
Respiratory Medicine, DOI 10.1007/978-1-4939-3749-3_16

Mechanisms of Injury

The most common causes of disability and death from trauma are cerebral, cervical, thoracic, and abdominal injuries [1, 2]. The outcome of trauma patients is primarily impacted by severity of the injury to the brain and other neural structures [4].

Traumatic Brain Injury

Traumatic brain injury (TBI) is most commonly seen in young children 0–4 years of age and older adolescents [5], males [5], and those living in urban areas and from lower socioeconomic status [6]. Other risk factors include attention-deficit disorder and behavioral difficulties [7]. In the United States, falls are the overall leading cause of TBI [5]. In adolescents, TBI most commonly results from motor vehicle occupant accidents [8], while assault or abuse is the most common cause in infants. Outcome of inflicted TBI is poor with a mortality rate of up to 30 %. Furthermore, it is associated with significant morbidity with long-term neurologic sequelae [9].

Head injuries are very common in childhood due to several factors. Children have a greater head to body ratio, and their brain is less myelinated, and hence they are more easily injured. In addition, the cranial bones are thinner and thus afford less protection [10]. Severe head injury results in increased risk of developing intra-cranial hypertension and "malignant brain edema" [11, 12] making the child vulnerable to secondary brain injury and severe neurologic dysfunction.

Pulmonary problems frequently complicate moderate to severe traumatic brain injury. Most pulmonary complications are directly related to the trauma itself such as pneumothorax and flail chest but can also result from the severe neurologic deficits due to the TBI. Respiratory complications associated with neurologic injury include aspiration pneumonia, atelectasis, and prolonged mechanical ventilation [13]. Pediatric trauma patients older than 10 years of age with head injury and an injury severity score over 25 may be at risk for ventilator-associated pneumonia [14]. The incidence of dysphagia is high in children with severe TBI with Glasgow Coma Scale of ≤8.5 and a ventilation period of ≥1.5 days following MVA [15].

Karanjia et al. reported an overall rate of reintubation of 7.9 % following any type of neurologic injury in patients aged 12–92 years admitted to neurocritical care unit of a tertiary hospital. Of those with primary brain injury, the overall rate of reintubation within 72 h was 6.1 %. The most common cause of reintubation was respiratory distress secondary to altered mental status. These patients had prolonged hypoventilation, indicating a respiratory control abnormality. Atelectasis and decreased minute ventilation are common and result in ventilation perfusion mismatch and eventual respiratory failure. Aspiration and nosocomial pneumonias were also identified as risk factors for reintubation [16].

Spinal Cord Injury

Traumatic spine injuries in children are relatively rare although the true incidence is underestimated due to on-scene mortality or death during transport [17, 18]. The most common mechanism of injury is motor vehicle accidents, accounting for 62 % in one series [18]. Non-accidental trauma accounted for 20 % of injuries in children aged 0–3 years [18]. In younger children, spine injuries most commonly involve the high cervical spine (0–C4) [17, 18], while C4–C8 lesions are more common in older children and adolescents [19]. Infants and younger children are more susceptible to cervical spine injuries due to their disproportionately large head, underdeveloped neck musculature, and decreased motor control [20]. The majority of spinal fractures have associated injuries, most commonly involving the thorax [18] followed by abdominal, head, skeletal, and neurologic injuries.

Traumatic injuries to the spinal cord result in paralysis of the muscles innervated by segments caudal to the involved spinal cord segment. More than half of all spinal cord injury (SCI) syndromes involve the cervical cord resulting in interruption of descending neural pathways that control ventilatory muscles [21]. Injury to one of the eight cervical segments of the spinal cord results in tetraplegia, while lesions involving thoracic, lumbar, or sacral regions result in paraplegia. The higher and more complete the motor level of injury, the greater the respiratory muscle impairment [22]. Injuries above the level of the phrenic motoneurons (C3–C5) cause complete paralysis of the diaphragm as well as other muscles of inspiration and expiration and often lead to the need for mechanical ventilation. In one study of adult patients, those with injuries of C5 and above had severe respiratory failure requiring tracheostomy. Furthermore, all surviving patients with injury at the level of C4 and above still needed ventilatory support at discharge [23]. The presence of associated injuries also contributes to need for ventilatory support [23]. In cervical injury below C5, the diaphragm may still function but the intercostal muscles may be paralyzed. Furthermore, the abdominal muscles when paralyzed eliminate the ability to cough.

Spinal cord injury results in decreased lung compliance, chest wall distortion, and impairment in both inspiratory and expiratory muscle function. There is a reduction in vital capacity to 20–50 % predicted, inefficiency in ventilation, and markedly impaired cough [22]. Scanlon et al. reported that the reduction in lung compliance occurs within a month of injury [24]. Although chest wall compliance is also reduced [24], the abdominal wall is highly compliant [25]. Thus inefficient ventilation (high energy cost for the ventilation achieved) occurs, resulting in risk of respiratory muscle fatigue that is exacerbated when there is an increase in respiratory load as with pneumonia or airway obstruction [26].

Partial recovery of respiratory muscle performance may occur over the year following injury with improvement in FEV1 and FVC [27]. This is dependent on the level and completeness of the injury, the extent of spontaneous recovery, and associated factors such as history of chest injury or operation, asthma, wheezing, or maximal inspiratory pressure [28]. Although partial recovery of ventilatory function in the acute phase of cervical cord injury is frequently seen, many patients enter rehabilitation facilities on mechanical ventilation, and some will require long-term mechanical ventilation.

Thoracic Injuries

Chest trauma in children often indicates severe injury. Thoracic injuries occur infrequently but, when present, occur in association with head and abdominal injuries [29]. Chest injuries may accompany spinal trauma in children and adolescents [18]. Due to the elasticity of the chest, rib fractures are rare and the energy is transmitted to the thoracic contents. Therefore, pulmonary contusion-laceration is the most commonly reported injury after severe blunt chest trauma in children. Other injuries include hemopneumothorax, ruptured diaphragm, and tracheobronchial injury [29]. In adults, pulmonary contusion of 20 % of the lung volume is a risk factor for respiratory failure and acute respiratory distress syndrome [30]. However, this may not occur in children. Hamrick reported that in children, a similar degree of pulmonary contusion did not result in the same morbidity as adult population. In this series, none of the children with pulmonary contusions required intubation, none died, and the mean length of hospital stay was 3.9 days [31]. Therefore, unlike adults, children who recover from pulmonary contusion-laceration usually do not suffer from significant respiratory problems [32].

Development of Chronic Respiratory Failure Following Trauma

To sustain spontaneous ventilation, adequate function of all components of the respiratory system, i.e., neurologic control of breathing, ventilatory muscles, and lung mechanics, must be present. When any of these components is impaired, the child's ability to breathe spontaneously may be impaired and respiratory failure may ensue. Specifically, when ventilatory muscle power and central respiratory drive are sufficiently decreased and thus unable to overcome the respiratory load, respiratory failure results (Fig. 16.1). If the cause of this imbalance is not reversed, chronic respiratory failure occurs and chronic ventilator support will therefore be required [33]. Children who survive trauma or neurologic injury are at risk for developing chronic respiratory failure as listed in Table 16.1.

The outcome of patients suffering from trauma is generally good with many patients weaned off mechanically assisted ventilation. In the acute phase, the goal is for the child to be weaned from the ventilator by addressing potential barriers to weaning. Keeping the respiratory system balance in mind (Fig. 16.1), this can be achieved by directing the therapy toward reducing the respiratory load, improving ventilatory muscle power, and increasing central respiratory drive.

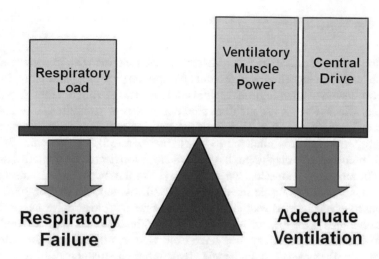

Fig. 16.1 The respiratory balance. In normal individuals, adequate ventilation occurs when the ventilatory muscle power and central drive are greater to overcome the respiratory load, tipping the balance to the right. However, when ventilatory muscle power and central drive are decreased and/or the respiratory load is increased, the ventilatory muscle power and central drive may not be adequate to overcome the respiratory load. Thus, the balance will tip to the left, and respiratory failure will result

Table 16.1   Factors contributing to chronic respiratory failure following trauma

Increased respiratory load	Reduced ventilatory muscle power	Decreased central respiratory drive
Aspiration pneumonia	Tetraplegia/paraplegia	Seizure
Ventilator-associated pneumonia	Cerebral palsy	Encephalopathy
Atelectasis	Scoliosis	Intracranial hypertension
Airway obstruction	Hypoxia	Metabolic alkalosis
Hemopneumothorax	Hypercapnia	Intracranial hemorrhage
Flail chest	Acidosis	Narcotics; anxiolytics
Obesity	Hyperinflation	
	Malnutrition	
	Narcotics; anxiolytics	

Reduce the Respiratory Load

In order to reduce the respiratory load, the pulmonary mechanics must be optimized. Strategies include treatment of infection with appropriate antibiotics; prevention of ventilator-associated pneumonia and aspiration pneumonia, addressing pneumo- or hemothorax; and promotion of appropriate airway clearance with chest physiotherapy, inhaled bronchodilators, and use of anti-inflammatory agents. Acute respiratory distress syndrome when present must be aggressively managed. When diuretics are used careful attention to electrolyte balance is required as metabolic alkalosis can hinder respiratory drive.

Increase Ventilatory Muscle Power

Attention to the optimization of ventilatory muscle function is an important adjunct to the treatment of any child with prolonged respiratory failure, particularly in those who have sustained neurologic and spinal cord injuries. Ventilatory muscle power is adversely affected by many conditions commonly present in children suffering from trauma and neurologic injury. Fatigue of the ventilatory muscles occurs when muscle energy production is hindered [34–38]. Hypoxia [38], hypercapnia [39], and acidosis predispose to diaphragm fatigue. Malnutrition decreases oxidative energy-producing enzymes in muscle. Hyperinflation places the diaphragm at a mechanical disadvantage because muscle fibers are short and develop less tension [40]. If the child has received assisted ventilation for some time, muscle atrophy and decreased oxidative capacity may occur from disuse [35]. Thus, a child who suffered from trauma and neurologic injury may have decreased ventilatory muscle endurance associated with hypoxia, hypercapnia, hyperinflation, malnutrition, and disuse. Therefore, therapy should be directed toward adequate oxygenation and ventilation, removal of airway obstruction and hyperinflation, adequate nutrition, and ventilatory muscle training [34, 35]. Pharmacologic neuromuscular blockade, sedation, and pain medications may also decrease ventilatory muscle function. When possible, these medications should be weaned as tolerated [41].

Ventilator weaning techniques should be designed to improve ventilatory muscle power in an attempt to raise the child's fatigue threshold (Fig. 16.2). The authors recommend a sprint weaning approach similar to athletic training of any other skeletal muscle [35]. Athletes train for performance by bursts of muscle activity (training stress) followed by rest periods. To achieve this, we adjust the ventilator settings to completely meet the child's ventilatory demands by the use of a physiologic ventilator rate for age and the attainment of normal noninvasive monitoring of gas exchange ($S_pO_2 \geq 95\%$ and end-tidal Pco_2 [$P_{ET}co_2$] of 30–35 Torr). The goal is to provide total ventilatory muscle rest. The patient is then removed from the ventilator for short periods of time during wakefulness. The authors refer to this time off the ventilator as a sprint. The child is carefully monitored noninvasively during sprints to prevent hypoxia or hypercapnia, using pulse oximetry and $P_{ET}co_2$ monitoring. Increased supplemental oxygen may be required during sprinting. The sprint is terminated for $S_pO_2 < 95\%$, $PETco_2 > 45$–50 Torr, or if the child shows signs of respiratory distress, cyanosis, tachypnea, retractions, diaphoresis, or tachycardia. However, it is important to remember that the child who has a respiratory control disorder may not exhibit respiratory distress. The length of each sprint is increased daily as tolerated. Initially, sprinting should be performed only during wakefulness, as ventilatory muscle function and central respiratory drive are more intact during wakefulness than during sleep. When the child is weaned off the ventilator completely during wakefulness, sprint during sleep is initiated [41]. Prior to weaning off the ventilator during sleep, we perform a polysomnogram off the ventilator to determine adequacy of gas exchange. We cannot overemphasize the importance of complete ventilatory support during rests. Because sprint weaning simulates athletic

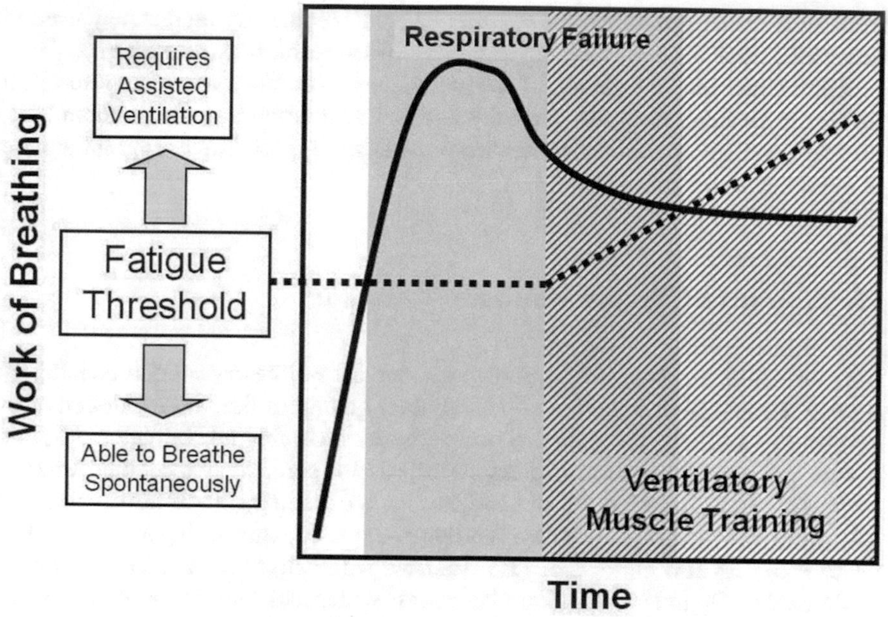

Fig. 16.2 Ventilatory muscle training. Mechanically assisted ventilation (shaded area) is required when the work of breathing (*Y* axis) exceeds the fatigue threshold. Ventilatory muscle training may increase the work of breathing that the patient can perform (hatched area), raising the fatigue threshold until it exceeds the work of breathing required. Respiratory failure overlaps ventilatory muscle training until the fatigue threshold exceeds the required work of breathing. Then, the child can perform the work of breathing required to breathe spontaneously and can be weaned from the ventilator

training, better success has been observed with this form of ventilator weaning particularly when ventilatory muscle fatigue is thought to be a component. In effect, this technique raises the fatigue threshold, so that a child can perform an increased level of work of breathing and sustain adequate spontaneous ventilation [35].

Improve Central Respiratory Drive

In general central respiratory stimulants are not effective. Swaminathan demonstrated no effect of theophylline on ventilatory responses to hypercapnia or hypoxia in normal subjects [42]. Since central respiratory drive can be inhibited by chronic metabolic alkalosis, electrolyte balance should be maintained, with maintenance of serum chloride concentrations >95 mEq/dL and avoiding alkalosis. Chronic hypoxia and/or hypercapnia may cause habituation of chemoreceptors, leading to a decrease in central respiratory center stimulation, and decreased central respiratory drive. Narcotic analgesia and benzodiazepine anxiolytics may need to be weaned prior to sprint weaning as these are also respiratory depressants.

Appropriate implementation of the techniques as outlined above may result in successful weaning from mechanically assisted ventilation in these children [41]. However, some may continue to require ventilatory support despite appropriate use of the above techniques [33].

Philosophy of Chronic Ventilatory Support

For some children who survive trauma, weaning off ventilatory support completely is not a realistic goal. In order to optimize their quality of life, these children must have energy available for other physical activities including rehabilitation. For this reason, it is important that ventilators are adjusted to completely meet their ventilatory demands. The authors adjust ventilators to provide a $P_{ET}CO_2$ of 30–35 Torr and a $S_pO_2 \geq 95\%$. For children who are ventilator dependent only during sleep, ventilating to $PCO_2 \leq 35$ Torr during sleep is associated with better spontaneous ventilation while awake. Optimal ventilation also avoids atelectasis and the development of coexisting lung disease. It has also been our experience that children who receive chronic ventilatory support actually have fewer complications and generally do better clinically, with some degree of hyperventilation during assisted ventilation. Since hypoventilation is more severe during sleep than during wakefulness, nocturnal assisted ventilation often prevents the development of pulmonary hypertension and other complications of chronic intermittent hypoxia and hypercapnia [43]. Nocturnal ventilation allows ventilatory muscle rest and improves endurance for spontaneous breathing while awake; therefore, it is actually associated with an enhanced quality of life [44].

Modes of Ventilation

Portable Positive Pressure Ventilator via Tracheostomy

Positive pressure ventilation (PPV) via tracheostomy is a common method of providing assisted ventilation [44, 45]. For home mechanical ventilation, we advocate the use of relatively small, uncuffed tracheostomy tubes for the following reasons: (a) minimize the risk of tracheomalacia or tracheal mucosal damage, (b) allow an expiratory leak so that the child may speak, (c) allow use of a one-way, positive-closure speaking valve to enable the child to phonate and prevent aspiration during swallowing, and (d) provide a margin of safety because the child may still be able to ventilate around the tracheostomy tube should the tracheostomy plug. The disadvantage of using small, uncuffed tracheostomy tubes includes the presence of leaks, which can be large and variable, especially in small children. Periodic assessment of the degree of leak around the tracheostomy tube and upsizing the tube as the child grows is required. While we advocate a small, uncuffed tracheostomy tube, some patients require a customized length or an extension from the stoma site. In spite of pressure-limited ventilation, a few children, especially the older ones, might need cuffed tubes to decrease the leak and allow better ventilation during sleep. During wakefulness, the cuffed tubes can be deflated to allow speech. Occasionally, the cuffed tubes do not even need to be inflated to decrease the air leak and to improve ventilation. Placing a deflated cuffed tracheostomy tube may increase the resistance above the tracheostomy enough to decrease the leak and achieve adequate ventilation [41, 44].

Noninvasive Positive Pressure Ventilation

Noninvasive positive pressure ventilation (NPPV) can be used in children who require ventilatory support only during sleep and who have relatively mild intrinsic lung disease. NPPV is usually delivered via a nasal mask but nasal prongs or face mask can also be used [16, 45–48].

Patients with primary brain injury and encephalopathy who have intact cough and gag reflexes may benefit from trial of noninvasive ventilatory support to reduce atelectasis and facilitate alveoli recruitment [46]. In one study, the implementation of nighttime bi-level NPPV was successful in limiting atelectasis without apparent increase in the risk of aspiration pneumonia [16]. Noninvasive ventilator support has been used to prevent endotracheal intubation in adults with acute spinal cord injury [49] and support the terminal phase of weaning from mechanical ventilation [49, 50].

NPPV is best suited for those who require only ventilator support at night. Noninvasive ventilation is not usually used 24 h/day, because the mask interferes with daily activities and social interaction; therefore, it would not be helpful in patients who require rehabilitation during the day. Moreover, the risk of skin breakdown increases significantly with prolonged mask use. Because of the risk of aspiration, children who are unable to remove their own masks should not have full-face masks unless they are closely observed. Although, NPPV is not ideal in those who need 24-h ventilatory support, it may be considered as a palliative tool.

Noninvasive bi-level ventilation is not as powerful as PPV via tracheostomy. Thus, these children may require intubation and more sophisticated ventilatory support during acute illnesses.

Diaphragm Pacing via Phrenic Nerve Stimulation and Diaphragm Muscle Pacing

Diaphragm pacing (DP) may provide adequate ventilatory support in patients who become quadriplegic or have central hypoventilation following trauma [51]. Diaphragm pacing requires a functional phrenic nerve, hence, may not be effective in patients with C3–C5 spinal cord injury. Each hemidiaphragm is innervated by a phrenic nerve, which is formed from the C3–C5 cervical roots. With C3–C5 spinal cord injury, damage to the phrenic motoneurons and axons may occur resulting in inadequate phrenic nerve function [52]. Therefore patients with C3–C5 spinal cord injury may not be ideal candidates for DP by phrenic nerve stimulation The involvement of the phrenic nerve may only be determined at the time of surgery. Thus, when this is considered in patients with C3–C5 spinal cord injury, patient and parents must be aware that there is the possibility that diaphragm pacing by phrenic nerve stimulation may not work.

Diaphragm pacing involves direct simulation of the phrenic nerve with subsequent diaphragm movement producing respiration. It involves surgical implantation of the phrenic nerve electrode thoracoscopically or via cervical approach. At our center, thoracic placement of the phrenic nerve electrodes is done thoracoscopically [53]. The electrode wires are connected to two implanted radiofrequency receivers which are usually positioned superficially over the anterior chest wall or abdomen. Two antennas are positioned over each receiver and connected to an external radio transmitter [53, 54]. As opposed to a traditional mechanical ventilator, diaphragm pacing uses the child's own diaphragm as the "ventilator" pump. The external transmitter, which is portable and battery operated, generates electrical energy similar to radio frequency via an external antenna that is placed over the receiver. The receiver converts the energy to electrical current that is then conducted to the phrenic nerve, stimulating diaphragm contraction.

Le Pimpec-Barthes et al. reported ventilator weaning in 18/20 patients who were full-time ventilator dependent (19 from posttraumatic tetraplegia, 1 with CCHS). One elderly woman with a 4-year history of tetraplegia was not able to be weaned. She exhibited profound diaphragmatic amyotrophy during preoperative testing. One patient with severe malnutrition despite aggressive enteral and parenteral management recovered only partially and eventually gave up stimulation attempts. All the patients weaned from mechanical ventilation have reported improved quality of life, improved mobility, and better quality sleep [55].

Based on our experience with diaphragm pacing in patients with congenital central hypoventilation syndrome, we do not prescribe full-time use of the diaphragm pacers via phrenic nerve stimulation because of the risk of diaphragm fatigue. Thus, the patients with high cervical spinal cord injury may use diaphragm pacing during the day, but they will need to be on the ventilator via tracheostomy at night. Moreover, we have observed failure with diaphragm pacing in patients who are obese or who have become overweight. In those who require ventilatory support via diaphragm pacers only during sleep, decannulation of the tracheostomy has been possible. Virtually all of these patients have snoring and must be monitored for obstructive sleep apnea. If present we have adjusted the pacer settings by decreasing the tidal volume to decrease the force of inspiration with each diaphragm contraction and thus generate less negative pressure and less chance of collapse [54].

Another form of diaphragm pacing is provided via intramuscular diaphragm pacing. In this method, intramuscular electrodes are implanted laparoscopically in each diaphragm with leads tunneled subcutaneously to an exit site in the chest, where they are brought out through the skin and connected to external stimulator. In their series, Onders et al. showed good outcomes in adults who sustained cervical SCI as children and received intramuscular diaphragm pacing as adults. Of these patients, eight tolerated the surgical implantation, four utilized the pacing full time, four paced during day only, and two were still actively conditioning their diaphragms [56]. Similar to adults, Onders et al. also reported successful outcome in ventilator-dependent pediatric spinal cord-injured patients who were placed on intramuscular DP. Two patients went to full-time pacing without mechanical ventilation. One of the patients received implantation on day 1 and never returned to positive pressure mechanical ventilation and, after 3 weeks of full-time pacing, was weaned off DP and was decannulated. The other four paced for 8–23 h a day but were still conditioning and progressively weaning from the ventilator [57]. In addition to independence from the ventilator, intramuscular diaphragm pacing has been reported to decrease secretions and need for suctioning [58].

Respiratory Treatments

Pulmonary complications can be minimized by instituting strategies that improve airway clearance such as chest physiotherapy, use of cough assist device, inhaled bronchodilators, and use of anti-inflammatory agents.

Bronchodilators/Beta Adrenergic Agonists

Bronchodilators are an important component in the care of children who survive trauma. Several studies support the role of bronchodilators to help improve airway clearance, cough effectiveness, and respiratory symptoms. Patients with tetraplegia may have unsuspected small airway obstruction. Spungen et al. found that administration of B2 agonist metaproterenol sulfate to 34 subjects with chronic tetraplegia resulted in significant increase in FEV_1 ($\geq 12\%$ and 200 mL) in 41 % of subjects [59]. This heightened responsiveness is postulated to be due to interruption of sympathetic innervations to the lung resulting in parasympathetic (bronchoconstrictive) predominance [60]. In addition, a significant increase in FEV_1 and in sGaw is seen following inhalation of the anti-cholinergic agent ipratropium bromide [61, 62]. Patients with tetraplegia also demonstrate airway hyperresponsiveness in response to methacholine, histamine, and ultrasonically nebulized distilled water [63, 64]. Grimm reported that patients with tetraplegia who responded to antihistamine were found to have reduced airway caliber on spirometric measurements. The proposed mechanisms for reduced baseline airway caliber relative to lung size in patients with tetraplegia include unopposed parasympathetic activity secondary to the loss of sympathetic innervation to the lungs and/or the inability to stretch the airway smooth muscle with deep inhalation [64]. Long-term administration of a long-acting *B*2 adrenergic agonist improved pulmonary function parameters and static mouth pressure among subjects with tetraplegia [60]. During the 4-week period of salmeterol administration, FVC, FEV_1, PEF, MIP, and MEP improved indicating improvement in respiratory muscle strength which may increase cough effectiveness [60] and lead to prevention of atelectasis and pneumonia.

Assisted cough: Patients with spinal cord injuries may have impaired cough and will have accumulation of secretions that can lead to atelectasis and pneumonias. Several methods are available to deal with secretions in association with chest physiotherapy. One of these methods is the use of mechanical insufflation-exsufflation device (cough assist) via face mask or tracheostomy tube. This device provides a positive pressure breath followed by negative pressure to help mobilize airway mucus and secretions during exhalation. In those without an artificial airway, mouth application may result in discomfort during the negative pressure phase or cause collapse of the oropharyngeal muscles. The cough assist device can be used frequently, particularly during an acute respiratory illness. The use of the device has resulted in reduced hospitalization and improved quality of life in children with neuromuscular disorders and their families ([65]). It is recommended in children with neuromuscular disorders with impaired cough [66, 67] and may have a role in patients who survive trauma and neurologic injury.

Respiratory Muscle Training

Respiratory muscle training targeted at both endurance and strength has been found to provide improvement and enhance performance in patients with tetraplegia [68–70]. This involves both resistive inspiratory muscle training [69] and expiratory muscle training [68]. Neck breathing, an alternative method of voluntary respiration using neck accessory muscles, has been found to be successful in liberating quadriplegic children with acute C2 injury from the ventilator up to 12 h (average of 3.5 h). To accomplish neck breathing in one report, neck strengthening was begun as soon as the patient was considered medically stable. Strengthening of the neck muscles was done through manual resistive exercises and through activities using oral motor control such as driving an electric wheelchair or a computer or video game mouth sticks. When the patient was able to generate 10–15 cm H_2O of negative pressure, successful neck breathing was accomplished [71].

A glossopharyngeal breathing technique using the muscles of the mouth, throat, and larynx as an accessory respiratory system has been described. In this method, inspiration is achieved through the active generation of positive pressure in the upper airway by means of a series of pumping motions by the tongue and pharynx. The larynx rhythmically opens and closes for each stroke. After a series of strokes, the larynx subsequently relaxes and passive expiration occurs [72].

Nutrition

Malnutrition decreases strength by decreasing muscle mass and decreases endurance by decreasing muscle oxidative enzymes. When adequate nutrition cannot be achieved safely by oral feedings, gastrostomy tube may be indicated, as malnutrition will further weaken the ventilatory muscles.

Because of limited mobility and physical activity, patients who survive trauma are at increased risk of obesity. Patients with spinal cord injury (SCI) typically have lean body mass in the lower extremities, with increased abdominal and lower extremity fat tissue accumulation [73, 74]. Adults with SCI have been shown to have increased prevalence of obesity [75]. Furthermore, Nelson et al. found metabolic syndrome in adolescents with SCI [76, 77]. Therefore, regular involvement of a dietitian is necessary and should be part of the care of patients with quadriplegia following SCI.

Dysphagia Evaluation

Studies have shown that patients with traumatic brain injury [78], tetraplegia [79], those with tracheostomies [80], and trauma patients treated with halo-vest fixation [81] are at risk for dysphagia. Swallowing dysfunction can lead to hypoxemia, chemical pneumonitis, mechanical obstruction, atelectasis, and bronchospasm. Therefore, it is imperative that these patients undergo early and accurate evaluation. This can be performed by bedside evaluation with a speech pathologist or occupational therapist followed by videofluoroscopic endoscopic swallow study or modified barium swallow study as necessary. When dysphagia is identified, patients should then be followed closely by speech or occupational therapist for feeding therapy. Some patients may benefit with the use of Passy-Muir valve (PMV), a one-way silicone diaphragm check valve that fits over the end of the tracheostomy tube. The valve opens during inspiration and closes during exhalation, and the exhaled air passes through the upper airway including the vocal cords, thus allowing for phonation. It has been found to decrease the incidence of aspiration and improve swallowing function in some patients with tracheostomy [82] but not in others [79]. When severe dysphagia is present, placement of gastrostomy or jejunal tube may be required.

Follow-Up Studies and Monitoring

Polysomnography

In patients who are ventilator dependent, it is important to regularly check and readjust settings to ensure adequacy of ventilation. These evaluations are usually performed by polysomnogram. If the child is relatively stable, daytime polysomnograms may be adequate. Sleep studies may also be used to predict the success of sprint weaning during sleep when sprinting schedules are advancing in the home. When a sleep laboratory is not available, an overnight hospital admission with continuous recording of S_pO_2 and $P_{ET}CO_2$ may be sufficient to assess the adequacy of ventilator settings.

Echocardiogram

Ventilator-dependent patients are at risk for pulmonary hypertension and cor pulmonale because home mechanical ventilation may not completely meet the ventilatory requirements at all times. Because clinical right heart failure may not be recognized right away, we suggest periodic echocardiogram for following right heart function. When pulmonary hypertension is identified, it should be assumed that it is due to inadequate ventilation until proven otherwise and the patient should be hospitalized for continuous noninvasive monitoring of gas exchange and ventilator adjustments.

Monitoring for Sleep Issues and Sleep-Related Breathing Disorders

Children with traumatic brain injury are at increased risk of sleep disturbances including sleep apnea, periodic limb movements in sleep, narcolepsy, and parasomnias [83, 84]. Patients with spinal cord injury may be at high risk for sleep-related breathing disorders that include obstructive and central apneas, hypoxemia, and hypoventilation ([85–87]). This may be due to loss of tone and paralysis of intercostal and abdominal muscles and impaired diaphragm function, use of medications such as benzodiazepine and baclofen that may have depressant effects on the respiratory system, obesity, increased abdominal girth, and increased neck circumference [85, 87, 88]. When sleep apnea is suspected by the presence of snoring, observed apneas, night waking, choking, and daytime sleepiness, patients should undergo polysomnography to determine the presence and severity of a sleep-related breathing disorder. Tran et al. report high incidence of obstructive sleep apnea in adults without daytime sleepiness as early as 7 weeks after spinal cord injury. The authors did not find correlation with body mass index, neck circumference, or SpO_2 nadir and therefore suggest consideration for earlier screening even in those who may be asymptomatic [89].

Monitoring for Scoliosis and Restrictive Lung Disease

Children who sustain SCI before puberty experience a higher incidence of scoliosis which may result in restrictive lung disease and therefore must be monitored ([90–92]). In one series, up to 96 % of children had scoliosis, with most having a curve of ≥40° and had undergone surgical correction [93]. In addition to close follow-up by an orthopedist, pulmonary function tests should be performed to monitor for the presence of restrictive lung disease, when feasible.

Conclusion

Children who survive trauma or severe neurologic injury are at risk for respiratory complications due to ventilatory muscle weakness and/or decreased respiratory drive. Ventilatory muscle weakness when severe results in part-time or full-time ventilator dependence. Those who require part-time ventilatory support can be ventilated by noninvasive positive pressure ventilation, while those requiring full-time support are best ventilated by positive pressure ventilation via tracheostomy. Swallowing dysfunction is not uncommon and can lead to aspiration pneumonia. Those who can breathe spontaneously have a high index of suspicion for sleep-related breathing disorder.

References

1. Buschmann C, Kuhne CA, Losch C, Nast-Kolb D, Ruchholtz S. Major trauma with multiple injuries in German children: a retrospective review. J Pediatr Orthop. 2008;28:1–5.
2. Schalamon J, Sarkola T, Nietosvaara Y. Injuries in children associated with the use of nonmotorized scooters. J Pediatr Surg. 2003;38:1612–5.
3. Matsushima K, Schaefer EW, Won EJ, Nichols PA, Frankel HL. Injured adolescents, not just large children: difference in care and outcome between adult and pediatric trauma centers. Am Surg. 2013;79:267–73.
4. van der Sluis CK, Kingma J, Eisma WH, ten Duis HJ. Pediatric polytrauma: short-term and long-term outcomes. J Trauma. 1997;43:501–6.
5. Faul M, Xu L, Wald MM, Coronado V, Dellinger AM. Traumatic brain injury in the United States: National Estimates of Prevalence and Incidence, 2002–2006. Injury Prev. 2010;16:A268.
6. Yates PJ, Williams WH, Harris A, Round A, Jenkins R. An epidemiological study of head injuries in a UK population attending an emergency department. J Neurol Neurosurg Psychiatry. 2006;77:699–701.
7. Keenan HT, Bratton SL. Epidemiology and outcomes of pediatric traumatic brain injury. Dev Neurosci. 2006;28:256–63.
8. Asemota AO, George BP, Bowman SM, Haider AH, Schneider EB. Causes and trends in traumatic brain injury for United States adolescents. J Neurotrauma. 2013;30:67–75.
9. Barlow KM. Traumatic brain injury. Handb Clin Neurol. 2013;112:891–904.
10. Kissoon N, Dreyer J, Walia M. Pediatric trauma: differences in pathophysiology, injury patterns and treatment compared with adult trauma. CMAJ. 1990;142:27–34.

11. Bruce DA, Alavi A, Bilaniuk L, Dolinskas C, Obrist W, Uzzell B. Diffuse cerebral swelling following head injuries in children: the syndrome of "malignant brain edema". J Neurosurg. 1981;54:170–8.

12. Bruce DA, Raphaely RC, Goldberg AI, Zimmerman RA, Bilaniuk LT, Schut L, Kuhl DE. Pathophysiology, treatment and outcome following severe head injury in children. Childs Brain. 1979;5:174–91.

13. Wiercisiewski DR, McDeavitt JT. Pulmonary complications in traumatic brain injury. J Head Trauma Rehabil. 1998;13:28–35.

14. Taira BR, Fenton KE, Lee TK, Meng H, Mccormack JE, Huang E, Singer AJ, Scriven RJ, Shapiro MJ. Ventilator- associated pneumonia in pediatric trauma patients. Pediatr Crit Care Med. 2009;10(4):491–4.

15. Morgan A, Ward E, Murdoch B, Kennedy B, Murison R. Incidence, characteristics and predictive factors for dysphagia after pediatric traumatic brain injury. J Head Trauma Rehabil. 2003;18(3):239–51.

16. Karanjia N, Nordquist D, Stevens R, Nyquist P. A clinical description of extubation failure in patients with primary brain injury. Neurocrit Care. 2011;15:4–12.

17. Cirak B, Ziegfeld S, Knight VM, Chang D, Avellino AM, Paidas CN. Spinal injuries in children. J Pediatr Surg. 2004;39:607–12.

18. Rush JK, Kelly DM, Astur N, Creek A, Dawkins R, Younas S, Warner Jr WC, Sawyer JR. Associated injuries in children and adolescents with spinal trauma. J Pediatr Orthop. 2013;33:393–7.

19. DeVivo MJ, Vogel LC. Epidemiology of spinal cord injury in children and adolescents. J Spinal Cord Med. 2004;27 Suppl 1:S4–10.

20. Jones TM, Anderson PA, Noonan KJ. Pediatric cervical spine trauma. J Am Acad Orthop Surg. 2011;19:600–11.

21. Zimmer MB, Nantwi K, Goshgarian HG. Effect of spinal cord injury on the respiratory system: basic research and current clinical treatment options. J Spinal Cord Med. 2007;30:319–30.

22. Brown R, DiMarco AF, Hoit JD, Garshick E. Respiratory dysfunction and management in spinal cord injury. Respir Care. 2006;51:853–68; discussion 869–70.

23. Como JJ, Sutton ER, McCunn M, Dutton RP, Johnson SB, Aarabi B, Scalea TM. Characterizing the need for mechanical ventilation following cervical spinal cord injury with neurologic deficit. J Trauma. 2005;59:912–6. discussion 916.

24. Scanlon PD, Loring SH, Pichurko BM, McCool FD, Slutsky AS, Sarkarati M, Brown R. Respiratory mechanics in acute quadriplegia. Lung and chest wall compliance and dimensional changes during respiratory maneuvers. Am Rev Respir Dis. 1989;139:615–20.

25. Goldman JM, Williams SJ, Denison DM. The rib cage and abdominal components of respiratory system compliance in tetraplegic patients. Eur Respir J. 1988;1:242–7.

26. Urmey W, Loring S, Mead J, Slutsky AS, Sarkarati M, Rossier A, Brown R. Upper and lower rib cage deformation during breathing in quadriplegics. J Appl Physiol. 1986;60:618–22.

27. Bluechardt MH, Wiens M, Thomas SG, Plyley MJ. Repeated measurements of pulmonary function following spinal cord injury. Paraplegia. 1992;30:768–74.

28. Jain NB, Brown R.Tun CG, Gagnon D, Garshick E. Determinants of Forced Expiratory Volume in 1 Second (FEV-1), Forced Vital Capacity (FVC), and FEV1/FVC in Chronic Spinal Cord Injury. Arch Phys Med Rehabil. 2006;87(10):1327–1333.

29. Shorr RM, Crittenden M, Indeck M, Hartunian SL, Rodriguez A. Blunt thoracic trauma. Analysis of 515 patients. Ann Surg. 1987;206:200–5.

30. Hamrick MC, Duhn RD, Ochsner MG. Critical evaluation of pulmonary contusion in the early post-traumatic period: risk of assisted ventilation. Am Surg. 2009;75:1054–8.

31. Hamrick MC, Duhn RD, Carney DE, Boswell WC, Ochsner MG. Pulmonary contusion in the pediatric population. Am Surg. 2010;76:721–4.

32. Haxhija EQ, Nores H, Schober P, Hollwarth ME. Lung contusion-lacerations after blunt thoracic trauma in children. Pediatr Surg Int. 2004;20:412–4.

33. Make BJ, Hill NS, Goldberg AI, Bach JR, Criner GJ, Dunne PE, Gilmartin ME, Heffner JE, Kacmarek R, Keens TG, McInturff S, O'Donohue Jr WJ, Oppenheimer EA, Robert

D. Mechanical ventilation beyond the intensive care unit. Report of a consensus conference of the American College of Chest Physicians. Chest. 1998;113:289S–344.

34. Keens TG, Bryan AC, Levison H, Ianuzzo CD. Developmental pattern of muscle fiber types in human ventilatory muscles. J Appl Physiol. 1978;44:909–13.

35. Keens TG, Chen V, Patel P, O'Brien P, Levison H, Ianuzzo CD. Cellular adaptations of the ventilatory muscles to a chronic increased respiratory load. J Appl Physiol. 1978;44:905–8.

36. Nickerson BG, Keens TG. Measuring ventilatory muscle endurance in humans as sustainable inspiratory pressure. J Appl Physiol. 1982;52:768–72.

37. Randolph AG, Meert KL, O'Neil ME, Hanson JH, Luckett PM, Arnold JH, Gedeit RG, Cox PN, Roberts JS, Venkataraman ST, Forbes PW, Cheifetz IM, Pediatric Acute Lung I, Sepsis Investigators N. The feasibility of conducting clinical trials in infants and children with acute respiratory failure. Am J Respir Crit Care Med. 2003;167:1334–40.

38. Roussos CS, Macklem PT. Diaphragmatic fatigue in man. J Appl Physiol. 1977;43:189–97.

39. Juan G, Calverley P, Talamo C, Schnader J, Roussos C. Effect of carbon dioxide on diaphragmatic function in human beings. N Engl J Med. 1984;310:874–9.

40. Muller NL, Bryan AC. Chest wall mechanics and respiratory muscles in infants. Pediatr Clin North Am. 1979;26:503–16.

41. Keens TG, Kun S, Ward SLD. Chronic respiratory failure. In: Nichols DG, editor. Roger's textbook of pediatric intensive care. Garland: Lippincott, Williams & Wilkins; 2008. p. 753–66.

42. Swaminathan S, Paton JY, Ward SL, Sargent CW, Keens TG. Theophylline does not increase ventilatory responses to hypercapnia or hypoxia. Am Rev Respir Dis. 1992;146:1398–401.

43. Gilgoff IS, Kahlstrom E, MacLaughlin E, Keens TG. Long-term ventilatory support in spinal muscular atrophy. J Pediatr. 1989;115:904–9.

44. Gilgoff RL, Gilgoff IS. Long-term follow-up of home mechanical ventilation in young children with spinal cord injury and neuromuscular conditions. J Pediatr. 2003;142:476–80.

45. Srinivasan S, Doty SM, White TR, Segura VH, Jansen MT, Davidson Ward SL, Keens TG. Frequency, causes, and outcome of home ventilator failure. Chest. 1998;114:1363–7.

46. Bach JR. Noninvasive respiratory management of high level spinal cord injury. J Spinal Cord Med. 2012;35:72–80.

47. Berry RB, Chediak A, Brown LK, Finder J, Gozal D, Iber C, Kushida CA, Morgenthaler T, Rowley JA, Davidson-Ward SL, NPPV Titration Task Force of the American Academy of Sleep Medicine. Best clinical practices for the sleep center adjustment of noninvasive positive pressure ventilation (NPPV) in stable chronic alveolar hypoventilation syndromes. J Clin Sleep Med. 2010;6:491–509.

48. Fauroux B, Boffa C, Desguerre I, Estournet B, Trang H. Long-term noninvasive mechanical ventilation for children at home: a national survey. Pediatr Pulmonol. 2003;35:119–25.

49. Tromans AM, Mecci M, Barrett FH, Ward TA, Grundy DJ. The use of the BiPAP biphasic positive airway pressure system in acute spinal cord injury. Spinal Cord. 1998;36:481–4.

50. deBoisblanc MW, Goldman RK, Mayberry JC, Brand DM, Pangburn PD, Soifer BE, Mullins RJ. Weaning injured patients with prolonged pulmonary failure from mechanical ventilation in a non-intensive care unit setting. J Trauma. 2000;49:224–30; discussion 230–21.

51. Bolikal P, Bach JR, Goncalves M. Electrophrenic pacing and decannulation for high-level spinal cord injury: a case series. J Spinal Cord Med. 2012;35:170–4.

52. DiMarco AF. Phrenic nerve stimulation in patients with spinal cord injury. Respir Physiol Neurobiol. 2009;169:200–9.

53. Shaul DB, Danielson PD, McComb JG, Keens TG. Thoracoscopic placement of phrenic nerve electrodes for diaphragmatic pacing in children. J Pediatr Surg. 2002;37:974–8; discussion 974–78.

54. Chen ML, Tablizo MA, Kun S, Keens TG. Diaphragm pacers as a treatment for congenital central hypoventilation syndrome. Expert Rev Med Devices. 2005;2:577–85.

55. Le Pimpec-Barthes F, Gonzalez-Bermejo J, Hubsch JP, Duguet A, Morelot-Panzini C, Riquet M, Similowski T. Intrathoracic phrenic pacing: a 10-year experience in France. J Thorac Cardiovasc Surg. 2011;142:378–83.

56. Onders RP, Elmo MJ, Ignagni AR. Diaphragm pacing stimulation system for tetraplegia in individuals injured during childhood or adolescence. J Spinal Cord Med. 2007;30 Suppl 1:S25–9.
57. Onders RP, Ponsky TA, Elmo M, Lidsky K, Barksdale E. First reported experience with intramuscular diaphragm pacing in replacing positive pressure mechanical ventilators in children. J Pediatr Surg. 2011;46:72–6.
58. Onders RP. Functional electrical stimulation: restoration of respiratory function. Handb Clin Neurol. 2012;109:275–82.
59. Spungen AM, Bauman WA, Lesser M, McCool FD. Breathing pattern and ventilatory control in chronic tetraplegia. Lung. 2009;187:375–81.
60. Grimm DR, Schilero GJ, Spungen AM, Bauman WA, Lesser M. Salmeterol improves pulmonary function in persons with tetraplegia. Lung. 2006;184:335–9.
61. Almenoff PL, Alexander LR, Spungen AM, Lesser MD, Bauman WA. Bronchodilatory effects of ipratropium bromide in patients with tetraplegia. Paraplegia. 1995;33:274–7.
62. Schilero GJ, Grimm DR, Bauman WA, Lenner R, Lesser M. Assessment of airway caliber and bronchodilator responsiveness in subjects with spinal cord injury. Chest. 2005;127:149–55.
63. Grimm DR, Arias E, Lesser M, Bauman WA, Almenoff PL. Airway hyperresponsiveness to ultrasonically nebulized distilled water in subjects with tetraplegia. J Appl Physiol. 1999;86:1165–9.
64. Grimm DR, Chandy D, Almenoff PL, Schilero G, Lesser M. Airway hyperreactivity in subjects with tetraplegia is associated with reduced baseline airway caliber. Chest. 2000;118:1397–404.
65. Moran FCE, Spittle A, Delany C, Tobertson CF, Massie J. Effect of home mechanical ventilation in-exsufflation on hospitalization and lifestyle in neuromuscular disease, a pilot study. J Pediatr Child Health. 2013;49(3):233–7.
66. Finder JD. A 2009 Perspective on the 2004 American Thoracic Society statement, "Respiratory care of the patient with duchenne muscular dystrophy". Pediatrics. 2009;123:S239–41.
67. Schroth MK. Special considerations in the respiratory management of spinal muscular atrophy. Pediatrics. 2009;123:S245–49.
68. Roth EJ, Stenson KW, Powley S, Oken J, Primack S, Nussbaum SB, Berkowitz M. Expiratory muscle training in spinal cord injury: a randomized controlled trial. Arch Phys Med Rehabil. 2010;91:857–61.
69. Rutchik A, Weissman AR, Almenoff PL, Spungen AM, Bauman WA, Grimm DR. Resistive inspiratory muscle training in subjects with chronic cervical spinal cord injury. Arch Phys Med Rehabil. 1998;79:293–7.
70. Wang TG, Wang YH, Tang FT, Lin KH, Lien IN. Resistive inspiratory muscle training in sleep-disordered breathing of traumatic tetraplegia. Arch Phys Med Rehabil. 2002;83:491–6.
71. Gilgoff IS, Barras DM, Jones MS, Adkins HV. Neck breathing: a form of voluntary respiration for the spine-injured ventilator-dependent quadriplegic child. Pediatrics. 1988;82:741–5.
72. Collier CR, Dail CW, Affeldt JE. Mechanics of glossopharyngeal breathing. J Appl Physiol. 1956;8:580–4.
73. Bauman WA, Spungen AM. Metabolic changes in persons after spinal cord injury. Phys Med Rehabil Clin N Am. 2000;11:109–40.
74. Liusuwan A, Widman L, Abresch RT, McDonald CM. Altered body composition affects resting energy expenditure and interpretation of body mass index in children with spinal cord injury. J Spinal Cord Med. 2004;27 Suppl 1:S24–8.
75. Gupta N, White KT, Sandford PR. Body mass index in spinal cord injury—a retrospective study. Spinal Cord. 2006;44:92–4.
76. Nelson MD, Widman LM, Abresch RT, Stanhope K, Havel PJ, Styne DM, McDonald CM. Metabolic syndrome in adolescents with spinal cord dysfunction. J Spinal Cord Med. 2007;30 Suppl 1:S127–39.
77. McDonald CM, Abresch-Meyer AL, Nelson MD, Widman LM. Body mass index and body composition measures by dual X-ray absorptiometry in patients aged 10 to 21 years with spinal cord injury. J Spinal Cord Med. 2007;30 Suppl 1:S97–104.
78. Schurr MJ, Ebner KA, Maser AL, Sperling KB, Helgerson RB, Harms B. Formal swallowing evaluation and therapy after traumatic brain injury improves dysphagia outcomes. J Trauma. 1999;46:817–21; discussion 821–13.

79. Shem K, Castillo K, Wong S, Chang J. Dysphagia in individuals with tetraplegia: incidence and risk factors. J Spinal Cord Med. 2011;34:85–92.
80. Murray KA, Brzozowski LA. Swallowing in patients with tracheotomies. AACN Clin Issues. 1998;9:416–26; quiz 456–18.
81. Bradley 3rd JF, Jones MA, Farmer EA, Fann SA, Bynoe R. Swallowing dysfunction in trauma patients with cervical spine fractures treated with halo-vest fixation. J Trauma. 2011;70:46–8; discussion 48–50.
82. Elpern EH, Borkgren Okonek M, Bacon M, Gerstung C, Skrzynski M. Effect of the Passy-Muir tracheostomy speaking valve on pulmonary aspiration in adults. Heart Lung. 2000;29:287–93.
83. Guilleminault C, Faull KF, Miles L, van den Hoed J. Posttraumatic excessive daytime sleepiness: a review of 20 patients. Neurology. 1983;33:1584–9.
84. Stores G, Stores R. Sleep disorders in children with traumatic brain injury: a case of serious neglect. 2013. Developmental medicine and child neurology.
85. Burns SP, Kapur V, Yin KY, Buhrer R. Factors associated with sleep apnea in men with spinal cord injury: a population- based case-control study. Spinal Cord. 2001;39:15–22.
86. Flavell H, Marshall R, Thornton AT, Clements PL, Antic R, McEvoy RD. Hypoxia episodes during sleep in high tetraplegia. Arch Phys Med Rehabil. 1992;73:623–7.
87. McEvoy RD, Mykytyn I, Sajkov D, Flavell H, Marshall R, Antic R, Thonrton AT. Sleep apnea in patients with quadriplegia. Thorax. 1995;50:613–9.
88. Berlowitz DJ, Brown DJ, Campbell DA, Pierce RJ. A longitudinal evaluation of sleep and breathing in the first year after cervical spinal cord injury. Arch Phys Med Rehabil. 2005;86:1193–9.
89. Tran K, Hukins C, Geraghty T, Eckert B, Fraser L. Sleep-disordered breathing in spinal cord-injured patients: a short-term longitudinal study. Respirology. 2009;15:272–6.
90. Betz RR. Unique management needs of pediatric spinal cord injury patients: orthopedic problems in the child with spinal cord injury. J Spinal Cord Med. 1997;20:14–6.
91. Mulcahey MJ, Gaughan JP, Betz RR, Samdani AF, Barakat N, Hunter LN. Neuromuscular scoliosis in children with spinal cord injury. Top Spinal Cord Injury Rehabil. 2013;19:96–103.
92. Vogel L, Mulcahy MJ, Betz RR. The child with a spinal cord injury. Dev Med Child Neurol. 1997;39:202–7.
93. Schottler J, Vogel LC, Sturm P. Spinal cord injuries in young children: a review of children injured at 5 years of age and younger. Dev Med Child Neurol. 2012;54:1138–43.

Chapter 17
Care of the Child with Congenital Central Hypoventilation Syndrome

Fiona Healy and Carole L. Marcus

Pathophysiology

Genetics

In 2003, it was discovered that CCHS is caused by a defect in the *PHOX2B* homeobox gene and that inheritance is autosomal dominant [1, 2]. *PHOX2B* maps to chromosome 4p12 and encodes for a transcription factor that plays a role in the regulation of neural crest cell migration and development of the autonomic nervous system [1, 2]. The transcription factor consists of 314 amino acids with two short and stable polyalanine repeats of nine and 20 residues, respectively. Approximately 90% of *PHOX2B* mutations in CCHS involve expansion of the 20-residue polyalanine region, adding 4–13 copies [3]. These polyalanine repeat expansion mutations (PARMs) produce genotypes of 20/24 to 20/33, whereas the normal genotype is 20/20. The remaining 10% of *PHOX2B* mutations in CCHS are nonpolyalanine repeat mutations (NPARMs) and include missense, nonsense, and frameshift mutations.

To date, there have been some associations made between the *PHOX2B* genotype and CCHS phenotype. Typically, a higher number of repeats are associated with a greater severity of the respiratory phenotype [3, 4]. Specifically, individuals with genotypes from 20/27 to 20/33 usually require ventilatory support during both wakefulness and sleep, while those with the 20/25 genotype usually require only

F. Healy, M.B.B.Ch. (✉)
Department of Respiratory Medicine, Children's University Hospital,
Temple Street, Dublin, Ireland
e-mail: marcus@email.chop.edu

C.L. Marcus, M.B.B.Ch.
Sleep Center, Children's Hospital of Philadelphia, University of Pennsylvania,
34th Street and Civic Center Boulevard, Philadelphia, PA 19104, USA
e-mail: fionamhealy@gmail.com

© Springer Science+Business Media New York 2016
L.M. Sterni, J.L. Carroll (eds.), *Caring for the Ventilator Dependent Child*,
Respiratory Medicine, DOI 10.1007/978-1-4939-3749-3_17

nocturnal ventilation [3, 5, 6]. Later-onset cases with milder hypoventilation have been documented with 20/24 or 20/25 genotypes and likely represent cases of variable penetrance of these mutations [5–7]. Most mutations occur de novo in CCHS, but 5–10 % are inherited from a mosaic typically unaffected parent [7].

Effect of Sleep State

Central alveolar hypoventilation is diagnosed when the arterial partial pressure of carbon dioxide (PCO_2) is >45 mmHg during wakefulness, due to decreased central ventilatory drive. This cutoff cannot be applied during sleep however, as PCO_2 levels are typically higher in this state. The regulation of arterial blood gases during sleep in healthy humans is maintained primarily by central chemoreceptors which respond to changes in the PCO_2 by detecting the pH of cerebrospinal fluid and peripheral chemoreceptors which respond to decreased arterial partial pressure of oxygen (PO_2) and increased PCO_2. During wakefulness, additional behavioral and arousal-related influences on breathing (from reticular activating system, forebrain, and mechanoreceptor afferents) also affect ventilatory control. In many situations, these non-chemoreceptive inputs to breathing result in relatively well-controlled arterial blood gases in patients with CCHS while awake and not engaged in vigorous exercise. This may explain why some patients with CCHS who breathe sufficiently during wakefulness (e.g., those with genotypes 20/24, 20/25, and some 20/26) only require ventilatory support during sleep.

Huang et al. studied nine children with CCHS during spontaneous breathing in both rapid eye movement (REM) and non-REM (NREM) sleep and demonstrated more severe hypoventilation during NREM periods, with greater decreases in minute ventilation [8]. It has been proposed that an intrinsic REM-related ventilatory drive could explain these findings, as shown by increased firing of single neuron recordings of medullary respiratory cells during REM compared to NREM sleep in healthy animals [9]. In addition, it is known that there are tonic excitatory inputs to the respiratory system during both REM and wakefulness that decline during NREM sleep. However, although patients with CCHS have better ventilation during REM than NREM sleep, they still have significant hypoventilation during REM sleep and thus require mechanical ventilation during all sleep stages including REM.

Mechanoreception

Additional proposed non-chemoreceptive inputs to breathing in patients with CCHS include mechanoreceptor pathways. Studies have confirmed that in children with CCHS, both passive motion during wakefulness and active exercise improve ventilation [10, 11]. In a study of treadmill exercise testing in five children with CCHS, exercise-induced hyperpnoea occurred [11]. CCHS subjects increased minute ventilation primarily by increasing respiratory rate, in association with increasing limb pacing frequency on the treadmill. Gozal et al. demonstrated that passive motion of the lower extremities during NREM sleep in six patients with CCHS resulted in increased respiratory frequency and decreased end-tidal CO_2 levels [12]. These findings suggest that CCHS patients may be at higher risk for hypoventilation when they are physically still. One study of five patients with CCHS also demonstrated that they increased ventilation with mental activities such as reading, solving arithmetic problems, or playing video games [13].

A study of seven patients with CCHS during wakefulness demonstrated upward shift of EEG signals just before inspiration (pre-inspiratory potential) suggestive of supplementary motor area activation [14]. These potentials were present in a variety of conditions including resting breathing, exposure to CO_2, and inspiratory mechanical constraints. In the control group, however, these pre-inspiratory potentials were generally absent except for during mechanical constraint. These findings indicate the existence of cortical mechanisms compensating for deficient generation of automatic breathing in CCHS.

Clinical Presentation

CCHS is characterized by the clinical presentation of alveolar hypoventilation with insensitivity to hypoxemia and hypercapnia, most pronounced during sleep. Infants with CCHS typically present in the newborn period with intermittent episodes of cyanosis or apnea, and most require mechanical ventilation immediately after birth. As their oxygen saturation falls and their carbon dioxide level rises, affected infants demonstrate no increase in respiratory rate or effort and usually do not arouse or appear distressed [15]. During sleep, infants will appear to have regular but shallow respirations with reduced chest wall movement, interspersed with periods of central apnea. Occasionally, infants may present in the first few months of life with acute life-threatening events or even frank respiratory arrest.

In many infants during the first few months of life, hypoventilation may be evident during both wakefulness and sleep. However, these patients may eventually breathe adequately while awake, probably reflecting the development of sleep-wake regulation or maturation of the respiratory and central nervous systems rather than an improvement in their CCHS [16]. Some affected patients may continue to display symptoms of hypoventilation during quiet activities while awake and may require daytime ventilatory support.

Symptoms of hypoventilation are more pronounced in times of illness or stress because patients with CCHS are unable to demonstrate respiratory responses to increased ventilatory demands. Thus, when faced with gas exchange abnormalities (e.g., during a respiratory tract infection), children with CCHS do not manifest signs of respiratory distress such as tachypnea, retractions, or nasal flaring. In some cases patients with CCHS can present late with symptoms of end-organ damage, such as cor pulmonale, seizures, developmental delay, or failure to thrive, from chronic, unrecognized hypoxemia and hypercarbia. In one survey of almost 200 children with CCHS, developmental delays, including motor, speech, and learning disabilities, were reported in 45 % [17].

Rarely, patients with CCHS survive into adulthood before presenting with symptoms of hypoventilation that are triggered by a minor respiratory tract infection or general anesthesia. Other potential presenting symptoms of adult cases include epileptic seizures, cognitive disabilities, and sleep apnea or in rare occasions after a child is diagnosed with CCHS [1]. In such late-onset cases, there is frequently a history of ventilatory disturbances in infancy that resolved spontaneously, e.g., breath-holding spells, and patients often have cognitive impairment [18].

Autonomic Dysfunction

Patients with CCHS often manifest symptoms of autonomic nervous system dysregulation including temperature instability, excessive sweating, decreased perception of discomfort and anxiety, and swallowing dysfunction. Periods of autonomic crises with and without elevated urinary catecholamines have also been described [19]. Although baseline heart rate does not differ from controls, the relative increase above the mean heart rate at rest with exercise is attenuated, and heart rate variability is decreased [20–22]. Cardiac arrhythmias, including sinus bradycardia and transient asystole up to 6.5 s, have also been reported [20]. One study of 39 patients with CCHS reported that among three children who had R-R intervals greater than 3 s and did not receive a cardiac pacemaker, two died suddenly [23]. Additionally, blood pressure in patients with CCHS is lower during wakefulness and higher during sleep compared to controls, indicating attenuation of the normal sleep-related blood pressure decrement [22]. Goldberg et al. documented ophthalmologic disorders in 27 of 37 children with CCHS, most of whom had miotic pupils that reacted poorly to light [24].

Abnormalities of neural crest origin, also known as neurocristopathies, may be present in patients with CCHS. Hirschsprung's disease is present in approximately 16 % of cases of CCHS [17]. This is often severe, with 50 % of cases having total colonic aganglionosis, compared to the general population with Hirschsprung's disease in whom 80 % have short segment forms [25]. Children with CCHS who receive mechanical ventilation for 24 h a day are more likely to have Hirschsprung's disease [17].

Case reports of tumors of neural crest origin, including mediastinal or abdominal neuroblastoma or ganglioneuromas, have been documented in association with CCHS [25–27]. Approximately 5 % of patients with CCHS will have neural crest tumors although tumor-related deaths are uncommon [17, 28]. The tumors can present at variable ages with neuroblastoma typically presenting before age two years and ganglioneuromas presenting later as incidental findings [28]. Tumors of neural crest origin occur more frequently in patients with NPARMS, specifically missense or frameshift homozygous mutations of the *PHOX2B* gene [29, 30]. Among patients with PARMs, only subjects with the 20/29 and 20/33 genotypes have been identified with neural crest tumors (ganglioneuromas and ganglioneuroblastomas) to date [7].

Late-Onset Central Hypoventilation Syndrome with Hypothalamic Dysfunction

Late-onset central hypoventilation syndrome with hypothalamic dysfunction (LO-CHS) has been reported in previously well children who present after infancy [31]. This syndrome was first described in 1965 and is distinct from CCHS [32]. Both CCHS and LO-CHS can be associated with diseases of neural crest origin; however, features of hypothalamic dysfunction are not seen in CCHS [31]. Features of hypothalamic function reported in LO-CHS include hyperphagia, hypersomnolence, thermal dysregulation, emotional lability, and endocrinopathies. The diagnostic term "rapid onset obesity with hypothalamic dysfunction, hypoventilation, and autonomic dysregulation (ROHHAD)" has also been used [33]. Clinical presentation can be varied with additional reported symptoms of thermal dysregulation, pain hyposensitivity, behavioral disorders, strabismus, pupillary anomalies, and tumors of neural crest origin [34]. A recent study of 23 children with this syndrome demonstrated negative *PHOX2B* gene sequencing in all cases [33]. Thus, this clinical presentation represents a syndrome clinically distinct from CCHS.

Evaluation and Diagnosis

A diagnosis of CCHS should be considered in all children with evidence of hypoventilation without underlying cardiopulmonary, metabolic, neuromuscular, or brainstem dysfunction. Initial genetic testing should be performed with the *PHOX2B* screening test, which will identify the mutation in 95 % of CCHS cases [7]. If the screening test is negative but the patient's phenotype supports the diagnosis of CCHS, a *PHOX2B* sequencing test may detect a subset of NPARMs [7]. Additionally, recent evidence indicates that further deletion/duplication analysis can identify another subset of patients affected (<1 %) [35].

Table 17.1 Differential diagnoses of congenital central hypoventilation syndrome

Metabolic	*Pulmonary*
Mitochondrial defects, e.g., Leigh's disease	Primary lung disease
Pyruvate dehydrogenase deficiency	Respiratory muscle weakness, e.g.,
Hypothyroidism	diaphragm paralysis, congenital myopathy
Neurologic	*Genetic*
Structural abnormalities, e.g., Arnold-Chiari malformation, Moebius syndrome	Prader-Willi syndrome
Vascular injury, e.g., central nervous system hemorrhage, infarct	Familial dysautonomia
Trauma	*Sedative drugs*
Tumor	

Differential diagnoses for CCHS are wide and varied and should be ruled out while genetic testing for CCHS is pending (Table 17.1). Investigations to consider include chest radiograph, echocardiogram, and fluoroscopy of the diaphragm to identify any primary cardiopulmonary diseases or respiratory muscle weakness. Pulmonary function testing may be performed in cooperative older children. Infant pulmonary function testing, however, should be considered with caution due to the increased risk of hypoventilation with sedation. Intracranial lesions resulting in central hypoventilation can be identified by magnetic resonance imaging of the brain. Metabolic screening should be considered when clinical signs suggest inborn errors of metabolism.

Assessment of Hypoventilation

Children with a suspected diagnosis of CCHS should have comprehensive studies of respiratory physiology during wakefulness, REM, and NREM sleep to assess the degree of hypoventilation and the level of ventilatory support required. Testing should include all aspects of routine polysomnography including end-tidal/transcutaneous CO_2 monitoring. Figure 17.1 shows different patterns on polysomnography that may be observed in children with CCHS [8, 36]. Ventilatory responses to hypoxia and hypercapnia during wakefulness and sleep can be measured to confirm the diagnosis and are usually flat [37]. This testing is performed primarily as a research tool but at times may be useful in establishing a diagnosis.

The severity or chronicity of the central hypoventilation should be assessed by screening the patient for chronic respiratory acidosis and compensatory metabolic alkalosis (bicarbonate levels) and polycythemia (hemoglobin levels). Echocardiogram (ECG) and serum brain-type natriuretic peptide levels will determine if there is any evidence of pulmonary hypertension or cor pulmonale as a result of chronic hypoxemia.

Screening for Autonomic Dysfunction

Patients with CCHS and symptoms suggestive of autonomic dysfunction should be investigated appropriately. Barium enema or rectal biopsy should be performed for patients with constipation or abdominal distension to rule out Hirschsprung's disease. Chest and abdominal imaging should be obtained early if there is any possibility of a neural crest tumor, particularly in patients with missense or frameshift mutations of the *PHOX2B* gene which correlate more frequently with this phenotype [29, 30].

Holter monitoring should be performed if there is clinical suspicion of cardiac arrhythmias, including bradycardias, that may necessitate pacemaker insertion. An ophthalmologic examination will identify any eye involvement and allow for early intervention to avoid interference with learning. Other measures of autonomic testing may be employed as clinically indicated, e.g. tilt testing to assess syncope [7].

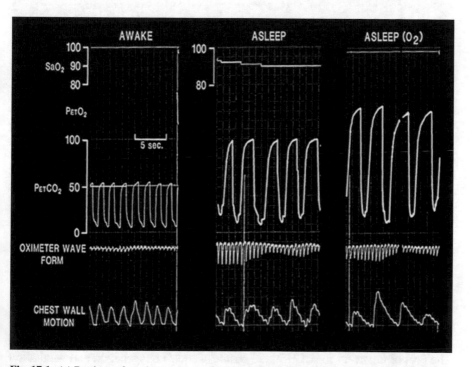

Fig. 17.1 (a) Portions of a polysomnogram from an infant with congenital central hypoventilation syndrome. In the *left panel*, the infant is awake with normal oxyhemoglobin saturation but is hypoventilating slightly. At sleep onset (*middle panel*), end-tidal carbon dioxide levels begin to rise and oxyhemoglobin levels begin to drop. When placed on supplemental oxygen (right panel), the oxyhemoglobin levels normalize, but end-tidal carbon dioxide levels continue to rise (Marcus CL. 2001. Sleep-disordered breathing in children. American Journal of Respiratory and Critical Care Medicine. 164: 16–30. Official Journal of the American Thoracic Society. Reprinted with permission of the American Thoracic Society. Copyright © 2013 American Thoracic Society). (b) Polysomnogram epoch from an 8-year-old subject with CCHS during NREM sleep is shown. Following ventilator disconnection (*arrow*), the subject had an immediate 24-s central apnea, followed by an arousal. Cardiac oscillations are present on the airflow and PCO_2 waveform channels. Y-axis parameters; time axis, clock time (in s) is shown, with the epoch number superimposed; C3-A2, C4-A1, O1-A2, and O2-A1 are EEG leads; LOC-A2 and ROCA1 are left and right electrooculograms, respectively; *CHIN* submental EMG signal, *CHEST* chest wall motion, *ABDM* abdominal wall motion, *PNEUMFLO* airflow measured with a pneumotachograph, *PN* pressure measured at the tracheostomy site, *CAP* end-tidal PCO_2 waveform, *ETCO_2* end-tidal PCO_2 value, *TCCO_2* transcutaneous PCO_2, *SAO_2* arterial oxygen saturation, *PWF* oximeter pulse waveform, *LLEG* left tibial EMG, *RLEG* right tibial EMG (Huang J et al. J Appl Physiol 2008. Am Physiol Soc, with permission)

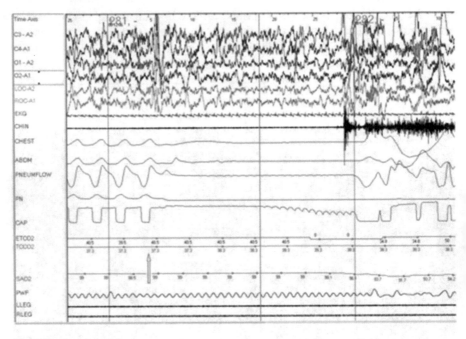

Fig. 17.1 (continued)

Management

Goals of Care

The goal of treatment for CCHS is to ensure adequate oxygenation and ventilation during both wakefulness and sleep. This will improve long-term prognosis by reducing the risks of cor pulmonale and neurological insult from chronic hypoxemia.

Ventilation

The natural history of CCHS is that ventilatory responses to hypoxemia and hypercarbia do not improve over time. All newly diagnosed infants and children will require some form of assisted ventilation in the home setting. The proportion of all patients with CCHS who require ventilatory support during both wakefulness and sleep varies from 6 to 33 % in different study populations [16, 21]. Oxygen administration alone will improve oxygen saturation (SpO_2) levels but will not prevent hypoventilation and the ensuing complications. Respiratory stimulants including theophylline, dexamphetamine, and clomipramine have not been shown to improve ventilatory drive in this patient population [38, 39]. Objective measurements of adequate ventilation, including pulse oximetry levels, should be monitored in the home. Ventilators are adjusted to maintain CO_2 levels ideally between 30 and 40 mmHg and $SpO_2 \geq 95\%$ [7]. Maintaining low-normal CO_2 levels ensures that patients with CCHS have some ventilatory reserve when challenged during their daily activities, e.g., exercise, and when ill with intercurrent infections. Ventilator settings should be adjusted regularly during polysomnography or hospital admission, particularly in young children who are growing rapidly or patients who are symptomatic. Establishing optimal ventilator settings will help prevent neurocognitive dysfunction and avoid the development of atelectasis.

A variety of modalities of home ventilation are available to the patient with CCHS including portable positive pressure ventilation via tracheostomy, noninvasive ventilation (NIV) via nasal mask, diaphragmatic pacing, and, rarely, negative pressure ventilation. The advantages and disadvantages of each modality should be discussed with the family prior to decision-making (Table 17.2). Factors that determine the choice of technique include efficacy, practicality, psychosocial acceptance, complications, and cost. Ideally, the choice of ventilation should provide optimal technology to meet the patient's lifestyle needs.

Transition of a patient with CCHS to a home portable ventilator should be established in the hospital under the supervision of an expert medical team. Discharge planning should include arrangements for the home ventilator, a backup ventilator, and home nursing support. In addition, a pulse oximeter and end-tidal CO_2 monitor in the home allow for objective measurements of any clinical deterioration or change in ventilatory requirements.

During early infancy and childhood, patients with CCHS typically require more ventilatory support than older children and adults. This is because younger infants typically sleep for longer periods, are more prone to infections, and overall have more immature respiratory systems, which contribute to more instability in ventilation. It should be highlighted, however, that although there may be some maturation of the respiratory system, the patient never develops ventilatory responses and cannot be weaned from nocturnal ventilatory support. In a study of 196 patients with CCHS, two-thirds were able to adequately maintain ventilatory homeostasis during waking hours by age 12 months, while another quarter of the children were older than one year before they achieved such an ability [17]. This study also revealed a reduced need for intervention by medical professionals with age [17]. A greater healthcare burden was present among the 24-h ventilator-dependent patients; however, the need for hospitalization decreased with age in all patients [17].

The weaning of daytime assisted ventilation is best accomplished by sprint weaning where the child is removed from the ventilator for short periods of time during wakefulness [15]. The child with CCHS may not exhibit any signs of respiratory distress and so must be carefully monitored noninvasively during sprints to prevent hypoxemia or hypercapnia. The duration and frequency of sprints may be increased as tolerated, but progress will be hampered if performed too rapidly or without meticulous supervision.

Table 17.2 Advantages and disadvantages of ventilator modalities for congenital central hypoventilation syndrome

	Noninvasive ventilation	Diaphragmatic pacing	Tracheostomy and positive pressure ventilation
Advantages	• No surgical procedure • Ventilator is simpler to operate • Less expensive • May permit tracheal decannulation	• Improved patient mobility • May permit tracheal decannulation	• Most reliable method for ensuring adequate ventilation Secure airway during illness • Can be used continuously • Can use higher settings than with noninvasive ventilation
Disadvantages	• Difficult to find appropriate interfaces for younger patients • Difficult to ensure placement of interfaces at sleep onset in young children without established sleep/wake cycles • Difficulty triggering machines in young children • Need to overcome the added load of upper airway resistance • Nasal symptoms, aerophagia, and skin breakdown • Limited portability	• Specialized surgical procedure • May need repeat surgery for mechanical failure • Risk of infection • Risk of upper airway obstruction if trachea decannulated • Must have access to team specialized in care of pacers	• Mobility with home ventilators is limited if used while awake • Complications of tracheostomies including recurrent laryngeal nerve injury, hemorrhage, infection, accidental decannulation, speech problems, tracheomalacia, and granulation tissue

Positive Pressure Ventilation via Tracheostomy

Positive pressure ventilation (PPV) via tracheostomy is the commonest mode of ventilation used, particularly in infants and younger children. Many physicians agree that it is the safest form of ventilation to ensure adequate ventilation and oxygenation during the first years of life while the respiratory and central nervous systems are maturing [7]. While beneficial in older children, use of NIV is avoided in younger infants because of potential problems including difficulty with mask fitting, difficulty with triggering/cycling NIV ventilators, and the propensity of infants to take frequent naps. Older patients with tracheostomies may opt for decannulation and transition to NIV. Home positive pressure ventilators are portable and can be battery operated, improving mobility for the patient. Uncuffed tracheostomy tubes are typically used to permit a leak large enough to use a Passy-Muir valve, which encourages speech development, and to avoid subglottic stenosis. Pressure plateau ventilation or pressure control modes can be used to accommodate leak, compensate for tubing compliance, and ensure sufficient lung inflation.

While PPV via tracheostomy is generally a safe technique, there are a number of longer-term complications associated with it, including delayed speech and language development, colonization and infection of the lower respiratory tract, and tracheal granulation and stenosis [40]. There is also the low ($\leq 6\%$) but definite risk of tracheostomy-related death from cannula obstruction or accidental decannulation [41]. Due to the risk of complications, these patients will require caregivers available at all times that are trained to change and manage tracheostomies. This can further increase financial and social burdens on the patients and their families.

Despite the disadvantages, an epidemiological survey involving 196 patients with CCHS from 19 countries reported that more than 60 % of patients with CCHS were ventilated via tracheostomy [17]. In this study, the transition to NIV typically occurred between the ages of 6 and 11 years. A recent Japanese study of 37 patients with CCHS reported a similar proportion of 57 % ventilated by tracheostomy [42].

Noninvasive Bi-level Positive Airway Pressure

This is a mode of NIV via nasal mask or nasal prongs that does not require tracheostomy. These machines provide variable continuous flow via a blower (fan) and have a fixed leak that prevents CO_2 retention and can compensate for leaks around the mask. When used in the timed/pressure control mode, they guarantee breath delivery in children with CCHS who cannot generate adequate large spontaneous breaths to trigger the ventilator [7]. NIV is not, however, suitable in isolation for patients requiring 24-h ventilation because it can interfere with daytime activity. Prolonged daily use of NIV can cause significant facial skin breakdown, nasal deformity, and injury to the eyes. Midfacial hypoplasia and dental malocclusion may occur in younger patients [43, 44]. One report of the use of NIV in two infants reported the development of class 3 dental malocclusion in both patients, after about 2 years, necessitating addition of negative pressure ventilation to reduce the duration of mask ventilation [45]. Presumably, midfacial hypoplasia is due to the chronic pressure exerted by the headgear and face mask unit against the malleable nasal, zygomatic, and maxillary areas in young patients and appears to be less of an issue with modern interfaces [44]. The severity of these complications can be reduced by alternating between nasal masks and nasal pillows, using customized masks, and avoiding tight-fitting interfaces [46]. Villa et al. described successful correction of midface hypoplasia with an orthodontic device in a 7-year-old child with CCHS who had been ventilated with a nasal mask from the age of 9 months [44].

Other potential problems encountered with use of NIV in children with CCHS include gastric overdistension resulting in gastroesophageal reflux. In addition, incorrect positioning of the nasal interface or oral leakage during sleep could cause pressure losses and reduce the effectiveness of NIV [47].

Another frequent challenge to the successful use of NIV is poor patient adherence to treatment. One study reported that adherence to NIV in children and adolescents with obstructive sleep apnea was related primarily to family and demographic factors rather than severity of apnea, pressure levels, or psychosocial functioning [48]. Important supportive mechanisms to promote NIV adherence include education of both parents and patients along with anticipatory guidance for common problems, side effects, and device troubleshooting [49]. Another intervention to promote NIV adherence is to ensure positive first experiences for patients with NIV, including during in-laboratory or in-hospital treatment trials [49].

The first successful case of NIV use for CCHS was reported in 1987 in a 6-year-old child who had previously received mechanical ventilation [50]. A 2004 survey of 196 patients with CCHS (age range 0.4–38 years, mean 10.2 years) reported that 55 (28.1 %) were using NIV alone [17].

Some patients have been successfully transitioned from PPV via tracheostomy to NIV support upon reaching school age when the clinical course is more stable and the child is able to accept mask ventilation and cooperate fully. Limitations to transition include the availability of suitable and comfortable nasal interfaces for the child. In cases where there is pressure loss because of open mouth breathing, the concomitant use of chin straps or full face masks can permit adequate ventilation. One must also consider that, when transitioning to NIV from PPV via tracheostomy, there will be the added load of upper airway resistance to overcome, which may necessitate higher ventilator settings. Evaluation of the upper airway for possible tonsillectomy and adenoidectomy may be indicated in patients requiring high settings. NIV generally does not provide pressures as high as those provided by invasive ventilators, and children may require intubation and greater levels of ventilatory support during acute respiratory illnesses.

Patients with CCHS may have life-threatening events if not adequately ventilated during sleep; thus, documentation of the adequacy of NIV settings is essential before chronic NIV treatment can be safely initiated [51]. As with PPV, optimal NIV settings should be determined and titrated periodically in the sleep laboratory. The American Academy of Sleep Medicine published guidelines for sleep center adjustment of NIV in patients with stable chronic alveolar hypoventilation syndromes including those with central respiratory control disturbances [51]. The underlying concept is that a successful NIV titration is one in which there is an optimized trade-off between increasing pressure to yield efficacy in supporting ventilation and decreasing pressure to minimize emergence of pressure-related side effects [51].

One recent case report described a 16-year-old female with CCHS who was successfully transitioned to a new modality of NIV, average volume-assured pressure support (AVAPS), that automatically adjusts the pressure support level in order to provide a consistent tidal volume [52]. AVAPS has been recently introduced as a new additional mode for bi-level pressure ventilation that automatically adjusts the pressure support level to provide a consistent tidal volume. Studies on its physiologic and clinical effects are few and more are needed [53, 54].

Negative Pressure Ventilation

Negative pressure ventilation (NPV) causes inspiration by generating a negative inspiratory pressure around the chest and abdomen. The popularity of NPV, however, has been limited by the risk of obstructive sleep apnea because of lack of synchrony between vocal fold opening and thoracic inspiratory efforts. In one report, additional mask CPAP was used successfully in cases of upper airway obstruction during NPV [55].

Negative pressure ventilators are bulky and not portable, and some necessitate that the patient remains in the supine position. In addition, the chest shells or wraps currently available can cause discomfort, skin breakdown, and leaks that make their use unacceptable in many cases. NPV has been used rarely since the advent of PPV and NIV. It may be an acceptable alternative for those requiring ventilation during sleep if other modes of ventilation are unsuitable. In rare cases, it has permitted decannulation in patients with CCHS.

Diaphragmatic Pacing

This mode of ventilation involves electrical stimulation of the phrenic nerve that results in diaphragmatic contraction. In 1972, Glenn et al. first demonstrated that electrical stimulation of the phrenic nerves resulted in rhythmic contraction of the diaphragm (pacing) and could provide full-time, long-term ventilatory support for an adult patient with acquired central hypoventilation [56]. In 1978, Hunt et al. reported the first three cases of diaphragmatic pacing in infants with CCHS [57].

Typically, pacing during the day and PPV by mask or tracheostomy at night affords more daytime mobility for active children who require ventilation 24 h per day. This can both improve quality of life and optimize neurodevelopmental progress. Pacing has not been used for 24 h a day because of a theoretical concern of damage to the phrenic nerves. Patients with CCHS who may best benefit from diaphragm pacing include those with no or mild intrinsic lung disease with preserved phrenic nerve-diaphragm axis integrity and presence of a tracheostomy at least during the initiation of pacing [58].

Diaphragmatic pacing requires surgical implantation of bilateral phrenic nerve electrodes, in the intrathoracic or intracervical segments of the nerve. The cervical approach in the lower neck is a less desirable site for placement because the phrenic nerve forms a complex of rootlets that only unite in the thorax. Thus, the cervical approach may only capture 75 % of the fibers in the neck [59]. Bilateral receivers are implanted subcutaneously that transmit radio frequency signals from a battery-operated external pulse generator to the phrenic nerve electrodes. The patient also wears an energy transfer coil on the skin over the receiver. When a signal arrives from the external pulse generator, it is converted via the subcutaneous receivers to an electrical current that stimulates the phrenic nerve (Fig. 17.2). Settings on the external generator include respiratory rate and electrical voltage and are adjusted to give enough tidal volume to allow for adequate oxygenation and ventilation.

The goal with diaphragm pacing is to minimize the electrical stimulation while providing optimal ventilation and oxygenation. Pacing is typically initiated 4–6 weeks after surgical implantation to allow tissue reaction around the electrodes to stabilize [15]. Training of the muscle fibers is necessary to sustain pacing for the required 12–16 h per day, and a period of 3–4 months is usually required to attain full pacing [15]. In patients with CCHS who also have cardiac pacemakers, it is important to minimize the potential for electromagnetic interference by ensuring that the cardiac pacemaker is bipolar [7].

Potential complications of pacing include equipment failure, infection (e.g., empyema), and late injury due to fibrosis or tension on the phrenic nerve [60]. In

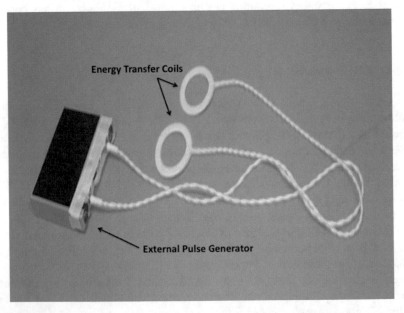

Fig. 17.2 (a) Diaphragmatic pacing device showing the external pulse generator and energy transfer coils. (Reprinted from Paediatric Respiratory Reviews, 2011 Dec; 12 (4):253–63. Healy F, Marcus CL. Congenital central hypoventilation syndrome in children, pages 253–63, Copyright 2011, with permission from Elsevier). (b) Patient with congenital central hypoventilation syndrome post tracheal decannulation who uses nocturnal diaphragmatic pacing. Here she is wearing the energy transfer coils of her diaphragmatic pacer and holding the external pulse generator during setup for a titration polysomnogram (Reprinted from Paediatric Respiratory Reviews, 2011 Dec; 12 (4):253–63. Healy F, Marcus CL. Congenital central hypoventilation syndrome in children, pages 253–63, Copyright 2011, with permission from Elsevier)

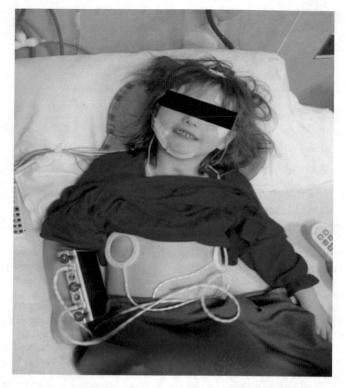

Fig. 17.2 (continued)

one study of 33 infants and children using diaphragmatic pacing, receiver failure was the most common cause of internal component failure [61]. However, the receiver can be replaced without thoracotomy because it is located in a subcutaneous pocket. Longevity of equipment should improve as hardware becomes more refined over time. Flageole et al. reported their longest survivor to date was paced for 21 years [59]. This patient had successfully tolerated seven separate procedures for receiver or wire replacement.

Pacing at night may permit tracheal decannulation. However, in some decannulated patients, obstructive sleep apnea occurs because vocal fold opening does not occur with a paced inspiration (Fig. 17.3). In some cases this may be overcome by adjusting settings on the pacers to lengthen inspiratory time and/or decrease the force of inspiration. If the obstruction persists, then these patients may be better managed by NIV. Patients should be monitored by polysomnography to ensure that they do not have obstructive sleep apnea related to diaphragmatic pacing.

All patients with CCHS who rely on diaphragm pacing should have an additional backup diaphragm pacer transmitter already set to their physiological requirements. An additional advantage of a second transmitter is that, for children who are paced during the day, the backup transmitter can be set to deliver optimal settings for exercise. This allows the child to use one transmitter during school and the other

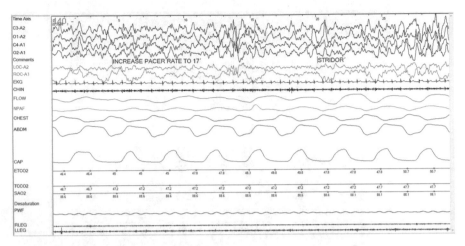

Fig. 17.3 Thirty-second epoch from a titration polysomnogram image from the patient with congenital central hypoventilation syndrome in Fig. 17.2b who had previously been decannulated and was using nocturnal diaphragmatic pacing. During the study the patient experienced persistent partial upper airway obstruction while paced, with stridor, paradoxical breathing, and oxyhemoglobin desaturation. *C3-A2*, *O1-A2*, *C4-A1*, *O2-A1* electroencephalogram channels, *LOC-A2* and *ROCA1* left and right electrooculograms, *CHIN* submental EMG, *EKG* electrocardiogram, *NPAF* nasal pressure airflow, *CHEST* thoracic movement, *ABDM* abdominal movement, *CAP* capnography, *ETCO₂* end-tidal carbon dioxide level (torr), *SAO₂* arterial oxygen saturation, *PWF* oximeter pulse waveform, *TCCO₂* transcutaneous carbon dioxide level (torr), *RLEG* right tibial EMG, *LLEG* left tibial EMG (Reprinted from Paediatric Respiratory Reviews, 2011 Dec; 12 (4):253–63. Healy F, Marcus CL. Congenital central hypoventilation syndrome in children, pages 253–63, Copyright 2011, with permission from Elsevier)

transmitter during a moderate level of age-appropriate activity (settings for each should be ascertained during physiologic assessments at a center with expertise in diaphragmatic pacing) [7].

Diaphragmatic pacers can work well, but patients must have access to teams with the necessary expertise in maintaining them. This includes staff with the ability to set the pacers with a digital oscilloscope and surface electromyogram recordings. In addition, the implantation of the internal components (receivers, connecting wires, and phrenic nerve electrodes) requires thoracic surgery and should only be implanted by experienced pediatric surgeons at a center with the appropriate expertise [7].

Ongoing Care and Monitoring

Screening for Medical Comorbidities Associated with CCHS

Children with CCHS require input by a wide variety of medical specialists due to the array of associated medical conditions including autonomic dysfunction and sequelae of ventilatory insufficiency and hypoxemia. Neurocognitive assessments should be considered as patients with CCHS have an increased risk of learning disabilities and developmental delay [62, 63]. Most children with CCHS have adequate growth and nutrition, but some may have swallowing incoordination requiring temporary gastrostomies [15].

Genetic Counseling

Genetic counseling should be offered to the parents of children diagnosed with CCHS irrespective of whether a genetic mutation is identified or not. This will provide information on the nature, autosomal dominant inheritance pattern, and implications of this disorder to help them make informed medical and personal decisions. If a specific PHOX2B mutation is identified in their child, parents should be offered testing to determine their own risk for later-onset CCHS or mosaicism [28]. Risk to siblings and other family members will depend on the genotype status of the parents.

Home Care and Nursing Support

The majority of care for children with CCHS occurs in the home setting where parents can easily be overwhelmed by sophisticated medical equipment and coordination of appointments with multiple medical professionals. Children with CCHS are a particularly vulnerable group who require skilled care and monitoring, particularly at sleep onset when they could suffer severe hypoventilation or even complete respiratory arrest if ventilation is not adequately supported. Additionally, these children do not typically develop fever, tachypnea, or dyspnea in response to respiratory tract infections, even pneumonia, and thus careful assessment is necessary during illness [13, 64]. Caregivers need to be well educated about CCHS, and nursing support, if available, can be very helpful. One study reported that, of 196 families with a child with CCHS, 49.5 % had no nursing support at night [17]. Access to other skilled healthcare professionals including social workers, speech therapists, physical therapists, and special education teachers may be needed to optimize care.

Social Issues and Quality of Life

Most children with CCHS will have a good quality of life if diagnosed early and managed rigorously. There should be minimal restrictions on daytime activity; however, children with CCHS lack the appropriate ventilatory and autonomic responses to heavy or extended exercise [65]. If swimming, they should be carefully supervised regardless of the presence or absence of a tracheostomy (swimming is not recommended for those with tracheostomies) [7]. Children with CCHS do not derive discomfort from breath-holding and are therefore at heightened risk of drowning.

Normal risk-taking behavior during adolescence places CCHS patients in great danger. Sedative medications and central nervous system depressants such as alcohol or illicit drugs should be avoided as much as possible, as they worsen hypoventilation. Chen et al. reported three cases of young adults with CCHS who had severe adverse events related to alcohol use, including coma and death [66]. Parents and patients should be counseled about these specific risks prior to and throughout adolescence. Patients should wear MedicAlert bracelets to warn paramedical and medical staff in case of emergency.

In the majority of cases, CCHS does not cause significant levels of psychological distress in caregivers, who typically report good coping resources and high levels of motivation to provide care [17, 63]. Some studies do, however, report higher levels of marital discord [63].

Perioperative Care

Children with CCHS will require ventilatory support during sedation or general anesthesia. Anesthetic care for the child with CCHS can be challenging. To avoid the need for additional ventilation during wakefulness and prolonged hospitalization, anesthetic drugs with the shortest half-life should be chosen, e.g., remifentanil, nitrous oxide, and sevoflurane [67]. For other procedures, the use of regional anesthesia techniques may avoid the central effects of anesthetic drugs. Cardiovascular complications of CCHS including cor pulmonale and autonomic dysfunction may also impact perioperative care. Metabolic alkalosis should be prevented as this can further inhibit central respiratory drive. Drugs with negative chronotropic effects or direct effects on blood pressure should be avoided.

Pregnancy

Increasing numbers of patients with CCHS are now progressing to parenthood themselves [68, 69]. Although most current cases of CCHS represent de novo mutations in the PHOX2B gene, some cases are inherited in an autosomal dominant fashion. If both parent and children are affected, this creates greater challenges for the parent who must monitor the ventilatory needs of both themselves and their child. Prenatal testing by amniocentesis for PHOX2B allows for anticipated cases to be delivered in appropriate tertiary centers that can manage ventilation of both mother and child. Pregnant women with CCHS will require frequent physiological monitoring because they do not have the central respiratory drive to meet the increased respiratory load caused by the enlarging uterus [68]. Diaphragmatic pacing is poorly tolerated after Cesarian section due to the abdominal incision, and alternative means of ventilation will be required [68].

Long-Term Prognosis

Long-term follow-up of patients with CCHS and neurodevelopmental outcome reveal a broad range of results with a great deal of variability, usually correlating with the degree of severity of their CCHS [15]. Mortality rates ranging from 8 to 38 % have been documented in various CCHS patient cohorts [21, 42, 58, 63]. The main causes of death include cor pulmonale, pneumonia, and aspiration.

With an increasing awareness of the disease entity, patients will be recognized and treated earlier than in the past. Advancements in home ventilation and monitoring abilities as well as vigilant ongoing patient assessment and equipment maintenance by medical teams will further improve prognosis. As these children survive to adulthood, the development of transition programs with age-appropriate support will contribute to independent lifestyles, careers, and family lives for this complex population.

Future Directions

As the prognosis for patients with CCHS improves, there remains, however, the need to ensure that ventilatory requirements are addressed with ongoing research into new, more acceptable forms of artificial ventilation. The deficiencies in current methods of ventilation are most apparent in those children who require support 24 h a day. During varied levels of daytime activity and exercise, these patients may become hypercapnic and hypoxemic but cannot adequately compensate because of fixed artificial ventilatory support with either diaphragmatic pacers or a mechanical ventilator.

At present the only effective therapeutic option for patients diagnosed with CCHS is mechanical ventilation. One potential treatment was recently reported in two women with CCHS who demonstrated improved ventilatory responses to hypoxia and hypercapnia after taking the progestin contraceptive, desogestrel [70]. The exact mechanism of action of desogestrel remains unclear, but it has been postulated that it may stimulate or activate "alternative" central and/or peripheral chemosensitive neural circuits [70]. Further trials are warranted to determine the true potential of this treatment option.

Since the discovery of the *PHOX2B* mutation, there has been increasing interest in the possibility of a genetic therapy for CCHS. The severity of the CCHS phenotype correlates with the length of polyalanine expansions, which ultimately lead to the formation of toxic intracytoplasmic aggregates and impaired *PHOX2B*-mediated transactivation [71]. A recent study by Zanni et al. identified two molecules, 17-AAG and curcumin, that were effective in vitro in counteracting these pathological effects [71]. The ultimate goal of such research is to identify medications that, if initiated in early infancy or even in utero, could modify disease progression and avoid the need for mechanical ventilation, permitting significant improvements in quality of life, morbidity, and mortality for these patients.

Continuing investigation of the genetic intricacies of this syndrome is needed, with ongoing attempts to correlate the genotype-phenotype relationship and improve patient care and prognosis. In addition, the presumed genetic etiology of patients with late-onset central hypoventilation and hypothalamic dysfunction remains to be determined. As with any complex illness, further research, including autopsy studies using new molecular technologies, will help to define the anatomical and physiological features of this syndrome.

References

1. Amiel J, Laudier B, Attie-Bitach T, Trang H, de Pontual L, Gener B, et al. Polyalanine expansion and frameshift mutations of the paired-like homeobox gene PHOX2B in congenital central hypoventilation syndrome. Nat Genet. 2003;33(4):459–61.
2. Weese-Mayer DE, Berry-Kravis EM, Zhou L, Maher BS, Silvestri JM, Curran ME, et al. Idiopathic congenital central hypoventilation syndrome: analysis of genes pertinent to early autonomic nervous system embryologic development and identification of mutations in PHOX2b. Am J Med Genet A. 2003;123A(3):267–78.
3. Antic NA, Malow BA, Lange N, McEvoy RD, Olson AL, Turkington P, et al. PHOX2B mutation-confirmed congenital central hypoventilation syndrome: presentation in adulthood. Am J Respir Crit Care Med. 2006;174(8):923–7.
4. Matera I, Bachetti T, Puppo F, Di Duca M, Morandi F, Casiraghi GM, et al. PHOX2B mutations and polyalanine expansions correlate with the severity of the respiratory phenotype and associated symptoms in both congenital and late onset Central Hypoventilation syndrome. J Med Genet. 2004;41(5):373–80.
5. Repetto GM, Corrales RJ, Abara SG, Zhou L, Berry-Kravis EM, Rand CM, et al. Later-onset congenital central hypoventilation syndrome due to a heterozygous 24-polyalanine repeat expansion mutation in the PHOX2B gene. Acta Paediatr. 2009;98(1):192–5.
6. Weese-Mayer DE, Berry-Kravis EM, Zhou L. Adult identified with congenital central hypoventilation syndrome—mutation in PHOX2b gene and late-onset CHS. Am J Respir Crit Care Med. 2005;171(1):88.
7. Weese-Mayer DE, Berry-Kravis EM, Ceccherini I, Keens TG, Loghmanee DA, Trang H. An official ATS clinical policy statement: congenital central hypoventilation syndrome: genetic basis, diagnosis, and management. Am J Respir Crit Care Med. 2010;181(6):626–44.
8. Huang J, Colrain IM, Panitch HB, Tapia IE, Schwartz MS, Samuel J, et al. Effect of sleep stage on breathing in children with central hypoventilation. J Appl Physiol. 2008;105(1):44–53.
9. Orem JM, Lovering AT, Vidruk EH. Excitation of medullary respiratory neurons in REM sleep. Sleep. 2005;28(7):801–7.
10. Gozal D, Marcus CL, Ward SL, Keens TG. Ventilatory responses to passive leg motion in children with congenital central hypoventilation syndrome. Am J Respir Crit Care Med. 1996;153(2):761–8.
11. Paton JY, Swaminathan S, Sargent CW, Hawksworth A, Keens TG. Ventilatory response to exercise in children with congenital central hypoventilation syndrome. Am Rev Respir Dis. 1993;147(5):1185–91.
12. Gozal D, Simakajornboon N. Passive motion of the extremities modifies alveolar ventilation during sleep in patients with congenital central hypoventilation syndrome. Am J Respir Crit Care Med. 2000;162(5):1747–51.
13. Shea SA, Andres LP, Paydarfar D, Banzett RB, Shannon DC. Effect of mental activity on breathing in congenital central hypoventilation syndrome. Respir Physiol. 1993;94(3):251–63.

14. Tremoureux L, Raux M, Hudson AL, Ranohavimparany A, Straus C, Similowski T. Does the supplementary motor area keep patients with Ondine's curse syndrome breathing while awake? PLoS One. 2014;9(1), e84534.
15. Chen ML, Keens TG. Congenital central hypoventilation syndrome: not just another rare disorder. Paediatr Respir Rev. 2004;5(3):182–9.
16. Lesser DJ, Ward SL, Kun SS, Keens TG. Congenital hypoventilation syndromes. Semin Respir Crit Care Med. 2009;30(3):339–47.
17. Vanderlaan M, Holbrook CR, Wang M, Tuell A, Gozal D. Epidemiologic survey of 196 patients with congenital central hypoventilation syndrome. Pediatr Pulmonol. 2004;37(3):217–29.
18. Trochet D, de Pontual L, Straus C, Gozal D, Trang H, Landrieu P, et al. PHOX2B germline and somatic mutations in late-onset central hypoventilation syndrome. Am J Respir Crit Care Med. 2008;177(8):906–11.
19. Commare MC, Francois B, Estournet B, Barois A. Ondine's curse: a discussion of five cases. Neuropediatrics. 1993;24(6):313–8.
20. Silvestri JM, Hanna BD, Volgman AS, Jones PJ, Barnes SD, Weese-Mayer DE. Cardiac rhythm disturbances among children with idiopathic congenital central hypoventilation syndrome. Pediatr Pulmonol. 2000;29(5):351–8.
21. Trang H, Dehan M, Beaufils F, Zaccaria I, Amiel J, Gaultier C. The French Congenital Central Hypoventilation Syndrome Registry: general data, phenotype, and genotype. Chest. 2005;127(1):72–9.
22. Trang H, Boureghda S, Denjoy I, Alia M, Kabaker M. 24-hour BP in children with congenital central hypoventilation syndrome. Chest. 2003;124(4):1393–9.
23. Gronli JO, Santucci BA, Leurgans SE, Berry-Kravis EM, Weese-Mayer DE. Congenital central hypoventilation syndrome: PHOX2B genotype determines risk for sudden death. Pediatr Pulmonol. 2008;43(1):77–86.
24. Goldberg DS, Ludwig IH. Congenital central hypoventilation syndrome: ocular findings in 37 children. J Pediatr Ophthalmol Strabismus. 1996;33(3):175–80.
25. Rohrer T, Trachsel D, Engelcke G, Hammer J. Congenital central hypoventilation syndrome associated with Hirschsprung's disease and neuroblastoma: case of multiple neurocristopathies. Pediatr Pulmonol. 2002;33(1):71–6.
26. Swaminathan S, Gilsanz V, Atkinson J, Keens TG. Congenital central hypoventilation syndrome associated with multiple ganglioneuromas. Chest. 1989;96(2):423–4.
27. Haddad GG, Mazza NM, Defendini R, Blanc WA, Driscoll JM, Epstein MA, et al. Congenital failure of automatic control of ventilation, gastrointestinal motility and heart rate. Medicine (Baltimore). 1978;57(6):517–26.
28. Weese-Mayer DE, Marazita ML, Rand CM, Berry-Kravis EM. Congential Central Hypoventilation Syndrome. In: Pagon RA, Adam MP, Ardinger HH, Wallace SE, Amemiya A, Bean LJH et al, editors. GeneReviews [Internet]. Seattle (WA): University of Washington, Seattle; 1993–2016.
29. Berry-Kravis EM, Zhou L, Rand CM, Weese-Mayer DE. Congenital central hypoventilation syndrome: PHOX2B mutations and phenotype. Am J Respir Crit Care Med. 2006;174(10):1139–44.
30. Trochet D, O'Brien LM, Gozal D, Trang H, Nordenskjold A, Laudier B, et al. PHOX2B genotype allows for prediction of tumor risk in congenital central hypoventilation syndrome. Am J Hum Genet. 2005;76(3):421–6.
31. Katz ES, McGrath S, Marcus CL. Late-onset central hypoventilation with hypothalamic dysfunction: a distinct clinical syndrome. Pediatr Pulmonol. 2000;29(1):62–8.
32. Fishman LS, Samson JH, Sperling DR. Primary alveolar hypoventilation syndrome (Ondine's curse). Am J Dis Child. 1965;110:155–61.
33. Ize-Ludlow D, Gray JA, Sperling MA, Berry-Kravis EM, Milunsky JM, Farooqi IS, et al. Rapid-onset obesity with hypothalamic dysfunction, hypoventilation, and autonomic dysregulation presenting in childhood. Pediatrics. 2007;120(1):e179–88.
34. Abaci A, Catli G, Bayram E, Koroglu T, Olgun HN, Mutafoglu K, et al. A case of rapid-onset obesity with hypothalamic dysfunction, hypoventilation, autonomic dysregulation, and neural crest tumor: ROHHADNET syndrome. Endocr Pract. 2013;19(1):e12–6.

35. Jennings LJ, Yu M, Rand CM, Kravis N, Berry-Kravis EM, Patwari PP, et al. Variable human phenotype associated with novel deletions of the PHOX2B gene. Pediatr Pulmonol. 2012;47(2):153–61.
36. Marcus CL. Sleep-disordered breathing in children. Am J Respir Crit Care Med. 2001;164(1):16–30.
37. Paton JY, Swaminathan S, Sargent CW, Keens TG. Hypoxic and hypercapnic ventilatory responses in awake children with congenital central hypoventilation syndrome. Am Rev Respir Dis. 1989;140(2):368–72.
38. Frank Y, Kravath RE, Inoue K, Hirano A, Pollak CP, Rosenberg RN, et al. Sleep apnea and hypoventilation syndrome associated with acquired nonprogressive dysautonomia: clinical and pathological studies in a child. Ann Neurol. 1981;10(1):18–27.
39. Proulx F, Weber ML, Collu R, Lelievre M, Larbrisseau A, Delisle M. Hypothalamic dysfunction in a child: a distinct syndrome? Report of a case and review of the literature. Eur J Pediatr. 1993;152(6):526–9.
40. Jiang D, Morrison GA. The influence of long-term tracheostomy on speech and language development in children. Int J Pediatr Otorhinolaryngol. 2003;67 Suppl 1:S217–20.
41. Kremer B, Botos-Kremer AI, Eckel HE, Schlondorff G. Indications, complications, and surgical techniques for pediatric tracheostomies—an update. J Pediatr Surg. 2002;37(11):1556–62.
42. Hasegawa H, Kawasaki K, Inoue H, Umehara M, Takase M. Epidemiologic survey of patients with congenital central hypoventilation syndrome in Japan. Pediatr Int. 2012;54(1):123–6.
43. Fauroux B, Lavis JF, Nicot F, Picard A, Boelle PY, Clement A, et al. Facial side effects during noninvasive positive pressure ventilation in children. Intensive Care Med. 2005;31(7):965–9.
44. Villa MP, Pagani J, Ambrosio R, Ronchetti R, Bernkopf E. Mid-face hypoplasia after long-term nasal ventilation. Am J Respir Crit Care Med. 2002;166(8):1142–3.
45. Tibballs J, Henning RD. Noninvasive ventilatory strategies in the management of a newborn infant and three children with congenital central hypoventilation syndrome. Pediatr Pulmonol. 2003;36(6):544–8.
46. Simonds AK. Home ventilation. Eur Respir J. 2003;47:38s–46.
47. Migliori C, Cavazza A, Motta M, Bottino R, Chirico G. Early use of Nasal-BiPAP in two infants with Congenital Central Hypoventilation syndrome. Acta Paediatr. 2003;92(7):823–6.
48. DiFeo N, Meltzer LJ, Beck SE, Karamessinis LR, Cornaglia MA, Traylor J, et al. Predictors of positive airway pressure therapy adherence in children: a prospective study. J Clin Sleep Med. 2012;8(3):279–86.
49. Sawyer AM, Gooneratne NS, Marcus CL, Ofer D, Richards KC, Weaver TE. A systematic review of CPAP adherence across age groups: clinical and empiric insights for developing CPAP adherence interventions. Sleep Med Rev. 2011;15(6):343–56.
50. Ellis ER, McCauley VB, Mellis C, Sullivan CE. Treatment of alveolar hypoventilation in a six-year-old girl with intermittent positive pressure ventilation through a nose mask. Am Rev Respir Dis. 1987;136(1):188–91.
51. Berry RB, Chediak A, Brown LK, Finder J, Gozal D, Iber C, et al. Best clinical practices for the sleep center adjustment of noninvasive positive pressure ventilation (NPPV) in stable chronic alveolar hypoventilation syndromes. J Clin Sleep Med. 2010;6(5):491–509.
52. Vagiakis E, Koutsourelakis I, Perraki E, Roussos C, Mastora Z, Zakynthinos S, et al. Average volume-assured pressure support in a 16-year-old girl with congenital central hypoventilation syndrome. J Clin Sleep Med. 2010;6(6):609–12.
53. Ambrogio C, Lowman X, Kuo M, Malo J, Prasad AR, Parthasarathy S. Sleep and non-invasive ventilation in patients with chronic respiratory insufficiency. Intensive Care Med. 2009;35(2):306–13.
54. Storre JH, Seuthe B, Fiechter R, Milioglou S, Dreher M, Sorichter S, et al. Average volume-assured pressure support in obesity hypoventilation: a randomized crossover trial. Chest. 2006;130(3):815–21.
55. Hartmann H, Jawad MH, Noyes J, Samuels MP, Southall DP. Negative extrathoracic pressure ventilation in central hypoventilation syndrome. Arch Dis Child. 1994;70(5):418–23.

56. Glenn WW, Holcomb WG, McLaughlin AJ, O'Hare JM, Hogan JF, Yasuda R. Total ventilatory support in a quadriplegic patient with radiofrequency electrophrenic respiration. N Engl J Med. 1972;286(10):513–6.

57. Hunt CE, Matalon SV, Thompson TR, Demuth S, Loew JM, Liu HM, et al. Central hypoventilation syndrome: experience with bilateral phrenic nerve pacing in 3 neonates. Am Rev Respir Dis. 1978;118(1):23–8.

58. Weese-Mayer DE, Hunt CE, Brouillette RT, Silvestri JM. Diaphragm pacing in infants and children. J Pediatr. 1992;120(1):1–8.

59. Ali A, Flageole H. Diaphragmatic pacing for the treatment of congenital central alveolar hypoventilation syndrome. J Pediatr Surg. 2008;43(5):792–6.

60. DiMarco AF. Phrenic nerve stimulation in patients with spinal cord injury. Respir Physiol Neurobiol. 2009;169(2):200–9.

61. Weese-Mayer DE, Morrow AS, Brouillette RT, Ilbawi MN, Hunt CE. Diaphragm pacing in infants and children. A life-table analysis of implanted components. Am Rev Respir Dis. 1989;139(4):974–9.

62. Zelko FA, Nelson MN, Leurgans SE, Berry-Kravis EM, Weese-Mayer DE. Congenital central hypoventilation syndrome: neurocognitive functioning in school age children. Pediatr Pulmonol. 2010;45(1):92–8.

63. Marcus CL, Jansen MT, Poulsen MK, Keens SE, Nield TA, Lipsker LE, et al. Medical and psychosocial outcome of children with congenital central hypoventilation syndrome. J Pediatr. 1991;119(6):888–95.

64. Idiopathic congenital central hypoventilation syndrome: diagnosis and management. American Thoracic Society. Am J Respir Crit Care Med. 1999;160(1):368–73.

65. Silvestri JM, Weese-Mayer DE, Flanagan EA. Congenital central hypoventilation syndrome: cardiorespiratory responses to moderate exercise, simulating daily activity. Pediatr Pulmonol. 1995;20(2):89–93.

66. Chen ML, Turkel SB, Jacobson JR, Keens TG. Alcohol use in congenital central hypoventilation syndrome. Pediatr Pulmonol. 2006;41(3):283–5.

67. Strauser LM, Helikson MA, Tobias JD. Anesthetic care for the child with congenital central alveolar hypoventilation syndrome (Ondine's curse). J Clin Anesth. 1999;11(5):431–7.

68. Sritippayawan S, Hamutcu R, Kun SS, Ner Z, Ponce M, Keens TG. Mother-daughter transmission of congenital central hypoventilation syndrome. Am J Respir Crit Care Med. 2002;166(3):367–9.

69. Silvestri JM, Chen ML, Weese-Mayer DE, McQuitty JM, Carveth HJ, Nielson DW, et al. Idiopathic congenital central hypoventilation syndrome: the next generation. Am J Med Genet. 2002;112(1):46–50.

70. Straus C, Trang H, Becquemin MH, Touraine P, Similowski T. Chemosensitivity recovery in Ondine's curse syndrome under treatment with desogestrel. Respir Physiol Neurobiol. 2010;171(2):171–4.

71. Di Zanni E, Bachetti T, Parodi S, Bocca P, Prigione I, Di Lascio S, et al. In vitro drug treatments reduce the deleterious effects of aggregates containing polyAla expanded PHOX2B proteins. Neurobiol Dis. 2012;45(1):508–18.

Index

© Springer Science+Business Media New York 2016
L.M. Sterni, J.L. Carroll (eds.), *Caring for the Ventilator Dependent Child*,
Respiratory Medicine, DOI 10.1007/978-1-4939-3749-3

Printed in the United States
By Bookmasters